Handbook of Methods for Designing, Monitoring, and Analyzing Dose-Finding Trials

Chapman & Hall/CRC
Handbooks of Modern Statistical Methods

Series Editor

Garrett Fitzmaurice

Department of Biostatistics
Harvard School of Public Health
Boston, MA, U.S.A.

Aims and Scope

The objective of the series is to provide high-quality volumes covering the state-of-the-art in the theory and applications of statistical methodology. The books in the series are thoroughly edited and present comprehensive, coherent, and unified summaries of specific methodological topics from statistics. The chapters are written by the leading researchers in the field, and present a good balance of theory and application through a synthesis of the key methodological developments and examples and case studies using real data.

The scope of the series is wide, covering topics of statistical methodology that are well developed and find application in a range of scientific disciplines. The volumes are primarily of interest to researchers and graduate students from statistics and biostatistics, but also appeal to scientists from fields where the methodology is applied to real problems, including medical research, epidemiology and public health, engineering, biological science, environmental science, and the social sciences.

Published Titles

Handbook of Mixed Membership Models and Their Applications
Edited by Edoardo M. Airoldi, David M. Blei,
Elena A. Erosheva, and Stephen E. Fienberg

Handbook of Statistical Methods and Analyses in Sports
Edited by Jim Albert, Mark E. Glickman, Tim B. Swartz, Ruud H. Koning

Handbook of Markov Chain Monte Carlo
Edited by Steve Brooks, Andrew Gelman,
Galin L. Jones, and Xiao-Li Meng

Handbook of Big Data
Edited by Peter Bühlmann, Petros Drineas,
Michael Kane, and Mark van der Laan

Chapman & Hall/CRC
Handbooks of Modern
Statistical Methods

Handbook of Methods for Designing, Monitoring, and Analyzing Dose-Finding Trials

Edited by

John O'Quigley
French National Institute for Health and Medical Research
Faculty of Mathematics,
University Pierre and Marie Curie, Paris, France

Alexia Iasonos
Memorial Sloan Kettering Cancer Center
New York, USA

Björn Bornkamp
Novartis
Basel, Switzerland

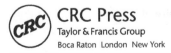

CRC Press
Taylor & Francis Group
Boca Raton London New York

CRC Press is an imprint of the
Taylor & Francis Group, an **informa** business
A CHAPMAN & HALL BOOK

CRC Press
Taylor & Francis Group
6000 Broken Sound Parkway NW, Suite 300
Boca Raton, FL 33487-2742

First issued in paperback 2019

© 2017 by Taylor & Francis Group, LLC
CRC Press is an imprint of Taylor & Francis Group, an Informa business

No claim to original U.S. Government works

ISBN-13: 978-1-4987-4610-6 (hbk)
ISBN-13: 978-0-367-33068-2 (pbk)

**Visit the Taylor & Francis Web site at
http://www.taylorandfrancis.com**

**and the CRC Press Web site at
http://www.crcpress.com**

Contents

III   Phase II Dose-Finding Trials   187

Editors

John O'Quigley is a professor of mathematics and research director at the French National Institute for Health and Medical Research based at the Faculty of Mathematics, University Pierre and Marie Curie, in Paris, France. He is author of the text *Proportional Hazards Regression* and has published extensively in the field of dose finding.

Alexia Iasonos is an associate attending biostatistician at the Memorial Sloan Kettering Cancer Center in New York. She has over one hundred publications in the leading statistical and clinical journals on the methodology and design of early-phase clinical trials. Dr. Iasonos has wide experience in the actual implementation of model-based, early-phase trials and has taught courses in international scientific meetings.

Björn Bornkamp is a statistical methodologist at Novartis in Basel, Switzerland, researching and implementing dose-finding designs in Phase II clinical trials. He is one of the co-developers of the MCP-Mod methodology for dose finding and main author of the DoseFinding R package. He has published numerous papers on dose finding, nonlinear models, and Bayesian statistics, and in 2013, he won the Royal Statistical Society award for statistical excellence in the pharmaceutical industry.

Preface

This volume covers recent developments in the design and analysis of dose-finding clinical trials. While the theory is closely examined, the unifying driving force is the clinical applications themselves. Given the high failure rate of Phase III confirmatory clinical trials, together with an increasing need to look at new agents in a timely manner, it has become apparent that poor accuracy in the early-phase trials can have significant consequences further down the line in the overall drug development. The aim of recent developments in early-phase trials is to greatly improve this accuracy and to achieve this while strictly respecting ethical requirements governing clinical trials in human subjects. In the long term, the end result will be a speedier and more reliable drug development process so that patients can more quickly see the real benefit from scientific advances in the laboratory.

In Phase I first-in-human trials, little is known on how the probability of encountering adverse events relates to dose when the drug is given to humans based on preclinical data. One objective of a trial is to learn more about this relationship, although we are severely hampered by the need to avoid overdosing. Further, underdosing is also a concern for oncology patients who participate in these trials, if there is no hope of benefit one should not offer to include patients in the trial. We need a trade-off between information gained via experimentation at various dose levels and the requirements of the treated patients themselves on a particular study. The statistical setting is thus unusual. This presents a considerable statistical challenge and has formed the basis of several of the model-based approaches that are discussed here. Challenges in Phase II dose-finding studies include the fact that efficacy information evaluated on the different dose levels is limited not only by a typically rather low sample size but also by the fact that biomarker, or short-term, endpoints are used compared to more definitive endpoints used in more extensive and longer-term Phase III clinical trials.

Explicitly characterizing the relation between the amount of a given drug and its effect, i.e., how the body reacts to given doses of the drug, has not traditionally been an objective of Phase I trials. Even some Phase II dose-finding trials do not aim to do this. As a result of this lack of precision, the goals of the older, or classical, standard dose-finding designs, such as the well-known 3 + 3, are not clear. In the absence of clear goals, it is not possible to say whether or not any proposed statistical methodology works well or is even fit for its purpose. In Phase II dose-finding clinical trials, a major focus has traditionally been statistical testing based on pairwise comparisons of the efficacy endpoint, which is not aligned with the goal of determining the efficacy dose–response curve. An aim in this current volume is to make very clear and explicit early on the goals of an early-phase study under different settings, and then to critically investigate how any statistical approach can meet these goals. In practice, the level of clinical complexity can increase rapidly, for example, studies in targeted therapies, combination therapies, bridging between different patient populations or several heterogeneous groups, and errors in recording adverse events. The several authors in this volume, through the many different approaches presented, never lose sight of the initial motivation and the study's objective. No statistical complexity, for its own sake, is presented, and the methods described are being currently used to provide answers in applied clinical research. The material presented here, along with references to further work, provides an overview of various existing methods that can help a practicing statistician select an appropriate clinical trial design to match the objective of the study.

Contributors

Björn Bornkamp
Clinical Development and Analytics
Novartis Pharma AG
Basel, Switzerland

Frank Bretz
Clinical Development and Analytics
Novartis Pharma AG
Basel, Switzerland

Ying Kuen K. Cheung
Mailman School of Public Health
Columbia University
New York, New York

Mark R. Conaway
Department of Public Health Sciences
University of Virginia
Charlottesville, Virginia

Vladimir Dragalin
Quantitative Sciences
Janssen Research & Development
Beerse, Belgium

Emily V. Dressler
Division of Cancer Biostatistics
Markey Cancer Center
University of Kentucky
Lexington, Kentucky

Lei Gao
Research and Development
Sanofi US
Cambridge, Massachusetts

Sofia Friberg Hietala
Pharmetheus AB
Uppsala, Sweden

Alexia Iasonos
Department of Epidemiology and
    Biostatistics
Memorial Sloan Kettering Cancer Center
New York, New York

Franz König
Section of Medical Statistics
Medical University of Vienna
Vienna, Austria

Markus R. Lange
Clinical Development and Analytics
Novartis Pharma AG
Basel, Switzerland

Shing Lee
Mailman School of Public Health
Columbia University
New York, New York

Efthymios Manolis
European Medicines Agency
London, United Kingdom

Tobias Mielke
Innovation Center
ICON Clinical Research
Cologne, Germany

Arzu Onar-Thomas
Department of Biostatistics
St. Jude Childrens Research Hospital
Memphis, Tennessee

John O'Quigley
Laboratory of Theoretical and Applied
    Statistics
University Pierre and Marie Curie
Paris, France

José Pinheiro
Model-Based Drug Development
Janssen Research & Development
Raritan, New Jersey

Heinz Schmidli
Clinical Development and Analytics
Novartis Pharma AG
Basel, Switzerland

Oleksandr Sverdlov
Biostatistical Sciences and
Pharmacometrics
Novartis Institutes for Biomedical Research
Cambridge, Massachusetts

Flora Musuamba Tshinanu
School of Pharmacy
University College London
London, United Kingdom

Fridtjof Thomas
Division of Biostatistics, Department of
    Preventive Medicine
University of Tennessee Health Science
    Center
Memphis, Tennessee

Nolan A. Wages
Department of Public Health Sciences
University of Virginia
Charlottesville, Virginia

Graham M. Wheeler
Cancer Research UK and UCL Cancer
    Trials Centre
University College London
London, United Kingdom

Xiaolei Xun
Clinical Development and Analytics
Novartis Pharma
Shanghai, China

Donglin Yan
College of Public Health, Department of
    Biostatistics
University of Kentucky
Lexington, Kentucky

Ying Yuan
Department of Biostatistics
The University of Texas MD Anderson
    Cancer Center
Houston, Texas

Liangcai Zhang
Department of Statistics
Rice University
Houston, Texas

Part I

Phase I Designs

1

Overview of Phase I Designs

Graham M. Wheeler

University College London

CONTENTS

Though many differing approaches for conducting phase I trials have been proposed over the past three decades, they all aim to target a specific dose level while minimizing the risk of patients in the trial experiencing intolerable toxicities. Here, we cover the two main types of phase I designs—rule-based and model-based—and provide an overview of the many designs available. We also discuss other design aspects, such as start-up rules and stopping rules, and summarize how clinical practice has changed over the years when it comes to designing a phase I trial.

1.1 Introduction

The primary objective of a phase I clinical trial is to investigate the safety profile of a novel drug or drug combination and identify a tolerable dose schedule that is likely to benefit patients (Chang and Chow, 2006). For cytotoxic therapies in oncology, such trials are conducted using a small number of cancer patients for whom standard therapies have not worked (Horstmann et al., 2005). Due to the possibility of experimental treatments causing severe side effects, trials are conducted as *dose-escalation studies*. In general, patients are recruited into the trial and treated in small cohorts of one, two, or three, with the first cohort treated at an exceedingly low dose level considered safe in humans (Von Hoff et al., 1984; Eisenhauer et al., 2000). The number and severity of toxic reactions, as defined by the National Cancer Institute's Common Terminology Criteria for Adverse Events [NCI CTCAE (National Cancer Institute, 2009)], observed in patients undergoing treatment are recorded, and based on the results for the current cohort (and possibly previous cohorts), the next cohort of patients will be treated at either a higher dose level, a lower dose level, or the same dose level. The trial continues in this manner until all available patients have been treated, or some other stopping criterion is satisfied, such as a target number of patients have been consecutively dosed at one dose level, or the proportion of patients experiencing severe toxicity at a dose level exceeds a prespecified threshold (see Section 1.4.2).

Commonly, toxicity frequency and severity data are reduced to a single binary outcome known as *dose-limiting toxicity* (DLT) (Le Tourneau et al., 2009), and this response is used to determine whether dose escalation occurs or not. What constitutes a DLT will vary from trial to trial (Le Tourneau et al., 2011), but it is often the case that a DLT is said to have occurred in a patient if at least one toxicity [grade 3 or higher under the NCI CTCAE (NCI, 2009)] in a particular body system or organ of interest is observed in the first cycle of treatment (Babb and Rogatko, 2004).

The main objective of phase I trials is to identify the *maximum tolerated dose* (MTD) of the new drug. Although definitions of the MTD vary (Le Tourneau et al., 2009), it is often defined as the dose that, at the end of the trial, has an estimated probability of causing a DLT as close to some predetermined *target toxicity level* (TTL) as possible (Babb and Rogatko, 2004). In oncology, the TTL is fixed often at some probability between 0.20 and 0.35 (Neuenschwander et al., 2008; Le Tourneau et al., 2009). An alternative definition of the MTD is the dose with no more than a certain proportion (e.g., 33%) of patients at that dose experiencing DLT. If an MTD is successfully identified in a phase I trial, the drug is then taken forward into a phase II trial, with the MTD or a slightly lower dose designated as the recommended phase II dose (RP2D) (Le Tourneau et al., 2012).

The rationale for targeting a dose level that is potentially harmful with small probability is due to the belief that the higher the dose of a cytotoxic drug, the better the speed or extent of tumor response (Marshall, 2012). Therefore, the MTD of a cytotoxic drug is seen as a proxy for an efficacious dose level with limited toxicity potential. When considering molecularly targeted agents, which affect particular molecules required for cancer cells to mutate (carcinogenesis) rather than all cells, this may not necessarily be the case (Le Tourneau et al., 2009); in some cases, it has been observed that the dose–response relationship may be nonmonotonically increasing (Conolly and Lutz, 2004; Bretz et al., 2008). Most methods for phase I trials are based on the *assumption of monotonicity* (Box 1.1); that is, if a patient has a DLT at a given dose level, then the same patient would have had a DLT had they been given a higher dose level than the one they received. Conversely, had the patient not had a DLT at a given dose level, then the same patient would not have had a DLT had they been given a lower dose level than the one they received (O'Quigley and Zohar, 2006). This assumption can be summarized on a population level by saying that the probability of a DLT occurring in a patient is monotonically increasing with dose.

Box 1.1   The Assumption of Monotonicity

The probability of observing a dose-limiting toxicity (DLT) is monotonically increasing with dose.

Methods for conducting dose-escalation studies are usually dichotomized into two families: *rule-based designs*, where fixed rules applied to empirical counts of DLT/non-DLT responses govern the escalation and de-escalation of doses, and *model-based designs*, where statistical models are employed to describe the relationship between the dose given to a patient and the probability of DLT occurring (Rosenberger and Haines, 2002). O'Quigley and Zohar (2006) stated that any method considered for use in a phase I trial should aim to (1) minimize the number of patients treated at dose levels below the true MTD, (2) minimize the number of patients treated at dose levels above the true MTD, (3) minimize the number of patients used in the study in its entirety, and (4) be able to respond quickly to errors in initial guesses or incorrect dose allocations. In this chapter, we describe the main rule-based and model-based approaches for conducting phase I dose-escalation studies with a single binary DLT endpoint. We follow these up with discussions on modifications to these designs that have been used in clinical practice, the popularity of particular designs in clinical practice, and available software for various methods.

1.2 Rule-Based Designs

Rule-based designs have long been popular with clinicians in cytotoxic drug experimentation (Storer, 1989; Rogatko et al., 2007). The fundamental aspect of rule-based designs is that they do not require the dose–toxicity relationship to be modeled according to some function of dose level. Many of the methods proposed stem from the work on the *up-and-down design* by Dixon and Mood (1948), who sought to identify the mean or median height from which a weight may be dropped upon an explosive compound without detonation occurring. Over time, variations of the up-and-down design made their way into medical research.

1.2.1 The 3 + 3 design

The 3 + 3 design (Carter, 1973; Storer, 1989) is one of the first methods used to conduct dose-escalation studies in humans. The 3 + 3 design is the most commonly used design in phase I clinical trials (Rogatko et al., 2007; Penel et al., 2009; Le Tourneau et al., 2009, 2012) and has long been considered the routine method by clinicians for estimating the MTD of novel drugs in oncology (Penel et al., 2009).

For a trial of k dose levels of a new drug, denoted as $D = \{d_1, \ldots, d_k\}$, patients are treated in cohorts of three for the 3 + 3 design. The first cohort of patients are treated at d_1, the lowest dose level. If no patients in a cohort experience a DLT, then the next cohort is treated at the next highest dose level. If one out of the three patients experiences a DLT, then the next cohort is treated at the same dose level. If at dose level d_i at least two out of the three or six patients experience a DLT, the trial is terminated and d_{i-1} is deemed to be the MTD; if $d_{i-1} = d_0$, then no MTD is identified for safety reasons. The 3 + 3 design may be adapted so that excessive toxicity leads to dose de-escalation rather than trial termination (Storer, 1989; Dignam et al., 2006; Skolnik et al., 2008; Chow, 2011). That is, if d_i is deemed excessively toxic, and only three patients have received dose d_{i-1}, then another three patients are dosed at d_{i-1}. If at most one out of the six patients experiences a DLT, then the trial is terminated and d_{i-1} is the MTD; otherwise, the dose is de-escalated again under the same rules. If six patients had been treated at d_{i-1}, and d_i was deemed excessively toxic, then the trial would terminate and d_{i-1} would be recommended as the MTD. Figure 1.1 illustrates the trial schematic for the 3 + 3 design with dose de-escalation not permitted, and Figure 1.2 illustrates an example trial using data from a real

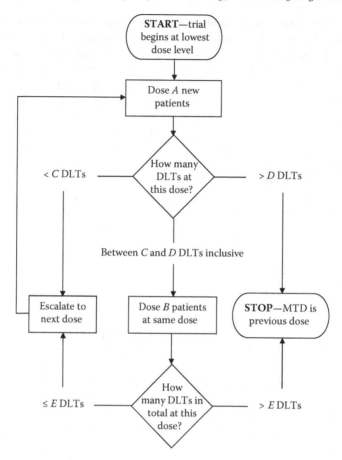

FIGURE 1.1
Design schematic of the $A + B$ design without dose de-escalation.

3 + 3 trial conducted by Park et al. (2005). The trial investigated the dose escalation of 5-fluorouracil (5-FU) in combination with a fixed dose of docetaxel in patients with advanced gastric cancer. Four dose levels were planned for experimentation: 250, 500, 750 and 1000 mg/m^2/day. In the first cohort, no patients experienced a DLT at the first dose level. The second cohort was given the dose level of 500 mg/m^2/day, at which one out of the three patients experienced a DLT. Therefore, the third cohort was also given the second dose level. No patients in the third cohort experienced a DLT, and so the fourth cohort was given the dose level of 750 mg/m^2/day. As two out of the three patients in the fourth cohort experienced a DLT, the trial was terminated after 12 patients and the MTD was identified as 500 mg/m^2/day.

There exist several variants of the traditional 3 + 3 design, including generic $A + B$ trials where A and B are positive integers that denote cohort sizes to be used in the trial (Lin and Shih, 2001). For example, a 2 + 4 trial would dose a cohort of two patients at a dose level and then add another four patients to that dose level if one of the initial two patients treated experienced a DLT. There are also $A + B + C$ designs where an extra cohort of C patients may be added onto a dose level if a predetermined number of DLTs are observed in $A + B$ patients. Examples include the 3 + 1 + 1 design, which offers more aggressive dose escalation than the 3 + 3 design (Storer, 2001), and the 3 + 3 + 3 design (Hamberg

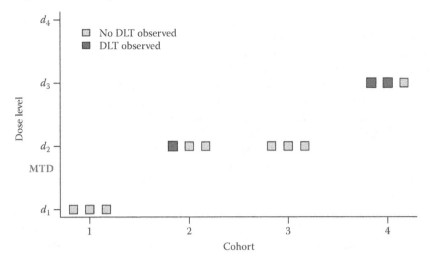

FIGURE 1.2
Example of dose-escalation pathway in a real $3 + 3$ trial (Park et al., 2005). After observing one DLT in cohort 2 at dose level d_2, cohort 3 were dosed at dose level d_2 also. After escalating to dose level d_3, excessive toxicity leads to termination of the trial and dose level d_2 is the final MTD.

and Verweij, 2009), which after observing two DLTs in six patients, doses another cohort of three patients at the same dose level.

The main advantages of the $3 + 3$ design are that neither a statistician nor highly technical computer software are required to help design or run the trial (Le Tourneau et al., 2009), and exact operating characteristics can be calculated (Lin and Shih, 2001; Wheeler et al., 2016). Additionally, the $3 + 3$ design may be ideal for screening drugs very quickly to identify a dose level that exhibits very little toxicity in a small number of patients (Rosenberger and Haines, 2002). However, the pitfalls associated with the $3 + 3$ design perhaps outweigh these benefits (Harrington et al., 2013). The $3 + 3$ design is a *memoryless* design (Ratain et al., 1993; O'Quigley and Zohar, 2006), i.e., dose-escalation decisions are based on the observed results at the current dose, and the distribution of toxicities in previous cohorts is ignored (Zohar and O'Quigley, 2009). Furthermore, many of the trial participants are treated at subtherapeutic doses due to the slow dose-escalation process that the algorithm enforces (O'Quigley et al., 1990; Ratain et al., 1993), and a new cohort cannot be enrolled until toxicity outcomes have been observed for all patients in the current cohort. A common misconception is that the MTD determined in a $3 + 3$ trial always has an expected toxicity rate of 33% since the dose selected as the MTD has an empirical toxicity rate of at most 33%. Large-scale simulation studies have shown that the expected toxicity rate at the estimated MTD depends on the number of doses under experimentation and is often much lower than 33% (Kang and Ahn, 2001, 2002; He et al., 2006; Chen et al., 2009). In fact, the $3 + 3$ design does not have a TTL to target per se, meaning that the design is searching for an unknown dose with an unspecified toxicity probability.

1.2.2 Rolling-6 design

In order to shorten trial duration for the $3 + 3$ design, Skolnik et al. (2008) proposed the *rolling-6 design*, in which dose-escalation/de-escalation decisions can be made for the next cohort of three patients, even when not all three patients in the previous cohort have a definitive DLT/no-DLT response. These decisions depend on the number of patients currently enrolled in the cohort, the number of patients with DLTs, and the number of patients enrolled but not yet evaluable for DLT. The trial is run as a 3 + 3 design, but with several modifications: if DLT data are unavailable for one or more of the three patients at dose d_i, or if one DLT is observed at d_i, then the fourth patient (the first patient in the next cohort) is also dosed at d_i; if two or more DLTs have been observed, even if the third patient is not yet evaluable for DLT, then the fourth patient is given dose d_{i-1}. These rules also apply to the fifth and sixth patients (patients 2 and 3 of the next cohort). Several comparative simulation studies have shown that trials using the rolling-6 design are shorter in duration than those using the 3 + 3 design, but on average require more patients to identify an MTD and are more likely to result in excessive numbers of DLTs (at least three per dose) occurring (Onar-Thomas and Xiong, 2010; Sposto and Groshen, 2011; Doussau et al., 2012). The design has been implemented in practice, particularly in pediatric oncology trials (Mossé et al., 2013; Hoffman et al., 2015). However, it still possesses many of the pitfalls of the 3 + 3 design, and model-based alternatives have been shown to offer much better performance (Onar-Thomas and Xiong, 2010; Zhao et al., 2011).

1.2.3   Accelerated titration designs

An alternative class of rule-based methods to the traditional 3 + 3 design are accelerated titration designs (Simon et al., 1997), which permit intrapatient dose escalation in order to reduce the total sample size and the number of patients treated at subtherapeutic doses. Under accelerated titration designs, dose-escalation/de-escalation decisions are made within patients as well as between patients/cohorts and are based on the toxicity observed in the current treatment cycles and/or the largest toxicity in the first treatment cycle. A drawback of such designs is that intrapatient dose escalation may lead to difficulty in the analysis of trial data since cumulative or delayed toxicities may be masked (Hansen et al., 2014). Simon et al. found that the number of high-grade toxicities increased under accelerated titration compared to a design without intrapatient dose escalation. Although not exhaustive, the 3 + 3 design and accelerated titration designs are the primary rule-based designs used in phase I oncology trials (Rogatko et al., 2007).

1.2.4   Pharmacologically guided dose escalation

Another variation is pharmacologically guided dose escalation (PGDE) (Collins et al., 1990), which relies on *in vivo* data to predict DLT outcomes in humans. Dose escalation of one-patient cohorts is based on whether the area under the curve (AUC) of drug concentration over time is less than some target level. When such a level is exceeded, or when DLTs begin to occur, the design switches to the traditional 3 + 3 design. The PGDE method has had mixed results in clinical practice, in that reliable phase II doses have been recommended for some cytotoxic compounds that have high interpatient variability/heterogeneity (Graham and Workman, 1992; Hansen et al., 2014).

1.2.5   Improvements to conventional rule-based designs

Ivanova et al. (2003) proposed various up-and-down rules that incorporate more trial information than approaches based on the 3 + 3 design (i.e., the most recent cohort) in order to guide dose escalation. Among these is the Narayana rule, derived from the unpublished work of Narayana (1953), which recommends dose escalation or de-escalation from the current dose level based on the empirical proportions of DLTs observed and the k most recent dose–toxicity outcomes at the current level. The authors also considered different procedures for estimating the MTD of a drug, including isotonic regression (Robertson et al., 1988), which adjusts the empirical DLT rates at different doses via the pooled adjacent violators algorithm (PAVA) to maintain monotonicity of toxicity in doses (Barlow et al., 1972).

The approaches discussed here aim to develop the early up-and-down design work of Dixon and Mood (1948) while keeping dose-escalation decisions dependent on the empirical DLT rates at each dose level. However, more statistical approaches for conducting dose-escalation studies have been proposed, which use mathematical models to quantify the relationship between the dose of a drug and the probability of a DLT occurring.

1.3   Model-Based Designs

Over the past two decades, there has been widespread interest in adaptive model-based designs for phase I clinical trials (Whitehead, 1997), particularly Bayesian designs, in order to overcome the shortcomings identified with the $3 + 3$ design and other rule-based methods. Model-based designs use statistical models to estimate the underlying dose–toxicity relationship and can easily incorporate all trial data as well as *a priori* beliefs into the dose–toxicity relationship to help determine dose allocation and MTD recommendation.

1.3.1   The continual reassessment method

One of the first model-based designs for phase I clinical trials was the *continual reassessment method* (CRM) (O'Quigley et al., 1990). Under the CRM, the dose–toxicity curve is assumed to have some monotonically increasing functional form (Table 1.1), which is characterized by a single parameter a and dose level d or a transformed set of dose levels based on the initial dose–toxicity probability guesses, known as the *dose–toxicity skeleton*. The models presented in Table 1.1 are the two simplest and most commonly used; other model structures have been proposed, but under certain conditions, these are equivalent to either the power or logistic model (Cheung, 2011). The models are parameterized with respect to $\exp(a)$ to ensure that the dose–toxicity function is increasing in dose. Transformed dose levels are used to ensure that the chosen model is a sensible fit for the dose–toxicity skeleton (the prior guesses for the dose–toxicity probabilities at each dose level) and can easily be computed by backward substitution (Cheung, 2011).

In a Bayesian setting, a prior belief about the shape of the dose–toxicity curve, along with any surrounding uncertainty, is expressed as a prior distribution on parameter a; this information may be elicited from clinical opinion and data from previous studies if available and calibrated so that it does not dominate over the data that are accrued during the trial (Legedza and Ibrahim, 2001; Rosenberger et al., 2005; Cheung, 2011). As the trial progresses, patient data are used to update the prior distribution on a to obtain a posterior belief about the shape of the dose–toxicity curve. Let $D = \{d_1, ..., d_k\}$ be the set of k dose

TABLE 1.1

Common models for one-parameter CRM.

Model	$\psi(d, a)$	Restrictions
Power	$d^{\exp(a)}$	$0 < d < 1$
Logistic	$\frac{\exp(a_1 + \exp(a)d)}{1 + \exp(a_1 + \exp(a)d)}$	a_1 fixed $-\infty < d < \infty$

labels, obtained from the dose–toxicity skeleton of a new drug under experimentation. Let $x_j \in D$ be the dose level that patient j receives and Y_j be the binary DLT outcome for patient j, i.e.,

$$Y_j = \begin{cases} 1 & \text{if patient } j \text{ experiences a DLT} \\ 0 & \text{otherwise} \end{cases} \tag{1.1}$$

Let $\Omega_j = \{x_1, y_1, \ldots, x_j, y_j\}$ denote the set of trial data (doses given and DLT outcomes) for the first j patients and $g(a)$ denote the prior distribution of a, which is defined on the set $\mathcal{A} = (-\infty, \infty)$. Then using Bayes' theorem (Bayes, 1763), we may obtain the posterior distribution of a, denoted as $f(a \mid \Omega_j)$:

$$f(a \mid \Omega_j) = \frac{g(a)L(a \mid \Omega_j)}{\int_{a \in \mathcal{A}} g(a)L(a \mid \Omega_j)\, da}, \tag{1.2}$$

where the likelihood $L(a \mid \Omega_j)$ is of the form

$$L(a \mid \Omega_j) = \prod_{l=1}^{j} \psi(x_l, a)^{y_l} \left[1 - \psi(x_l, a)\right]^{1-y_l}. \tag{1.3}$$

The posterior belief about the shape of the dose–toxicity curve, derived from the posterior distribution of a, allows us to select a dose level that has an estimated probability of DLT as close to the desired TTL as possible; we denote the TTL as θ here. O'Quigley et al. (1990) propose two different, but closely related, estimators. One obtains the posterior mean of a, denoted as $\hat{a}$, and uses this plug-in estimate to find x_{j+1}, the dose for the next patient, i.e.,

$$\hat{a} = \int_{a \in \mathcal{A}} a\, f(a \mid \Omega_j)\, da, \tag{1.4}$$

$$x_{j+1} = \arg \min_{d_i \in D} \left(\psi(d_i, \hat{a}) - \theta\right)^2. \tag{1.5}$$

The other approach integrates over the distribution of a to obtain a posterior mean estimate of $\psi(d_i, a)$ for $i = 1, \ldots, k$ and finds the dose with mean probability of DLT closest to θ:

$$x_{j+1} = \arg \min_{d_i \in D} \left(\int_{a \in \mathcal{A}} \psi(d_i, a)\, f(a \mid \Omega_j)\, da - \theta\right)^2. \tag{1.6}$$

Once the dose has been chosen for patient $j + 1$, the trial repeats the above computation based on the trial data set Ω_{j+1}, which is formed by the union of Ω_j and $\{x_{j+1}, y_{j+1}\}$, the dose and DLT outcome of patient $j + 1$. The trial is either stopped after an MTD estimate has been reached with a sufficient level of certainty or when a maximum number of patients have been treated (see Section 1.4.2). The CRM may also be used using maximum likelihood estimation to update the parameter a and determine dose escalation for future patients (O'Quigley and Shen, 1996). Rather than using a prior distribution $g(a)$ for a, the 3 + 3 design is used as a start-up rule until the first DLT response is observed (estimation of $\hat{a}$ requires at least one DLT response and one non-DLT response). After this, maximum likelihood estimation is used to estimate a, with dose escalation and MTD selection conducted as shown in Equation 1.5. An example of how the shape of the dose–toxicity curve changes with more data is shown in Figure 1.3.

There are several advantages to using the CRM instead of the 3 + 3 design. First, the CRM incorporates all trial information into the dose-escalation decision-making process, rather than just the current cohort as in the 3 + 3 design. Furthermore, an explicit TTL θ can be stated, which means that the MTD identified at the end of the trial has a meaning

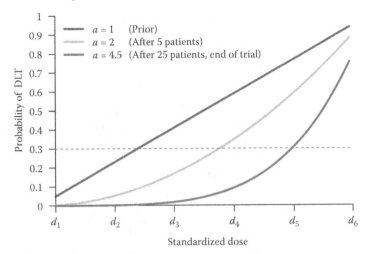

FIGURE 1.3

Example of how dose–toxicity curve changes with patient data, assuming a power model for the CRM design. Here, at the end of the trial seeking a dose with probability of DLT as close to $\theta = 0.30$ as possible, dose level d_5 is selected as the MTD.

to both statisticians and clinicians. The CRM provides faster dose escalation and more accurate convergence to the true MTD than the 3 + 3 design (O'Quigley et al., 1990; Le Tourneau et al., 2009), as shown in numerous simulation studies (O'Quigley, 1999; Thall and Lee, 2003; Iasonos et al., 2008; Onar et al., 2009; Onar-Thomas and Xiong, 2010). In its original form, the faster dose-escalation had the potential to lead to patients being assigned to high dose levels. The model and dose-escalation schematic of the CRM are easily adaptable to circumvent this problem, and several papers have proposed various changes to aspects of the original CRM design. In particular, it is now common practice to start the trial at the lowest dose under experimentation and to not escalate more than one dose level per patient (O'Quigley and Chevret, 1991; Faries, 1994; Goodman et al., 1995; Møller, 1995). There have also been investigations into how the prior distribution and dose–toxicity skeleton should be chosen (Cheung, 2011; Lee and Cheung, 2011; Iasonos and O'Quigley, 2012), as well as appropriate stopping rules for trials using the CRM (O'Quigley and Reiner, 1998; Zohar and Chevret, 2001) (Section 1.4.2) and how the CRM performs under model misspecification. While one can never truly know if they have chosen the correct model for the dose–toxicity curve, several studies have shown that while operating characteristics may be different under different model choices, a simple one-parameter CRM is likely to be more robust in targeting the correct MTD (Paoletti and Kramar, 2009; Iasonos et al., 2016).

1.3.2 Escalation with overdose control (EWOC)

In order to overcome concerns about quickly escalating doses and overdosing patients under the CRM, Babb et al. (1998) proposed the *escalation with overdose control* (EWOC) design. Under the EWOC design, the posterior distribution of the MTD is updated after each patient, and a chosen percentile of the MTD distribution is used to select doses for future patients. This percentile, denoted as α, is known as the *feasibility bound* and reflects how conservative investigators are in escalating dose levels between patients. The feasibility bound can be interpreted via a decision-theoretic loss function, which describes the relative preference of underdosing a patient compared to overdosing a patient. For some dose level d and MTD μ, the loss function for feasibility bound α is

$$\text{Loss}(d,\mu) = \begin{cases} \alpha(\mu - d) & \text{if } d \text{ is an underdose, i.e., } d \leq \mu \\ (1 - \alpha)(d - \mu) & \text{if } d \text{ is an overdose, i.e., } d \geq \mu. \end{cases} \tag{1.7}$$

In words, for any $\delta > 0$, the loss incurred by overdosing a patient (with respect to the MTD μ) by δ units is $\frac{1-\alpha}{\alpha}$ times greater than underdosing a patient by δ units (Babb et al., 1998; Babb and Rogatko, 2001). For $\alpha < 0.50$, the loss function in Equation 1.7 places a higher penalty on overdosing, whereas if $\alpha = 0.50$, one is indifferent between overdosing and underdosing patients. In order to conduct dose escalation, Babb et al. (1998) proposed a two-parameter logistic function to model the probability of DLT, given dose level d_i:

$$\psi(d_i, a_1, a_2) = \frac{\exp(a_1 + \exp(a_2)d_i)}{1 + \exp(a_1 + \exp(a_2)d_i)}, \tag{1.8}$$

where a_1 and a_2 are model parameters. If for MTD μ, we denote $\psi(\mu, a_1, a_2) = \theta$ and for the lowest dose level d_1, we denote $\psi(d_1, a_1, a_2) = \rho_0$ for some probability $\rho_0 \in (0, 1)$, one can transform these expressions and rewrite a_1 and a_2 as

$$a_1 = \frac{\mu \log\text{it}(\rho_0) - d_1 \log\text{it}(\theta)}{\mu - d_1} \quad \text{and} \quad a_2 = \log\left(\frac{\log\text{it}(\theta) - \log\text{it}(\rho_0)}{\mu - d_1}\right). \tag{1.9}$$

So, a_1 and a_2 can be expressed in terms of μ, the MTD, and ρ_0, the probability of toxicity at dose d_1. These parameters are more meaningful to clinicians and can be used in the Bayesian updating procedure by placing prior distributions upon μ and ρ_0 (Kadane et al., 1980; Babb et al., 1998). For prior distributions on μ and ρ_0, Babb et al. (1998) suggest a uniform distribution over the interval $[d_1, d_k]$ for μ and a uniform distribution over the interval $[0, \theta]$ for ρ_0, though others have been proposed (Tighiouart et al., 2005). Similar to Equation 1.2, the joint posterior distribution for μ and ρ_0 given trial data Ω_j and prior distribution $g(\mu, \rho_0)$, denoted as $f(\mu, \rho_0 \mid \Omega_j)$, can be obtained. With this, the marginal cumulative distribution function of μ, $H_j(\mu')$ is

$$H_j(\mu') = \mathbb{P}(\mu \leq \mu' \mid \Omega_j) = \int_{x_1}^{\mu'} \int_0^\theta f(\mu, \rho_0 \mid \Omega_j) \, d\rho_0 \, d\mu, \tag{1.10}$$

and the dose for patient $j + 1$, x_{j+1} is chosen as

$$x_{j+1} = \arg\min_{d_i \in D} \left\{ (H_j(d_i) - \alpha)^2 \right\}. \tag{1.11}$$

Figure 1.4 illustrates how dose is chosen based on the cumulative distribution function of the MTD; in this instance with $\alpha = 0.25$ (i.e., overdosing is three times worse than underdosing), d_2 is the closest dose level and so would be chosen as the dose for the next patient.

The EWOC model is more conservative in dose escalation relative to the CRM. However, in some cases, the MTD estimated at the end of the trial may be a dose level not used for any patient throughout the trial (Berry et al., 2010). To overcome this, several trials have let the feasibility bound α increase as more patients are accrued (Babb and Rogatko, 2001, 2004; Cheng et al., 2004; Chu et al., 2009; Tighiouart and Rogatko, 2010). As information accrues during the trial, one can afford to be less conservative and escalate more quickly in order to identify the MTD. This can be achieved by letting α increase toward some upper limit, say 0.50, at which point the EWOC approach with $\alpha = 0.50$ is equivalent to a CRM model that uses the posterior median of the MTD distribution to select the next dose level [see Appendix B.3.1 of Carlin and Louis (2009)]. However, the mechanism by which α changes during the trial requires careful consideration (Wheeler, 2016).

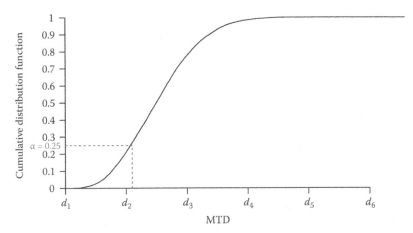

FIGURE 1.4
Example of dose selection for the EWOC approach with feasibility bound $\alpha = 0.25$.

1.3.3 Toxicity probability interval designs

The toxicity probability interval (TPI) (Ji et al., 2007) and modified TPI (mTPI) (Ji et al., 2010) designs are model-based alternatives to the $3+3$ design where posterior probabilities for the risk of DLT belonging to each of three intervals determine whether the dose for the next cohort is escalated, held at the current dose, or de-escalated. Each dose level's probability of causing a DLT is assigned a vague prior distribution (Ji et al., 2007, 2010, use beta distributions), and the number of patients and the number of DLTs at each dose are used to update these prior distributions, using what is known as a beta-binomial model. Three intervals, $U = [0, \theta - \epsilon_1)$, known as the underdosing interval, $P = [\theta - \epsilon_1, \theta + \epsilon_2]$, the proper dosing interval, and $O = (\theta + \epsilon_2, 1]$, the overdosing interval, are specified; the cutoffs ϵ_1 and ϵ_2 can be elicited from clinicians. Under the mTPI design at current dose level d_i, with the probability of DLT parameter p_i, the ratio between the area of the distribution p_i within each interval and its width is calculated. If the ratio is maximized for interval U, then the dose is escalated; if the ratio is maximized for interval P, then the dose stays at the same level; if the ratio is maximized for interval O, then the dose is de-escalated. The use of a beta-binomial model means that calculations to obtain the posterior probability distribution of DLT at each dose are computationally fast and simple. Furthermore, the simple escalate/stay/de-escalate rules are analogous to the $3+3$ design, which many clinicians are familiar with, except that under the mTPI design, a TTL can be explicitly targeted and estimates of p_i at the end of the trial (using isotonic regression, for example) can be used to choose the MTD. Ji and Wang (2013) conducted a simulation study that showed the mTPI design recommended the correct MTD more often and overdoses less often than the $3+3$ design, and the mTPI design can even be run using Microsoft Excel, making it accessible to those without advanced statistical programs.

1.3.4 Curve-free methods

Several approaches exist for dose-finding studies where an explicit model relating dose level to the probability of DLT is not required. Gasparini and Eisele (2000, 2001) proposed the use of a *product of beta prior* (PBP) approach, which induces a monotonic relationship between dose and probability of toxicity without specifying a particular model form. Given dose and toxicity outcome data for current patients in the trial, the dose for the next cohort of patients is that with a posterior probability of DLT closest to the TTL θ. A potential problem with the curve-free approach of Gasparini and Eisele (2000) is that it becomes stuck at a dose level and is unable to escalate even after observing many non-DLT responses (Cheung, 2002, 2011). Whitehead et al. (2010) also proposed a curve-free approach, where decisions to escalate are based on maximizing the probability of the risk of toxicity being equal to θ. In essence, discrete risks of toxicity are specified at the start of trial (say, 0.05, 0.10, 0.20, 0.30, and 0.60), and after observing dose and toxicity data, the posterior probability that the risk of toxicity is equal to each of the discrete risks is calculated. This form of design has been adapted for a trial of two agents in combination (Whitehead et al., 2012), including an extension with both toxicity and efficacy outcomes (Whitehead et al., 2011) (see Section 1.4.3). While curve-free methods do not assume a specific form for the relationship between dose and toxicity, separate assumptions are required to be made on the prior probabilities of DLT at each dose to be considered in the trial. O'Quigley (2002) provides a discussion on the equivalence of the CRM and the curve-free approach of Gasparini and Eisele (2000), in the sense that identical operating characteristics can be obtained from each method by specifying appropriate design quantities for each design.

1.3.5   Optimal design theory approaches

Haines et al. (2003) proposed the use of optimal design theory for dose-escalation decision making. In particular, Bayesian D-optimality was proposed, which chooses the dose level that minimizes the global variance of the model parameters, or equivalently, maximizes the information that can be obtained about the shape of the dose–toxicity relationship, subject to additional toxicity constraints. Other optimal design theoretic approaches for phase I trials have been proposed, particularly for trials with multiple outcomes and for combination therapies, though they require additional constraints or penalization in order to prevent unethical dose recommendations (Mats et al., 1998; Dragalin and Fedorov, 2006; Dragalin et al., 2008; Roy et al., 2009; Pronzato, 2010; Fedorov and Leonov, 2013; Azriel, 2014; Haines and Clark, 2014).

1.4   Modifications to Proposed Designs

The designs in Sections 1.2 and 1.3 are not necessarily fixed in how they are conducted. Methodologists and clinicians have proposed several modifications to these approaches in order to overcome potential design pitfalls, or because of specific requirements/constraints in their trials.

1.4.1   Start-up rules

A clinician may deem it problematic to immediately use a statistical model to determine dose escalation for the first few patients, especially if very little is known about how a novel drug behaves in human patients. For example, when using a Bayesian model, if the prior distributions for the model parameters are highly variable, one may not be comfortable in using these distributions to determine dose-escalation decisions until some data are obtained. Similarly, if one wishes to use maximum likelihood estimation methods to estimate parameters, we will not be able to obtain maximum likelihood estimates of the parameters until we observe heterogeneous DLT responses, i.e., at least one non-DLT response and at least one DLT response. Therefore, an initial dose-escalation rule may be used in order to obtain preliminary toxicity data before the statistical model is implemented. For example, the likelihood approach of the CRM (O'Quigley and Shen, 1996) uses the 3 + 3 design as a start-up rule until the first DLT outcome is observed, before then reverting to the CRM modeling approach described in Section 1.3.1. Iasonos and O'Quigley (2012) recommend using data from the first stage of the design to inform the structure of the skeleton to be used for the CRM in the second stage. Ivanova et al. (2003) proposed an alternative start-up rule that depends on the TTL, primarily aiming to conserve patient resources and enable the first dose given under the main design to be closer to the MTD. For optimal design approaches, Haines et al. (2003) constructed a constrained optimal design in the first stage, i.e., allocated a small number of patients across the dose levels so that information about the dose–toxicity curve was maximized, yet patients were not placed at toxic doses. After data on these patients were obtained, they proceeded with their sequential dose-escalation approach.

1.4.2 Stopping rules

As well as considerations for how to start a trial, the criteria for stopping a dose-escalation trial need to be stated. Stopping a trial before a maximum number of patients have been treated is considered for two reasons; either the MTD is judged to be outside of the planned set of doses to be experimented on (i.e., all doses are too toxic, or all doses have a probability of DLT well below the TTL), or the addition of more patients into the trial is unlikely to yield any more information that would change the current MTD estimate. There exist several different approaches for determining when it is suitable to stop a phase I trial. For example, Thall and Russell (1998) recommend terminating a trial if the posterior probability of all dose levels having a DLT rate above (or below) the TTL is at least 0.90, and this has been implemented as a safety constraint in many other dose-escalation designs (Yin et al., 2006). With respect to stopping a trial early when a suitably accurate MTD estimate has been obtained, several rules have been proposed, particularly for the CRM. These include stopping a trial when a fixed number of patients have been consecutively dosed at one dose level (Korn et al., 1994), when the width of the confidence interval for the MTD reaches a particular level (O'Quigley et al., 1990), or stopping when the probability that the next m patients to be dosed in the trial are given the same dose level exceeds some level (e.g., 0.90) (O'Quigley and Reiner, 1998; Zohar and Chevret, 2001; O'Quigley, 2002). The choice of one or more stopping rules for a trial is ultimately dependent on the number of patients available, as well as the statistical expertise at hand, the prior knowledge of the dose–toxicity relationship, and the number of dose levels under consideration.

1.4.3 Choice of endpoints

The methods discussed so far all use a single binary outcome for the occurrence of DLT. While conveniently simple, there are pitfalls to using such an endpoint. First, one has to wait for DLT outcomes to be recorded before making dose recommendations for the next cohort, thus potentially leading to long trial durations. Using a time-to-event (TITE) endpoint (see Chapter 3) can help to reduce trial duration, while still providing informed dose-escalation decision making. Also, toxicity outcomes are graded from 0 (no toxicity) to 5 (death), as per the NCI CTCAE (NCI, 2009), with intermediate gradings relating to the severity of a side effect. Rather than using a binary endpoint for DLT, a categorical endpoint for toxicity could be used so that recording of low-grade toxicities can provide information as to how toxic other doses might be; this can be done throughout the trial, or in the first stage of a two-stage design (Iasonos et al., 2011). Approaches incorporating toxicity gradings are discussed in Chapter 3. Furthermore, toxicities occurring in different body systems may be more or less important to clinicians, and one may wish to reduce the number of different DLTs or high-grade toxicities a patient might receive on treatment; approaches using multiple toxicity constraints have been developed to this end (Bekele and Thall, 2004; Lee et al., 2011).

In addition to using toxicity information, efficacy outcomes may also be used to inform dose-escalation and end-of-trial dose recommendation; it may be the case that a biologically optimal dose (BOD) is sought, rather than an MTD. Several joint-outcome models have been proposed, using binary, categorical, and continuous efficacy outcomes, and these are explored in Chapter 5.

1.4.4   Combination therapies and schedules

Combination therapies are used frequently in the treatment of cancer, and many designs for escalating two or more drugs together have been proposed, though not necessarily implemented (Harrington et al., 2013). Combination dose-escalation studies can present difficulties not observed in single-agent trials, such as modeling interactive treatment/toxicity effects between drugs, deciding on the escalation strategy, attributing toxicity to one specific drug or a combination of several, and in order to explore several combinations, more patients are likely to be required. Furthermore, it is possible to recommend multiple MTDs to take forward to phase II trials. Nevertheless, the aforementioned designs and modifications discussed in this chapter have all motivated the design of dose-escalation studies with multiple drugs, some of which include graded outcomes, efficacy endpoints, and attributing toxicity to specific agents; these are explored in Chapter 6. Furthermore, approaches for conducting dual-agent dose-escalation studies can be used for single-agent trials to optimize both dose and schedule of treatment administration; these designs are discussed in Chapter 7.

1.5   Usage of Different Designs in Clinical Practice

Several reviews have shown that model-based designs have been used rarely for conducting phase I dose-escalation studies. One review of 1,235 phase I dose-escalation studies testing new anticancer agents between 1991 and 2006 found that 1,215 (98.4%) of such trials used the traditional $3 + 3$ design or some variant, with only 17 trials (1.4%) using the CRM method and 3 trials using the EWOC design (Rogatko et al., 2007). Further, Le Tourneau et al. (2009) found that of 181 phase I clinical trials conducted between January 2007 and December 2008, 168 trials used the traditional $3 + 3$ design (1 of which featured intrapatient dose escalation) and 7 used the accelerated titration design. Of the remaining six trials, five used the modified CRM and one used the CRM design with a TITE endpoint (TITE-CRM) (see Chapter 3). In a review of single-agent phase I trials of molecularly targeted agents published between 2000 and 2010, Le Tourneau et al. (2012) found 6 (7.1%) out of 84 trials used a model-based design (specifically the modified CRM approach), and Rivoirard et al. (2016) assessed 228 radiochemotherapy phase I trials published between 1990 and 2015, finding 3 (1.3%) that used a model-based design (all TITE-CRM). With respect to planned phase I trials, a survey of 35 clinical trial units (CTUs) registered with the UK Clinical Research Collaboration showed that in the 7 CTUs involved in phase I trials, all ongoing studies were implementing the $3 + 3$ design, with only 1 study being planned with the CRM (Jaki, 2013). While these reviews generally indicate few phase I trials have used model-based designs, there is a growing movement for changes in clinical practice. In particular, Iasonos and O'Quigley (2014) found 53 trials published between 2003 and 2013 that implemented either the CRM, EWOC, or TITE-CRM designs, and recent papers have called for more early-phase cancer trials to use novel adaptive designs in practice (Petroni et al., 2017; Wong et al., 2016).

1.5.1 Barriers to adopting novel designs

The reluctance to use adaptive model-based designs for phase I dose-escalation studies has been attributed to numerous reasons, including lack of understanding of statistical methods, fears of lending control to statistical models, concerns about obtaining regulatory approval, lack of user-friendly software, or even just reluctance to break from traditional methods (Bailey et al., 2009; Gönen, 2009; Mandrekar et al., 2010; Harrington et al., 2013; Jaki, 2013). However, Bailey et al. (2009) described how in a phase I trial of nilotinib and imatinib in patients with imatinib-resistant gastrointestinal stromal tumors (GISTs), a close working relationship between the trial statisticians and clinicians with nontechnical training in related statistical concepts allowed all parties to be clear on interpreting trial findings and making dose-escalation decisions based on the model's recommendations. With respect to obtaining regulatory approval, the American Society of Clinical Oncology (ASCO), the US Food and Drug Administration (FDA), and the European Medicines Agency (EMA) have introduced guidance to encourage the use of Bayesian adaptive designs in oncology trials (Gaydos et al., 2006, 2012).

One of the more technical barriers to implementing adaptive model-based designs that Gönen (2009) highlighted was the specification of prior distributions for model parameters. However, for phase I trials, prior distributions can be obtained by working closely with clinical experts to elicit opinions about dose–toxicity relationships, by using information from past dose-escalation studies and other trials, and conducting sensitivity analyses and fine-tuning prior distributions so that unrealistic and unwanted model behavior is avoided (Legedza and Ibrahim, 2001; Geller, 2004; Rosenberger et al., 2005; Adamina et al., 2009; Cheung, 2011).

Perhaps the main reason for the infrequent use of novel adaptive designs in phase I trials is that an investigator insists on using a particular method (Jaki, 2013), either because the investigator has used it in past work or because previous studies in that disease area have used the same method. For phase I oncology trials, this means that the ubiquity of published trials using the 3 + 3 design will likely influence other investigators to use the 3 + 3 design also. Gönen (2009) also mentioned the challenge of motivating investigators to consider novel methods. While extensive simulation studies have shown several model-based designs to have much better operating characteristics than the standard 3 + 3 design (see Section 1.3.1), motivating investigators to consider new methods for future trials is dependent on overcoming all of the above barriers. Therefore, establishing good collaborative relationships between clinical and statistical experts [as discussed in the example trial of Bailey et al. (2009)] is likely to be fundamental to overcoming practical, technical, and motivational barriers (Harrington et al., 2013).

1.5.2 Available tools and software

Increases in computational power mean that advanced simulation studies to investigate model characteristics such as dose-escalation behavior and MTD recommendation can be conducted quickly with free, user-friendly software (Berry et al., 2010; Sweeting et al., 2013). Examples include the open software library of the MD Anderson Cancer Center*

---

* Division of Quantitative Sciences—Department of Biostatistics, The University of Texas MD Anderson Cancer Center, Software Download Site: https://biostatistics.mdanderson.org/SoftwareDownload

and the Comprehensive R Archive Network (CRAN) library[†], which provide open-source programs for, among many other things, conducting and simulating dose-escalation studies. More information on available software for designing and assisting with phase I dose-finding studies is presented in Chapter 10.

1.6   Summary

Over the past three decades, many approaches have been proposed for conducting phase I dose-escalation studies. These include both rule-based and model-based approaches that, as this chapter and the rest of this handbook will show, can be tailored to suit a wide range of trials defined by the disease and treatments under study, the endpoints of interest, the patient population, as well as the clinical, statistical, and computational expertise available. The uptake of novel designs that exhibit vast improvements upon the traditional up-and-down methods, such as the 3 + 3 design, has long been hindered by several barriers, but there is a growing movement to design new trials using these methods and for more widespread changes to be made to clinical practice. A collaborative effort between clinicians and statisticians can help to overcome the barriers documented, leading to well-designed trials that will benefit trial participants and future patients.

References

M. Adamina, G. Tomlinson, and U. Guller. Bayesian statistics in oncology: A guide for the clinical investigator. *Cancer*, 115(23):5371–5381, 2009. doi:10.1002/cncr.24628.

D. Azriel. Optimal sequential designs in phase I studies. *Computational Statistics and Data Analysis*, 71:288–297, 2014. doi:10.1016/j.csda.2013.05.010.

J. S. Babb and A. Rogatko. Bayesian methods for phase I cancer clinical trials. In N. L. Geller, editor, *Advances in Clinical Trial Biostatistics*, pp. 1–40. Marcel Dekker, New York, 2004.

J. S. Babb and A. Rogatko. Patient specific dosing in a cancer phase I clinical trial. *Statistics in Medicine*, 20(14):2079–2090, 2001. doi:10.1002/sim.848.

J. S. Babb, A. Rogatko, and S. Zacks. Cancer phase I clinical trials: Efficient dose escalation with overdose control. *Statistics in Medicine*, 17(10):1103–1120, 1998.

S. M. Bailey, B. Neuenschwander, G. Laird, and M. Branson. A Bayesian case study in oncology phase I combination dose-finding using logistic regression with covariates. *Journal of Biopharmaceutical Statistics*, 19(3):469–484, 2009. doi:10.1080/10543400902802409.

R. E. Barlow, D. J. Bartholomew, J. M. Bremner, and H. D. Brunk. *Statistical Inference under Order Restrictions*. Wiley, New York, 1972.

T. Bayes. An essay towards solving a problem in the doctrine of chances. *Philosophical Transactions of the Royal Society of London*, 53:370–418, 1763. doi:10.1098/rstl.1763.0053.

[†] Available at https://cran.r-project.org

B. N. Bekele and P. F. Thall. Dose-finding based on multiple toxicities in a soft tissue sarcoma trial. *Journal of the American Statistical Association*, 99(465):26–35, 2004. doi:10.1198/016214504000000043.

S. M. Berry, B. P. Carlin, J. J. Lee, and P. Mueller. *Bayesian Adaptive Methods for Clinical Trials*. Chapman & Hall/CRC Biostatistics Series, Taylor and Francis, Boca Raton, FL, 2010.

F. Bretz, J. Hsu, J. Pinheiro, and Y. Liu. Dose finding—A challenge in statistics. *Biometrical Journal*, 50(4):480–504, 2008. doi:10.1002/bimj.200810438.

B. P. Carlin and T. A. Louis. *Bayesian Methods for Data Analysis*, 3rd edn. Chapman & Hall/CRC, Boca Raton, FL, 2009.

S. K. Carter. Study design principles for the clinical evaluation of new drugs as developed by the chemotherapy programme of the National Cancer Institute. In M. Staquet, editor, *The Design of Clinical Trials in Cancer Therapy*, pp. 242–289. Éditions Scientifiques Europeenes, Brussels, Belgium, 1973.

M. Chang and S.-C. Chow. Power and sample size for dose response studies. In N. Ting, editor, *Dose Finding in Drug Development*, Chapter 14, pp. 220–242. Springer, New York, 2006.

Z. Chen, M. D. Krailo, J. Sun, and S. P. Azen. Range and trend of expected toxicity level (ETL) in standard A + B designs: A report from the Children's Oncology Group. *Contemporary Clinical Trials*, 30(2):123–128, 2009. doi:10.1016/j.cct.2008.10.006.

J. D. Cheng, J. S. Babb, C. Langer, S. Aamdal, F. Robert, L. R. Engelhardt, O. Fernberg, J. Schiller, G. Forsberg, and R. K. Alpaugh. Individualized patient dosing in phase I clinical trials: The role of escalation with overdose control in PNU214936. *Journal of Clinical Oncology*, 22(4):602–609, 2004. doi:10.1200/JCO.2004.12.034.

Y. K. Cheung. *Dose Finding by the Continual Reassessment Method*. Chapman & Hall/CRC Biostatistics Series, Taylor and Francis, Boca Raton, FL, 2011.

Y. K. Cheung. On the use of nonparametric curves in phase I trials with low toxicity tolerance. *Biometrics*, 58(1):237–240, 2002.

S.-C. Chow. *Controversial Statistical Issues in Clinical Trials*. Taylor and Francis, Boca Raton, FL, 2011.

P.-L. Chu, Y. Lin, and W. J. Shih. Unifying CRM and EWOC designs for phase I cancer clinical trials. *Journal of Statistical Planning and Inference*, 139(3):1146–1163, 2009. doi:10.1016/j.jspi.2008.07.005.

J. M. Collins, C. K. Grieshaber, and B. A. Chabner. Pharmacologically guided phase I clinical trials based upon preclinical drug development. *Journal of the National Cancer Institute*, 82(16):1321–1326, 1990. doi:10.1093/jnci/82.16.1321.

R. B. Conolly and W. K. Lutz. Nonmonotonic dose-response relationships: Mechanistic basis, kinetic modeling, and implications for risk assessment. *Toxicological Sciences*, 77(1):151–157, 2004. doi:10.1093/toxsci/kfh007.

J. Dignam, T. Karrison, and G. Bryant. Design and analysis of oncology clinical trials. In A. Chang, P. Ganz, D. Hayes, T. Kinsella, H. Pass, J. Schiller, R. Stone, and V. Strecher, editors, *Oncology: An Evidence-Based Approach*, pp. 112–126. Springer, New York, 2006.

W. Dixon and A. Mood. A method for obtaining and analyzing sensitivity data. *Journal of the American Statistical Association*, 43(241):109–126, 1948.

A. Doussau, B. Asselain, M. Le Deley, B. Geoerger, F. Doz, G. Vassal, and X. Paoletti. Dose-finding designs in pediatric phase I clinical trials: Comparison by simulations in a realistic timeline framework. *Contemporary Clinical Trials*, 33(4):657–665, 2012. 10.1016/j.cct.2011.11.015.

V. Dragalin and V. Fedorov. Adaptive designs for dose-finding based on efficacy-toxicity response. *Journal of Statistical Planning and Inference*, 136(6):1800–1823, 2006. 10.1016/j.jspi.2005.08.005.

V. Dragalin, V. Fedorov, and Y. Wu. Adaptive designs for selecting drug combinations based on efficacy-toxicity response. *Journal of Statistical Planning and Inference*, 138(2): 352–373, 2008. doi:10.1016/j.jspi.2007.06.017.

E. A. Eisenhauer, P. J. O'Dwyer, M. Christian, and J. S. Humphrey. Phase I clinical trial design in cancer drug development. *Journal of Clinical Oncology*, 18(3):684–692, 2000.

D. Faries. Practical modifications of the continual reassessment method for phase I cancer clinical trials. *Journal of Biopharmaceutical Statistics*, 4(2):147–64, 1994. doi:10.1080/10543409408835079.

V. V. Fedorov and S. L. Leonov. *Optimal Design for Nonlinear Response Models*. CRC Press, Boca Raton, FL, 2013.

M. Gasparini and J. Eisele. Correction: A curve-free method for phase I clinical trials. *Biometrics*, 57(2):659–660, 2001.

M. Gasparini and J. Eisele. A curve-free method for phase I clinical trials. *Biometrics*, 56 (2):609–615, 2000.

B. Gaydos, A. Koch, F. Miller, M. Posch, M. Vandemeulebroecke, and S. J. Wang. Perspective on adaptive designs: 4 years European Medicines Agency reflection paper, 1 year draft US FDA guidance—Where are we now? *Clinical Investigation*, 2(3):235–240, 2012. doi:10.4155/cli.12.5.

B. Gaydos, M. Krams, I. Perevozskaya, F. Bretz, Q. Liu, P. Gallo, D. Berry, C. Chuang-stein, J. Pinheiro, and A. Bedding. Adaptive dose-response studies. *Drug Information Journal*, 40:451–461, 2006.

N. L. Geller. *Advances in Clinical Trial Biostatistics*. Marcel Dekker, New York, 2004.

M. Gönen. Bayesian clinical trials: No more excuses. *Clinical Trials*, 6(3):203–204, 2009. doi:10.1177/1740774509105374.

S. N. Goodman, M. L. Zahurak, and S. Piantadosi. Some practical improvements in the continual reassessment method for phase I studies. *Statistics in Medicine*, 14(11):1149–1161, 1995. doi:10.1002/sim.4780141102.

M. A. Graham and P. Workman. The impact of pharmacokinetically guided dose escalation strategies in phase I clinical trials: Critical evaluation and recommendations for future studies. *Annals of Oncology*, 3(5):339–347, 1992.

L. M. Haines and A. E. Clark. The construction of optimal designs for dose-escalation studies. *Statistics and Computing*, 24:101–109, 2014. doi:10.1007/s11222-012-9356-2.

L. M. Haines, I. Perevozskaya, and W. F. Rosenberger. Bayesian optimal designs for phase I clinical trials. *Biometrics*, 59(3):591–600, 2003.

P. Hamberg and J. Verweij. Phase I drug combination trial design: Walking the tightrope. *Journal of Clinical Oncology*, 27(27):4441–4443, 2009. doi:10.1200/JCO.2009.23.6703.

A. R. Hansen, D. M. Graham, G. R. Pond, and L. L. Siu. Phase 1 trial design: Is 3 + 3 the best? *Cancer Control*, 21(3):200–208, 2014.

J. A. Harrington, G. M. Wheeler, M. J. Sweeting, A. P. Mander, and D. I. Jodrell. Adaptive designs for dual-agent phase I dose-escalation studies. *Nature Reviews Clinical Oncology*, 10(5):277–288, 2013. doi:10.1038/nrclinonc.2013.35.

W. He, J. Liu, B. Binkowitz, and H. Quan. A model-based approach in the estimation of the maximum tolerated dose in phase I cancer clinical trials. *Statistics in Medicine*, 25(12): 2027–2042, 2006. doi:10.1002/sim.2334.

L. M. Hoffman, M. Fouladi, J. Olson, V. M. Daryani, C. F. Stewart, C. Wetmore, M. Kocak, A. Onar-Thomas, L. Wagner, S. Gururangan, et al. Phase I trial of weekly MK-0752 in children with refractory central nervous system malignancies: A pediatric brain tumor consortium study. *Child's Nervous System*, 31(8):1283–1289, 2015. doi:10.1007/s00381-015-2725-3.

E. Horstmann, M. S. McCabe, L. Grochow, S. Yamamoto, L. Rubinstein, T. Budd, D. Shoemaker, E. J. Emanuel, and C. Grady. Risks and benefits of phase 1 oncology trials, 1991 through 2002. *The New England Journal of Medicine*, 352(9):895–904, 2005. doi:10.1056/NEJMsa042220.

A. Iasonos and J. O'Quigley. Adaptive dose-finding studies: A review of model-guided phase I clinical trials. *Journal of Clinical Oncology*, 32(23):2505–2511, 2014. doi:10.1200/JCO. 2013.54.6051.

A. Iasonos and J. O'Quigley. Interplay of priors and skeletons in two-stage continual reassessment method. *Statistics in Medicine*, 31(30):4321–4336, 2012. doi:10.1002/sim.5559.

A. Iasonos, N. A. Wages, M. R. Conaway, K. Cheung, Y. Yuan, and J. O'Quigley. Dimension of model parameter space and operating characteristics in adaptive dose-finding studies. *Statistics in Medicine*, 35(21):3760–3775, 2016. doi:10.1002/sim.6966.

A. Iasonos, A. S. Wilton, E. R. Riedel, V. E. Seshan, and D. R. Spriggs. A comprehensive comparison of the continual reassessment method to the standard 3 + 3 dose escalation scheme in phase I dose-finding studies. *Clinical Trials*, 5(5):465–477, 2008. doi:10.1177/1740774508096474.

A. Iasonos, S. Zohar, and J. O'Quigley. Incorporating lower grade toxicity information into dose finding designs. *Clinical Trials*, 8(4):370–379, 2011. doi:10.1177/1740774511410732..

A. Ivanova, A. Montazer-Haghighi, S. G. Mohanty, and S. D. Durham. Improved up-and-down designs for phase I trials. *Statistics in Medicine*, 22(1):69–82, 2003. doi:10.1002/sim.1336.

T. Jaki. Uptake of novel statistical methods for early-phase clinical studies in the UK public sector. *Clinical Trials*, 10(2):344–346, 2013. doi:10.1177/1740774512474375.

Y. Ji, Y. Li, and B. N. Bekele. Dose-finding in phase I clinical trials based on toxicity probability intervals. *Clinical Trials*, 4(3):235–244, 2007. doi:10.1177/1740774507079442.

Y. Ji, P. Liu, Y. Li, and B. N. Bekele. A modified toxicity probability interval method for dose-finding trials. *Clinical Trials*, 7(6):653–663, 2010. doi:10.1177/1740774510382799.

Y. Ji and S.-J. Wang. Modified toxicity probability interval design: A safer and more reliable method than the 3 + 3 design for practical phase I trials. *Journal of Clinical Oncology*, 31(14):1785–1791, 2013. doi:10.1200/JCO.2012.45.7903.

J. B. Kadane, J. M. Dickey, R. L. Winkler, W. S. Smith, C. Peters, M. Dickey, L. Winkler, and S. C. Peters. Interactive elicitation of opinion for a normal linear model. *Journal of the American Statistical Association*, 75(372):845–854, 1980.

S.-H. Kang and C. W. Ahn. The expected toxicity rate at the maximum tolerated dose in the standard phase I cancer clinical trial design. *Drug Information Journal*, 35(8): 1189–1199, 2001.

S.-H. Kang and C. W. Ahn. An investigation of the traditional algorithm-based designs for phase 1 cancer clinical trials. *Drug Information Journal*, 36:865–873, 2002.

E. L. Korn, D. Midthune, T. T. Chen, L. V. Rubinstein, M. C. Christian, and R. M. Simon. A comparison of two phase I trial designs. *Statistics in Medicine*, 13(18):1799–1806, 1994. doi:10.1002/sim.4780131802.

C. Le Tourneau, H. K. Gan, A. R. A. Razak, and X. Paoletti. Efficiency of new dose escalation designs in dose-finding phase I trials of molecularly targeted agents. *PlOS One*, 7(12):e51039, 2012. doi:10.1371/journal.pone.0051039.

C. Le Tourneau, J. J. Lee, and L. L. Siu. Dose escalation methods in phase I cancer clinical trials. *Journal of the National Cancer Institute*, 101(10):708–720, 2009. doi:10.1093/jnci/djp079.

C. Le Tourneau, A. R. A. Razak, H. K. Gan, S. Pop, V. Diéras, P. Tresca, and X. Paoletti. Heterogeneity in the definition of dose-limiting toxicity in phase I cancer clinical trials of molecularly targeted agents: A review of the literature. *European Journal of Cancer*, 47(10):1468–1475, 2011. doi:10.1016/j.ejca.2011.03.016.

S. M. Lee, B. Cheng, and Y. K. Cheung. Continual reassessment method with multiple toxicity constraints. *Biostatistics*, 12(2):386–398, 2011. doi:10.1093/biostatistics/kxq062.

S. M. Lee and Y. K. Cheung. Calibration of prior variance in the Bayesian continual reassessment method. *Statistics in Medicine*, 30(17):2081–2089, 2011. doi:10.1002/sim.4139.

A. T. R. Legedza and J. G. Ibrahim. Heterogeneity in phase I clinical trials: Prior elicitation and computation using the continual reassessment method. *Statistics in Medicine*, 20(6): 867–882, 2001.

Y. Lin and W. J. Shih. Statistical properties of the traditional algorithm-based designs for phase I cancer clinical trials. *Biostatistics*, 2(2):203–215, 2001. doi:10.1093/biostatistics/2.2.203.

S. J. Mandrekar, R. Qin, and D. J. Sargent. Model-based phase I designs incorporating toxicity and efficacy for single and dual agent drug combinations: Methods and challenges. *Statistics in Medicine*, 29(10):1077–1083, 2010. doi:10.1002/sim.3706.

J. L. Marshall. Maximum-tolerated dose, optimum biologic dose, or optimum clinical value: Dosing determination of cancer therapies. *Journal of Clinical Oncology*, 30(23):2815–2816, 2012. doi:10.1200/JCO.2012.43.4233.

V. A. Mats, W. F. Rosenberger, and N. Flournoy. Restricted optimality for phase I clinical trials. In N. Flournoy, W. F. Rosenberger, W. K. Wong, editors, *New Developments and Applications in Experimental Design*, IMS Lecture Notes—Monograph Series, Volume 34, pp. 50–61, 1998.

S. Møller. An extension of the continual reassessment methods using a preliminary up-and-down design in a dose finding study in cancer patients, in order to investigate a greater range of doses. *Statistics in Medicine*, 14(9):911–922, 1995.

Y. P. Mossé, M. S. Lim, S. D. Voss, K. Wilner, K. Ruffner, J.-F. Laliberté, D. Rolland, F. M. Balis, J. M. Maris, B. J. Weigel, et al. Safety and activity of crizotinib for paediatric patients with refractory solid tumours or anaplastic large-cell lymphoma: A Children's Oncology Group phase 1 consortium study. *The Lancet Oncology*, 14(6):472–480, 2013. doi:10.1016/S1470-2045(13)70095-0.

T. V. Narayana. Sequential procedures in probit analysis. Ph.D Thesis, University of North Carolina, 1953. http://www.stat.ncsu.edu/information/library/mimeo.archive/isms_1953_82.pdf.

National Cancer Institute (NCI). Common Terminology Criteria for Adverse Events v4.0, 2009. http://evs.nci.nih.gov/ftp1/CTCAE/.

B. Neuenschwander, M. Branson, and T. Gsponer. Critical aspects of the Bayesian approach to phase I cancer trials. *Statistics in Medicine*, 27(13):2420–2439, 2008. doi:10.1002/sim.3230.

A. Onar, M. Kocak, and J. M. Boyett. Continual reassessment method vs. traditional empirically based design: Modifications motivated by phase I trials in pediatric oncology by the Pediatric Brain Tumor Consortium. *Journal of Biopharmaceutical Statistics*, 19(3):437–455, 2009. doi:10.1080/10543400902800486.

A. Onar-Thomas and Z. Xiong. A simulation-based comparison of the traditional method, Rolling-6 design and a frequentist version of the continual reassessment method with special attention to trial duration in pediatric phase I oncology trials. *Contemporary Clinical Trials*, 31(3):259–270, 2010. doi:10.1016/j.cct.2010.03.006.

J. O'Quigley. Another look at two phase I clinical trial designs. *Statistics in Medicine*, 18 (20):2683–2690, 1999.

J. O'Quigley. Continual reassessment designs with early termination. *Biostatistics*, 3(1): 87–99, 2002.

J. O'Quigley and S. Chevret. Methods for dose finding studies in cancer clinical trials: A review and results of a Monte Carlo study. *Statistics in Medicine*, 10(11):1647–64, 1991. doi:10.1002/sim.4780101104.

J. O'Quigley, M. Pepe, and L. Fisher. Continual reassessment method: A practical design for phase 1 clinical trials in cancer. *Biometrics*, 46(1):33–48, 1990.

J. O'Quigley and E. Reiner. Miscellanea: A stopping rule for the continual reassessment method. *Biometrika*, 85(3):741–748, 1998.

J. O'Quigley and L. Z. Shen. Continual reassessment method: A likelihood approach. *Biometrics*, 52(2):673–684, 1996.

J. O'Quigley and S. Zohar. Experimental designs for phase I and phase I/II dose-finding studies. *British Journal of Cancer*, 94(5):609–13, 2006. doi:10.1038/sj.bjc.6602969.

X. Paoletti and A. Kramar. A comparison of model choices for the continual reassessment method in phase I cancer trials. *Statistics in Medicine*, 28(24):3012–3028, 2009. doi:10. 1002/sim.3682.

S. H. Park, S.-M. Bang, E. K. Cho, D. B. Shin, J. H. Lee, W. K. Lee, and M. Chung. Phase I dose-escalating study of docetaxel in combination with 5-day continuous infusion of 5-fluorouracil in patients with advanced gastric cancer. *BMC Cancer*, 5(87):1–5, 2005. doi:10.1186/1471-2407-5-87.

N. Penel, N. Isambert, P. Leblond, C. Ferte, A. Duhamel, and J. Bonneterre. "Classical 3 + 3 design" versus "accelerated titration designs": Analysis of 270 phase 1 trials investigating anti-cancer agents. *Investigational New Drugs*, 27(6):552–556, 2009. 10.1007/s10637-008-9213-5.

G. R. Petroni, N. A. Wages, G. Paux, and F. Dubois. Implementation of adaptive methods in early-phase clinical trials. *Statistics in Medicine*, 36(2):215–224, 2017. doi:10.1002/sim.6910.

L. Pronzato. Penalized optimal designs for dose-finding. *Journal of Statistical Planning and Inference*, 140:283–296, 2010. doi:10.1016/j.jspi.2009.07.012.

M. J. Ratain, R. Mick, R. L. Schilsky, and M. Siegler. Statistical and ethical issues in the design and conduct of phase I and II clinical trials of new anticancer agents. *Journal of the National Cancer Institute*, 85(20):1637–1643, 1993.

R. Rivoirard, A. Vallard, J. Langrand-Escure, M. Ben Mrad, G. Wang, J.-B. Guy, P. Diao, A. Dubanchet, E. Deutsch, C. Rancoule, and N. Magne. Thirty years of phase I radiochemotherapy trials: Latest development. *European Journal of Cancer*, 58:1–7, 2016. doi:10.1016/j.ejca.2016.01.012.

T. Robertson, F. T. Wright, and R. L. Dykstra. *Ordered Restricted Statistical Inference*. John Wiley & Sons, New York, 1988.

A. Rogatko, D. Schoeneck, W. Jonas, M. Tighiouart, F. R. Khuri, and A. Porter. Translation of innovative designs into phase I trials. *Journal of Clinical Oncology*, 25(31):4982–4986, 2007. doi:10.1200/JCO.2007.12.1012.

W. F. Rosenberger, G. C. Canfield, I. Perevozskaya, L. M. Haines, and P. Hausner. Development of interactive software for Bayesian optimal phase 1 clinical trial design. *Drug Information Journal*, 39:89–98, 2005.

W. F. Rosenberger and L. M. Haines. Competing designs for phase I clinical trials: A review. *Statistics in Medicine*, 21(18):2757–2770, 2002. doi:10.1002/sim.1229.

A. Roy, S. Ghosal, and W. F. Rosenberger. Convergence properties of sequential Bayesian D-optimal designs. *Journal of Statistical Planning and Inference*, 139(2):425–440, 2009. doi:10.1016/j.jspi.2008.04.025.

R. Simon, B. Freidlin, L. Rubinstein, S. G. Arbuck, J. Collins, and M. C. Christian. Accelerated titration designs for phase I clinical trials in oncology. *Journal of the National Cancer Institute*, 89(15):1138–1147, 1997.

J. M. Skolnik, J. S. Barrett, B. Jayaraman, D. Patel, and P. C. Adamson. Shortening the timeline of pediatric phase I trials: The rolling six design. *Journal of Clinical Oncology*, 26(2):190–195, 2008. doi:10.1200/JCO.2007.12.7712.

R. Sposto and S. Groshen. A wide-spectrum paired comparison of the properties of the rolling 6 and 3 + 3 phase I study designs. *Contemporary Clinical Trials*, 32(5):694–703, 2011. doi:10.1016/j.cct.2011.04.009.

B. E. Storer. Design and analysis of phase I clinical trials. *Biometrics*, 45(3):925–937, 1989.

B. E. Storer. An evaluation of phase I clinical trial designs in the continuous dose-response setting. *Statistics in Medicine*, 20(16):2399–2408, 2001. doi:10.1002/sim.903.

M. J. Sweeting, A. P. Mander, and T. Sabin. BCRM: Bayesian continual reassessment method designs for phase I dose-finding trials. *Journal of Statistical Software*, 54(13): 1–26, 2013.

P. F. Thall and S. Lee. Practical model-based dose-finding in phase I clinical trials: Methods based on toxicity. *International Journal of Gynecological Cancer*, 13:251–261, 2003.

P. F. Thall and K. E. Russell. A strategy for dose-finding and safety monitoring based on efficacy and adverse outcomes in phase I/II clinical trials. *Biometrics*, 54(1):251–264, 1998.

M. Tighiouart and A. Rogatko. Dose finding with escalation with overdose control (EWOC) in cancer clinical trials. *Statistical Science*, 25(2):217–226, 2010.

M. Tighiouart, A. Rogatko, and J. S. Babb. Flexible Bayesian methods for cancer phase I clinical trials. Dose escalation with overdose control. *Statistics in Medicine*, 24(14): 2183–2196, 2005. doi:10.1002/sim.2106.

D. D. Von Hoff, J. Kuhn, and G. M. Clark. Design and conduct of phase I trials. In M. E. Buyse, M. J. Staquet, R. J. Sylvester, editors, *Cancer Clinical Trials: Methods and Practice*, pp. 210–220. Oxford University Press, Oxford, 1984.

G. M. Wheeler, M. J. Sweeting, and A. P. Mander. AplusB: A web application for investigating A + B designs for phase I cancer clinical trials. *PLoS One*, 11(7):e0159026, 2016. doi:10.1371/journal.pone.0159026.

G. M. Wheeler. Incoherent dose-escalation in phase I trials using the escalation with overdose control approach. *Statistical Papers*, 1–11, 2016. doi:10.1007/s00362-016-0790-7.

J. Whitehead. Bayesian decision procedures with application to dose-finding studies. *International Journal of Pharmaceutical Medicine*, 11:201–208, 1997.

J. Whitehead, H. Thygesen, and A. Whitehead. A Bayesian dose-finding procedure for phase I clinical trials based only on the assumption of monotonicity. *Statistics in Medicine*, 29(17):1808–1824, 2010. doi:10.1002/sim.3963.

J. Whitehead, H. Thygesen, and A. Whitehead. Bayesian procedures for phase I/II clinical trials investigating the safety and efficacy of drug combinations. *Statistics in Medicine*, 30(16):1952–1970, 2011. doi:10.1002/sim.4267.

J. Whitehead, H. Thygesen, T. Jaki, S. Davies, S. Halford, H. Turner, N. Cook, and D. Jodrell. A novel Phase I/IIa design for early phase oncology studies and its application in the evaluation of MK-0752 in pancreatic cancer. *Statistics in Medicine*, 31(18): 1931–43, 2012. doi:10.1002/sim.5331.

K. M. Wong, A. Capasso, and S. G. Eckhardt. The changing landscape of phase I trials in oncology. *Nature Reviews Clinical Oncology*, 13(2):106–117, 2016. doi:10.1038/nrclinonc.2015.194.

G. Yin, Y. Li, and Y. Ji. Bayesian dose-finding in phase I/II clinical trials using toxicity and efficacy odds ratios. *Biometrics*, 62(3):777–784, 2006. doi:10.1111/j.1541-0420.2006.00534.x.

L. Zhao, J. Lee, R. Mody, and T. M. Braun. The superiority of the time-to-event continual reassessment method to the rolling six design in pediatric oncology phase I trials. *Clinical Trials*, 8(4):361–369, 2011. doi:10.1177/1740774511407533.

S. Zohar and S. Chevret. The continual reassessment method: Comparison of Bayesian stopping rules for dose-ranging studies. *Statistics in Medicine*, 20(19):2827–2843, 2001. doi:10.1002/sim.920.

S. Zohar and J. O'Quigley. Re: Dose escalation methods in phase I cancer clinical trials. *Journal of the National Cancer Institute*, 101(24):1732–1733; author reply 1733–1735, 2009. doi:10.1093/jnci/djp400.

2

Model-Based Designs for Safety

Emily V. Dressler and Donglin Yan

University of Kentucky

CONTENTS

2.1 Introduction

Traditional designs often utilize dichotomous toxicity outcomes for dose estimation, i.e., adverse events (AEs) are classified as either dose-limiting toxicities (DLTs) or non-DLTs based on prespecified criteria. While this is the most common choice for categorizing toxicities, an obvious flaw of dichotomizing outcomes is the loss of valuable information. Thus, ordinal grading and continuous toxicity scores have been proposed and developed for early-phase dose estimation algorithms.

Consider an ordinal scale that classifies AEs from 0 to 5, with 5 being the most severe toxicity response, 0 is no toxicity, and 1–2 are acceptable toxicities. Under the assumption of increasing probability of observing a toxicity as dose levels increase, a grade 0 toxicity and a marginal grade 2 toxicity are both considered as non-DLTs; however, a grade 0 indicates that the current dose level is probably less than optimal in terms of efficacy, while a marginal grade 2 could be a warning sign of potential DLTs with the next dose escalation. Given the small sample size in early-phase trials, incorporating ordinal toxicity or continuous scores could be advantageous by maximizing all available patient toxicity information.

In this chapter, we will introduce ordinal and continuous toxicity extensions for phase I clinical trials. This will include variations of algorithm-based designs, such as the 3 + 3 design, and model-based designs including the continual reassessment method (CRM) and escalation with overdose control (EWOC). We will present ordinal extensions of these designs with an example of how to design a trial and re-estimate dose levels as patients accrue based on the proportional odds CRM. Additionally, we will briefly discuss nonparametric methods that relax model assumptions in trial designs as well as designs incorporating continuous toxicities scores as an alternative to ordinal toxicity grading in these early-phase trials.

2.2   Algorithmic Designs

Although algorithmic designs are widely criticized for their-less-than desired statistical properties, they are still the most commonly used method in practice. Ordinal 3 + 3 designs were proposed with the hope of improving the existing 3 + 3 designs (Ivanova, 2006). By incorporating graded dose information, ordinal 3 + 3 designs utilize more information with toxicity grading, which may escalate faster than its traditional counterpart and hence allocate more patients to the optimal dose. We outline the various rules with an example cohort scenario for the up-and-down design below.

A toxicity outcome for a subject is denoted by a random variable Y, and Y has three possible values: $Y = 0$ being mild/no toxicity, $Y = 1$ being moderate toxicity, and $Y = 2$ being severe toxicity. Let $P_j(x)$ denote the probability of a subject experiencing grade j toxicity at dose level x. In this case, $P_1(x) + P_2(x) + P_3(x) = 1$. The goal is to find the dose so that $aP_2(x) + bP_3(x) = P_{DLT}$, where P_{DLT} is the predetermined target probability of DLT, and a and b are the weight constants of toxicity grade. For example, if $a = 1$ and $b = 2$, then each severe toxicity is counted as two moderate toxicities. A typical value for P_{DLT} in oncology trials is 25% or 30%.

Escalation Design: Suppose subjects are enrolled in groups of size m. The first group will start at the lowest dose. The next group will receive the next sequential dose if

$$\psi = \frac{a \times (\# \text{ of grade 2}) + b \times (\# \text{ of grade 3})}{m} \leq P_{DLT}$$

otherwise the trial is stopped.

Up-and-Down Design: Similar to the escalation design, the design begins at the lowest dose; however, now these designs allow dose levels to increase or decrease. Dose-finding rules are summarized as follows:

- Escalate if $\psi \leq P_{DLT} - \delta$.

- De-escalate if $\psi \geq P_{DLT} + \delta$.

- Otherwise, repeat the current dose.

δ is a prespecified constant, and $0 < \delta \leq P_{DLT}$. Consider that, for example, we test a cohort of $m = 3$ subjects, with prespecified assumptions of $P_{DLT} = 0.3$, $a = 1$, $b = 2$, and $\delta = 0.1$. This means that we count grade 3 toxicities twice as much as grade 2 toxicities in our rules. With a defined $\delta = 0.1$, our rules are to escalate when $\psi \leq 0.20$, de-escalate when $\psi \geq 0.40$, or repeat the same dose if ψ is between 0.20 and 0.40. If no subject in the cohort experienced a grade 2 or higher toxicity, $\psi = 0$, and the next cohort will receive a higher dose. If one subject experienced a grade 3 toxicity, $\psi = 0.667$, and the next cohort will receive a decreased dose. The current dose will be repeated if exactly one patient experienced grade 2 toxicity and the others experienced grade 1 or less, with $\psi = 0.333$.

Algorithmic designs still remain a popular choice in practice due to their simplicity in computation and implementation. We do not recommend these designs as a first option due to numerous research outlining deficiencies in estimating the target dose and treating too many patients at suboptimal and often nontherapeutic levels. The performance of a algorithmic design (Reiner et al., 1999; Lin and Shih, 2001) varies under different scenarios, but generally they have a low probability of correctly estimating the MTD, a large proportion of patients allocated to suboptimal doses, and an uncontrolled rate of the overall DLT incidences.

2.3   Modeling Ordinal Toxicities

As discussed in previous chapters, model-based designs have superior statistical properties over traditional algorithmic designs and have slowly been gaining use in early-phase trials. All model-based designs for safety follow a similar structure:

1. Choose an appropriate model for the safety outcome of interest.
2. Estimate model parameters.
3. Estimate the next dose to test from the model that meets your prespecified criteria.
4. Treat additional subjects and collect dose level treated and toxicity outcomes.
5. Repeat steps 2–4 until a prespecified stopping rule or sample size has been reached.

In this section, we will introduce two commonly used models to incorporate ordinal safety outcomes, the proportional odds model and the probit model, and their applications in early-phase trials.

2.3.1   Proportional odds model

One approach to incorporate ordinal toxicity grading into early-phase trial designs is to extend the original CRM from dichotomous outcome models, such as logistic regression, to those that can accommodate ordinal endpoints. In 2011, Van Meter et al. (2011) proposed a design utilizing the proportional odds model CRM. Utilized in both oncology clinical practice and trials outcomes, toxicity grades are often assigned in accordance with general guidelines by Common Terminology Criteria for Adverse Events version 4.0 (CTCAEv4.0). These guidelines classify AEs into grades 1–5: 1 as mild, 2 as moderate, 3 as severe, 4 as a life-threatening or disabling AE, and 5 as death related to AE (NCI, 2009). These guidelines provide specific criteria, outlined by each grade of severity, for all types of AEs. Grade 5 toxicities are not considered in this design since the trial would need to temporarily suspend for investigators and safety monitoring committees to meet and reassess continuation when a death is strictly related to an AE.

Although initially proposed in the context of oncology trials, the proportional odds model design could be applied to other medical conditions with varying numbers of toxicity categories. In the remainder of this section, we assume toxicity grades range from 0 to 4, with grades 3 and 4 representing DLTs equivalent to dichotomous rules. In the situation where patients experience more than one toxicity, we select the most severe toxicity grade observed for dose estimation purposes.

Suppose the following conditions are met:

1. Dose value for the ith patient, denoted by x_i, is on a continuous scale: $a \leq x_i \leq b$. Note: Trials with categorical dose levels can be a special case of this model, where observations are only collected at several discrete points and the estimated dose is rounded to the closest available discrete level.

2. Toxicities measured on the ith patient, denoted by Y_i, are on an ordinal scale:

$$Y_i = \begin{cases} 0 & \text{no toxicity} \\ i & \text{toxicity grade } i \end{cases}$$

where $Y_i = 3$ or 4 is considered DLTs.

3. The dose–response relationship is monotonically increasing.

The proportional odds model summarizes the dose–toxicity relationship by the following equation:

$$\text{For } j = 1, 2, 3, 4, \ \psi(x, \alpha, \beta) = \Pr[Y_i \geq j | x] = \frac{1}{1 + \exp(-(\alpha_j + \beta x))} \tag{2.1}$$

where $\alpha_4 > \alpha_3 > \cdots > \alpha_1$.

Equivalently, we can rewrite model (2.1) as the probability of each grade of toxicity:

$$\begin{cases} \Pr(Y_i = 0 | x) = 1 - \dfrac{1}{1 + \exp(-(\alpha_1 + \beta x))} \\[2mm] \Pr(Y_i = j | x) = \dfrac{1}{1 + \exp(-(\alpha_j + \beta x))} - \dfrac{1}{1 + \exp(-(\alpha_{j+1} + \beta x))}, \ \text{For } j = 1, 2, 3 \\[2mm] \Pr(Y_i = 4 | x) = \dfrac{1}{1 + \exp(-(\alpha_4 + \beta x))} \end{cases} \tag{2.2}$$

Figure 2.1 illustrates the dose–toxicity relationship described by the proportional odds model under two settings. The graph on the left represents a highly toxic drug, while the one on the right is less toxic. Assuming a 30% DLT rate, POM 1 recommends that the first dose to test is 1060 mg, while POM 2 suggests to start the trial at 2145 mg.

The dose–toxicity relationship from a proportional odds model can be interpreted in terms of odds ratios, which has nice clinical interpretations. The POM assumes that the odds of experiencing a more severe toxicity relative to a less severe toxicity are constant among all possible toxicity grades, which might not be reasonable for all clinical scenarios. Alternative models, such as continuation ratio (CR) models, have also been explored (Van Meter et al., 2012). While the approach is similar, CR models reasonably assume subjects have to pass through lower toxicity levels before reaching their highest grade.

2.3.2   Probit model

Another dose–toxicity model to consider for ordinal toxicities is the probit model. We first introduce a latent variable $Z_i = \alpha + \beta x_i + \epsilon_i$, with α and β model parameters and x_i denoting the dose level for the ith subject. Z_i can be viewed as the nonobservable true toxicity value caused by the drug at dose level x_i, and $\epsilon \sim \sigma N(0, 1)$ represents the variability between individual patients. The observed toxicity outcome, Y, is caused by Z_i exceeding a corresponding threshold. For instance, suppose we have ordinal toxicity grade ranging from 0 to 4, then there are four corresponding thresholds of the latent variable, $\gamma_1 < \gamma_2 < \cdots < \gamma_4$. The ith subject would have a grade 4 toxicity if $Z_i \geq \gamma_4$.

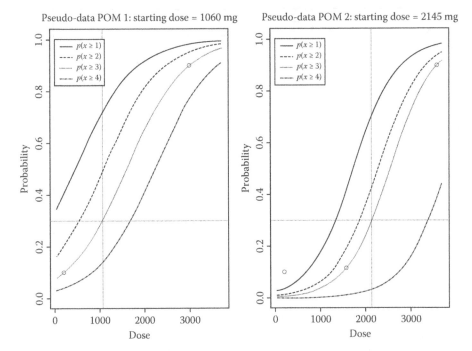

FIGURE 2.1
Examples of the proportional odds model.

The probability of subject i having a grade j or lower toxicity is

$$
\begin{aligned}
\Pr\left(Y_i < j | x\right) &= \Pr\left(Z_i < \gamma_j\right) \\
&= \Pr\left(\alpha + \beta x_i + \epsilon_i < \gamma_j\right) \\
&= \Pr\left(\epsilon_i < \gamma_j - \alpha + \beta x\right) \\
&= \phi\left(\frac{\gamma_j - (\alpha + \beta x)}{\sigma}\right)
\end{aligned}
\tag{2.3}
$$

where $\phi(\cdot)$ is the cumulative distribution function of standard normal distribution.

We fix the values of γ_1 and σ to 0 and 1, respectively, so that the model can have unique solutions without compromising the flexibility or validity of the probit model. Equation 2.3 can be rewritten as the probability of each grade of toxicity for subject i given the dose level x:

$$
\begin{cases}
\Pr\left(Y_i = 0 | x\right) = \phi(-(\alpha + \beta x)) \\
\Pr\left(Y_i = 1 | x\right) = \phi(\gamma_2 - (\alpha + \beta x)) - \phi(-(\alpha + \beta x)) \\
\Pr\left(Y_i = 2 | x\right) = \phi(\gamma_3 - (\alpha + \beta x)) - \phi(\gamma_2 - (\alpha + \beta x)) \\
\Pr\left(Y_i = 3 | x\right) = \phi(\gamma_4 - (\alpha + \beta x)) - \phi(\gamma_2 - (\alpha + \beta x)) \\
\Pr\left(Y_i = 4 | x\right) = 1 - \phi(\gamma_4 - (\alpha + \beta x))
\end{cases}
\tag{2.4}
$$

As an illustration of the probit model, suppose $\beta = 0.0256, \alpha = 1.1534, \gamma_2 = 0.769$, $\gamma_3 = 2.691$, and $\gamma_4 = 3.84$, then the probability of each grade of toxicity over dose can be visualized as shown in Figure 2.2. As dose level increases, the chance of having a higher-grade toxicity increases accordingly, which follows traditional monotonic increasing assumptions in early-phase trials.

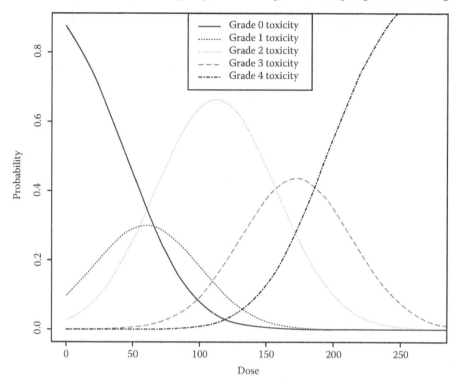

FIGURE 2.2
Example of the probit model.

2.4   Model Estimation

Once a model has been selected, there are two different statistical approaches to estimate the various parameters: maximum likelihood estimation (MLE) method and Bayesian estimation. We will conceptually introduce MLE and Bayesian estimation in the following subsections.

2.4.1   Maximum likelihood estimation

The concept behind the MLE can be loosely explained as choosing the parameters so that the observed data are the most likely to be observed. For example, suppose we are tossing a coin (maybe not a fair coin), and the probability of the result being "tails" is denoted by P. If we flip this coin 10 times and get 6 tails in the results, then $P = 0.6$ is more plausible than $P = 0.1$. Because $P = 0.6$ is more likely than any other values of P to generate 6 tails in the 10 flips, we say $P = 0.6$ maximized the likelihood of observing the result. Hence, $P = 0.6$ is the maximum likelihood estimator.

Suppose the dose–toxicity relationship can be described by the proportional odds model (2.2) with parameters α_j and β to be estimated. The MLE method assumes that α_j and β are constants unknown to us. If we knew the true values of α_j and β, we could write out the probability of each grade of toxicity for each individual patient. For example, if $\alpha_4 = 0.1$ and $\beta = 0.002$, then the probability of the ith subject having grade 4 toxicity when dose $= 100$ is

$$\Pr\left(Y_i = 4\right) = \frac{1}{1 + \exp(-(0.1 + 0.002 \times 100))} \approx 0.574.$$

Now suppose the first subject received dose $= 100$, the second subject received dose $= 50$, and we observed grade 4 and 3 toxicities for these two subjects, respectively. Assuming these two subjects are independent of each other, and holding α_3, α_4, and β constant, we can write the probability of observing this result as follows:

$$
\begin{aligned}
&\Pr\left(Y_1 = 4 | x_1 = 100 \text{ and } Y_2 = 3 | x_1 = 100, \text{and } x_2 = 50\right) \\
&= \Pr\left(Y_1 = 4 | x_1 = 100\right) \times \Pr\left(Y_2 = 3 | x_2 = 50\right) \\
&= \left[\frac{1}{1 + \exp(-(\alpha_4 + 100\beta))}\right] \left[\frac{1}{1 + \exp(-(\alpha_3 + 50\beta))} - \frac{1}{1 + \exp(-(\alpha_4 + 50\beta))}\right]
\end{aligned}
$$

The MLE estimators are parameters, α_j and β, that maximize the likelihood function given the observed *data*. MLE methods work best when the data have a reasonable size. For example, if we flip a coin only once and the result is tails, then the MLE of $P = \Pr\left(\text{"tails"}\right)$ is $\hat{P} = 1$. In the initial stage of a phase 1 trial, we may have only a few observations, so the MLE method will be unstable for small data. One solution is to start the trial with algorithm-based designs and switch to model-based methods after observing the first toxicity. Another solution is to use "data anchors" to stabilize initial parameter estimation. The "data anchor" is a set of pseudo-data generated based on clinicians' initial guess about the drug's dose–toxicity relationship. These initial guesses are not expected to be accurate since the pseudo-data will be dropped or down-weighted as more actual data are collected. In practice, the clinicians would need to identify a safe dose, where only 10% or less subjects will experience grade 3 or higher toxicity, and a dangerous dose, where 90% of the subjects will experience DLT, based on which pseudo-data can be generated. We provide an example of how to construct pseudo-data in Section 2.6.

2.4.2 Bayesian estimation

Bayesian estimation is quite different from MLE methods. First, unlike the MLE that treats model parameters as unknown constants, Bayesian estimations view both the data and model parameters as random variables. Before the trial, statisticians need to specify pretrial clinical information about the dose–toxicity relationship as a prior. The prior refers to the probability distribution of the model parameters before any data were collected, denoted by $p(\underline{\theta})$. The prior represents the range within which model parameters are most likely to take value. For example, $prior = p(\beta) \sim unif(0, 5)$ means that the prior distribution of β is a uniform distribution, with β having an equal chance to take any value between 0 and 5.

The process of choosing a proper prior is arguably the most challenging part for Bayesian models and requires intensive communication between clinicians and statisticians. More complicated methods have been published for systematic model calibration methods, and simulations should be performed to assess design characteristics (Lee and Cheung, 2009).

Once a prior has been specified, the next step is to collect data and combine prior assumptions and accrued observations into the posterior distribution. The *posterior*, denoted by $\Pi(\underline{\theta})$, is the distribution of model parameters after observing the *data*. It can be shown that

$$\Pi(\underline{\theta}) \propto p(\underline{\theta}) \times L(data|\underline{\theta})$$

where $L(data|\underline{\theta})$ is the likelihood function.

The posterior distribution is proportional to the product of the likelihood function and the prior, which is explained as the pooled knowledge of pretrial information and observed data. As more data are collected, the likelihood function will have more influence on the posterior. For the first enrolled patient, the dose estimation is solely based on the specified prior, as no observations have occurred. As such, some trial designs begin as an algorithmic design starting at a low dose and switch to model-based designs after observing the first toxicity case.

2.5   Dose Estimation

Now that the selected models have parameter estimates, we must choose a criteria by which the next dose to treat subjects is estimated. We present three approaches in the following.

2.5.1   Traditional DLT criteria

Traditionally, DLT refers to a severe AE that results in dose reduction or treatment discontinuation. These scenarios must be specified prior to any patient accruals, and different medical conditions will have varying definitions of DLT specific to the types of AEs expected for that particular disease. In oncology trials, a DLT is typically a grade 3 or higher toxicity according to CTCAE (NCI, 2009). Suppose the probability of DLT at dose x is denoted by π_x, then the MTD can be defined as the dose, denoted by d, that is associated with a prespecified probability π_d. Often oncology trials aim for $\pi_d = 30\%$ or 25%, i.e., the estimated MTD should have approximately 25% or 30% probability of any given subject experiencing a DLT.

Under this definition of DLT and MTD, rewriting $\Pr[Y \geq 3|x]$ from model (2.1), the estimated dose for the next patient using the proportional odds model is

$$\hat{x} = \left(\log \left(\frac{\pi_d}{1 - \pi_d} \right) - \hat{\alpha}_3 \right) / \hat{\beta} \tag{2.5}$$

Similarly, estimating the dose from the probit model (2.3),

$$\begin{aligned} \Pr(Y_i \geq 3|x) &= 1 - \Pr(Y_i < 3|x) \\ &= \Pr(Z_i < \gamma_3) \\ &= \phi \left(\frac{\gamma_3 - (\alpha + \beta x)}{\sigma} \right) \end{aligned} \tag{2.6}$$

And solving for x,

$$\hat{x} = (\psi^{-1}(1 - \pi_d) - \hat{\gamma}_3 - \hat{\alpha}) / \hat{\beta} \tag{2.7}$$

When sample size has reached the maximum quota or met stopping rules, $\hat{x}$ will be the estimated MTD.

2.5.2   Multiple constraints

The traditional definition of DLTs may not be optimal for utilizing all collected data and may be inappropriate for some studies. For example in a phase I trial in lymphoma patients (Ruan et al., 2011), the tested agent, Bortezomib plus standard CHOP-Rituximab, could cause neurological toxicity. In this trial, the DLT is defined as grade 3 or higher peripheral neuropathy. However, a grade 3 neuropathy may be resolved after discontinuation of the treatment, whereas a grade 4 neuropathy is irreversible and life-threatening. As a result, we might want to control the overall probability of a DLT so that the tolerance for grade 4 toxicity is much lower than that for grade 3 toxicity.

In order to constrain multiple toxicity grades, Lee et al. (2011) proposed an extension of the CRM that redefined criteria for DLTs and estimation of the MTD. The revised definition of MTD and the corresponding dose-finding methods are described in the following.

Let $\hat{x}$ denote MTD. For toxicity outcomes, T, and L prespecified toxicity constraints, define $\hat{x}$ as

$$\hat{x} = \arg\max\{\Pr\left(Y \geq t_l | x\right) \leq p_l, l = 1, \dots, L\},$$

where $t_1 < \cdots < t_L$ are the prespecified toxicity thresholds and $p_1 > \cdots > p_L$ are their corresponding target probabilities (Lee et al., 2011). $\hat{x}$ is the dose we assign to the next patient. As an example, consider a typical phase I cancer trial, where grade 3 and 4 toxicities are DLTs, and we want to restrict the probability of DLT to be less than 30%. Furthermore, we wish to constrain the probability of grade 4 toxicity to be less than 5%. Therefore, we have $L = 2$ toxicity constraints, and θ is defined as the maximum dose that satisfies both conditions above. This design will be further discussed in detail with examples in the next chapter.

2.5.3   Ordinal escalation with overdose control designs

EWOC is a well-known alternative to the CRM design (Babb et al., 1998). The main difference between EWOC and CRM is that EWOC's goal is to control the probability of overdosing. The prespecified probability of overdosing is referred to as the feasible bound, denoted by α in our notation. Here, overdosing is defined as a dose that exceeds the true MTD. Originally, EWOC incorporates dichotomized toxicity outcomes. Tighiouart proposed a modified EWOC to incorporate ordinal toxicities in the design (Tighiouart et al., 2012). In this extended EWOC design, the toxicities were classified into three ordinal categories: minimum, intermediate, and high toxicities. Proportional odds models were used to model dose–toxicity relationships. Details of this method are illustrated in the following.

Suppose toxicity grades are assigned according to the CTCAEv4.0, ranging from grades 0 to 4. Consider toxicities, Y,

$$Y_i = \begin{cases} 0, \text{ (minimum to mildly toxicity)} & \text{if grade} = 0, 1 \\ 1, \text{ (intermediate toxicity)} & \text{if grade} = 2 \\ 2, \text{ (DLT toxicity)} & \text{if grade} = 3, 4 \end{cases}$$

Assume the dose–toxicity relationship can be described by proportional odds model:

$$\Pr\left(Y_i \geq j | x\right) = F(\alpha_j + \beta x), j = 1, 2 \tag{2.8}$$

where α_j and β are model parameters and $\alpha_1 < \alpha_2$. $F(\cdot)$ is a monotonically increasing link function that ranges from 0 to 1. This equation models the cumulative probability of toxicity j and higher. The probability of individual toxicity level can be written as follows:

$$\Pr\left(Y_i = j\right) = \begin{cases} 1 - F(\alpha_1 + \beta x), & \text{if } j = 0 \\ F(\alpha_1 + \beta x) - F(\alpha_2 + \beta x) & \text{if } j = 1 \\ F(\alpha_2 + \beta x) & \text{if } j = 2 \end{cases}$$

The MTD, γ, is defined as the dose that is expected to produce θ percent DLTs: $\Pr(Y = 2|x = y) = F(\alpha_2 + \beta\gamma) = \theta$. The likelihood function after observing the first k subjects is

$$L(\alpha_1, \alpha_2, \beta | D_k) = \prod_{i=1}^{n} [1 - F(\alpha_1 + \beta x_i)]^{I(Y_i=0)}$$
$$\times [F(\alpha_1 + \beta x_i) - F(\alpha_2 + \beta x_i)]^{I(Y_i=1)}$$
$$\times F(\alpha_2 + \beta x_i)^{I(Y_i=2)}$$

where $I(\cdot)$ is the indicator function.

We can then reparametrize Equation 2.8 in terms of $\rho_0 = \Pr(Y_i = 2|x = X_{\min})$, the probability of a DLT for a patient i given dose $x = X_{\min}$, and $\rho_1 = \Pr(Y_i \geq 1|x = X_{\min})$, the probability of a grade 2 or higher toxicity for patient i given dose $x = X_{\min}$. As discussed in Babb et al. (1998), it can be shown as follows:

$$\alpha_1 = F^{-1}(\rho_1)\alpha_2 = F^{-1}(\rho_0)$$
$$\beta = \frac{1}{\gamma}(F^{-1}(\theta) - F^{-1}(\rho_0)) \tag{2.9}$$

For $0 \leq \rho_0 \leq \rho_1$ and $0 \leq \rho_0 \leq \theta$, define

$$F_1(\rho_0, \rho_1, \gamma; x) = F(F^{-1}(\rho_1) + (F^{-1}(\theta) - F^{-1}(\rho_0))\frac{x}{\gamma})$$
$$F_2(\rho_0, \rho_1, \gamma; x) = F(F^{-1}(\rho_0) + (F^{-1}(\theta) - F^{-1}(\rho_0))\frac{x}{\gamma}) \tag{2.10}$$

Thus, the likelihood is now

$$L(\rho_0, \rho_1, \gamma | D_k) = \prod_{i=1}^{n} [1 - F_1(\rho_0, \rho_1, \gamma; x_i)]^{I(Y_i=0)}$$
$$\times [(F_1(\rho_0, \rho_1, \gamma; x_i)) - F_2(\rho_0, \rho_1, \gamma; x_i)]^{I(Y_i=1)}$$
$$\times [F_2(\rho_0, \rho_1, \gamma; x_i)]^{I(Y_i=2)}$$

Using Bayesian estimation, we can obtain the posterior distribution for patient k:

$$\Pi(\rho_0, \rho_1, \gamma | D_k) \propto L(\rho_0, \rho_1, \gamma | D_k) \cdot prior(\rho_0, \rho_1, \gamma)$$

The dose for the next patient is estimated as $x_{k+1} = \Pi_k^{-1}(\alpha)$, where α is the feasibility bound. At the end of the trial with n patients, the final MTD can be estimated as $\hat{\gamma} = \Pi_n^{-1}(\alpha)$.

2.6   Example Using the Proportional Odds Model CRM

Previously, we discussed which models could be utilized to incorporate ordinal toxicities with varying methods of parameter estimation and dose selection criteria. In this section, we provide a phase I dose-finding example using the proportional odds model CRM with MLE estimation. This design identifies the next dose to treat based on traditional DLT criteria.

Consider a hypothetical drug that can be administered at any dose level between 0 and 150 mg/m². An investigator wishes to identify the MTD for a 33% target DLT rate while assessing cohorts of two patients at a time. To begin this design, we must first build "pseudo-data" to represent preclinical beliefs prior to the start of the trial. In this situation, we must inquire about dose levels that from a clinical perspective would result in very low and high DLT rates, given previous knowledge of the drug. From that conversation, we are told that 10% DLT rates will most likely occur at very low levels of the drug, approximately 5 mg/m², while excessive dose-limiting events (90%) should be seen at 140 mg/m². That is all the clinical information needed to start constructing proportional odds models.

To fit these models, we would also need the distribution of toxicities at the hypothesized 10% and 90% DLT rate dose levels. However, simulations over many scenarios have shown that we can distribute grades of toxicity at the low dose level as follows: 45% experiencing no toxicity, 35% grade 1, 10% grade 2, 8% grade 3, and 2% grade 4 toxicities. And, at the excessive toxicity level, we can specify 2% experiencing no toxicity, 3% grade 1, 5% grade 2, 40% grade 3, and 50% grade 4 toxicities. We use MLE methods to obtain $\hat{\alpha}_1 = 0.0170$, $\hat{\alpha}_2 = -1.5082$, $\hat{\alpha}_3 = -2.2931$, $\hat{\alpha}_4 = -4.3933$, and $\hat{\beta} = 0.0315$ (Figure 2.3).

Our criteria to estimate the next dose to test are based on the probability of a DLT (grade 3 or 4) no higher than our target DLT rate of 33%. Substituting the ML estimates into Equation 2.5, we can estimate the next dose to treat as follows:

$$\hat{x} = \left(\log \left(\frac{0.33}{1 - 0.33} \right) - (-2.2931) \right) / 0.0315 \approx 50$$

As shown in Figure 2.3, this proportional odds model would select the first dose to test at 50 mg/m², as that is the dose estimated to have approximately 33% grade 3 or 4 toxicities.

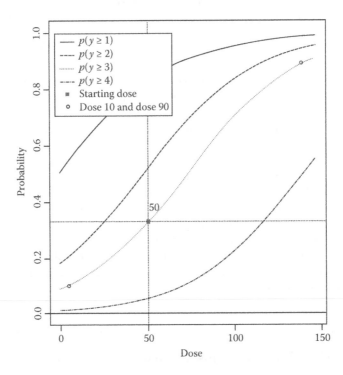

FIGURE 2.3
Initial proportional odds model: 10% DLT at 5 mg/m², 90% DLT at 140 mg/m², and starting dose = 50 mg/m².

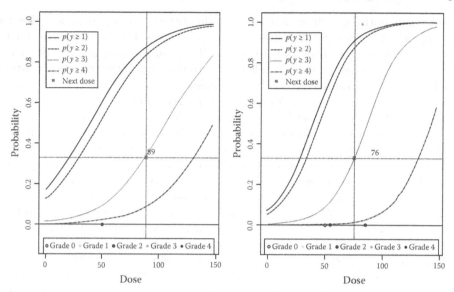

FIGURE 2.4

Accumulating data in the proportional odds CRM: the left graph is after two subjects accrued (one no toxicity and one grade 2) with the next dose estimated to 89 mg/m². The right graph is after four subjects accrued (an additional grade 2 toxicity and one grade 3) with the next dose estimated to 76 mg/m².

Additionally, the underlying dose–toxicity curves for the probability of experiencing a particular grade toxicity or one more severe are presented with the data anchors specified at 5 and 140 mg/m² for hypothesized 10% and 90% DLT rates, respectively.

  We now treat patients in cohorts of two and record all toxicities. We use the highest-grade toxicity for each patient to re-estimate our dose–toxicity curves after each cohort. Figure 2.4 illustrates the updated proportional odds models after each of the first two cohorts. For the cohort treated at 50 mg/m², the first subject experiences no toxicity and the second has a grade 2 toxicity. The updated dose–toxicity curve using toxicity information accrued from those two subjects is shown in the left graph. Because there was no severe toxicities, the proportional odds model shifts to the right and identifies the next dose to treat at 89 mg/m². We then treat two additional subjects at 89 mg/m², and we observe one grade 2 and one grade 3 toxicity in this cohort. After updating the proportional odds model again, the right graph in Figure 2.4 shows that the model now identifies a lower next dose to treat at 76 mg/m².

  This process would continue, where we accumulate the dose tested and toxicity grade observed for each cohort, update the proportional odds model, and re-estimate the next dose to treat based on traditional DLT criteria until we reach a prespecified sample size or stopping rule. The estimated dose identified from the last model with all toxicity information incorporated would be the estimated MTD from this trial. Software is currently available in the R package *ordcrm* (Dressler and Huang, 2016).

2.7   Alternative Toxicity Classifications

There are limitations to methods that monitor only one toxicity occurrence for each subject. First, different types and cumulative amounts of toxicities are not considered equally important in these models, as a patient suffering grade 3 neuropathy may be more concerning than a patient experiencing grade 3 fatigue. Second, the occurrence of one toxicity is not independent of the others as often seen in oncology trials; a patient with nausea is very likely to also have fatigue. The previous model-based methods, by using the maximum of various toxicities, essentially assume that all toxicities are equally important.

Others have explored alternative strategies to summarize a more comprehensive and cumulative toxicity outcome. Bekele and Thall proposed a toxicity scoring method: Total Toxicity Burden (TTB). The TTB is defined as the sum of the weights of all toxicities experienced by that patient (Bekele and Thall, 2004). To calculate the TTB, clinicians must list all potential types of toxicity and assign a severity weight to each grade 3 and 4 toxicity to quantify the overall clinical impact. Using a sarcoma trial as an example, we display the possible types of toxicity and the corresponding weights in Table 2.1. Note in this trial, fatigue of grade 4 is weighted less severe than grade 3 myelosuppression with fever since the later can lead to irreversible damage. Similarly, liver toxicity of grade 4 is considered more severe than that of grade 3 as it results in permanent organ damage.

After weights are assigned to each type and grade of toxicity, a target TTB needs to be determined by evaluating various hypothetical dose–toxicity scenarios. Based on these proposed scenarios, clinicians are asked to decide whether the next patient should receive a higher, lower, or equivalent dose level. Intensive communication between clinicians and statisticians is required to finalize a proper weighting scheme and a reasonable target TTB, which should be clinically meaningful for all possible scenarios. On the basis of TTB, the definition of DLT will be a patient's TTB exceeding the target TTB.

Another method for summarizing a patient's toxicity profile, called the Toxicity Index (TI) method, was proposed by Rogatko et al. (2004). Based on an analysis of 459 patients enrolled in phase I and II trials at Fox Chase Cancer Center from 1991 to 1999, the calculation of TI can be summarized as follows:

1. Subjects can have n types of toxicity with ordered toxicity severity as $X_1 \geq X_2 \geq X_3 \cdots \geq X_n$.

2. Calculate the weight of each type of toxicity as

$$w_i = \begin{cases} \sum_{j=1}^{n} \frac{1}{(X_j+1)}, & \text{if } i > 1 \\ 1 & \text{if } i = 1 \end{cases}$$

TABLE 2.1

Example of toxicity and assigned weights for TTB design.

	Type of Toxicity	Grade	Severity Weight
1	Myelosuppression without fever	3	1.0
	Myelosuppression with fever	4	1.5
2	Dermatitis	3	2.5
		4	6.0
3	Liver	2	2.0
		3	3.0
		4	6.0
4	Nausea/vomiting	3	1.5
		4	2.0
5	Fatigue	3	0.5
		4	1.0

3. Calculate TI as

$$TI = \sum_{i=1}^{n} w_i X_i$$
$$= X_1$$
$$+ \frac{X_2}{1 + X_1}$$
$$+ \frac{X_3}{(1 + X_1)(1 + X_2)}$$
$$+ \cdots$$
$$+ \frac{X_n}{(1 + X_1) \ldots (1 + X_{n-1})} \tag{2.11}$$

For example, suppose a subject can have three potential toxicities, A, B, and C, with toxicity grades of X_a, X_b, and X_c, respectively. If observed toxicities A and B are both grade 2 and toxicity C is a grade 4, then the ordered toxicity is $(X_1 = 4) \geq (X_2 = 2) \geq (X_3 = 2)$ so that the toxicity with the highest grade will have a weight of 1 with lower grades having less weight. From Equation 2.11, weights equal $w_1 = 1, w_2 = 1/(4 + 1) = 1/5$, and $w_3 = 1/[(4 + 1)(2 + 1)] = 1/15$ and TI is the sum of each toxicity grade weighted by w_i: $TI = [(1) \times (4)] + [(1/5) \times (2)] + [(1/15) \times (2)] \approx 4.53$.

A third approach for summarizing toxicity is known as TAME, which is the short form of (acute) Toxicity (**T**), Adverse long-term (late) effects (**A**), Mortality risk (**M**) generated by a treatment program, and End results (**E**) (Trotti et al., 2007). TAME is a more complex toxicity summary system compared to the two previous methods and is more suitable for trials with complicated toxicity profiles, such as aggressive treatments in cancer trials. Examples of these endpoints are given below.

T score for an individual patient is defined as the sum of the number of high-grade (3 or 4) acute events reported on that individual for a defined acute-risk interval. For a group of patients, we can calculate mean raw T values by taking the mean of all individual patient T scores.

A is the mean number of grade 3 and 4 late events for a treatment regimen during a defined late-toxicity risk period. For each individual patient, A score is the number of high-grade events reported for that individual during the defined late-risk interval.

M represents the risk of death attributed to treatment during a given risk period, typically defined as the cumulative incidence of death due to toxicity up to 30 days after completion of cancer treatment.

E is referred to as the end result defined for that trial.

TAME provides a comprehensive summary of the toxicity profile and systematically reflexes both long-term and short-term impacts of the treatments. In individual studies, T and A scores from individuals can be used for dose-finding trials. Additionally, TAME is a good standard when comparing different trial designs. Two dose-finding designs may have similar probability of identifying the MTD, but the TAME of these two methods is also an important factor to consider, as it summarizes the full toxicity profile of this drug over the course of treatment.

The last method we introduce is the toxicity burden score (TBS) system (Lee et al., 2012), which will be covered in more detail in the next chapter. In brief, TBS is a weighted sum of the grades of each type of toxicity, with weights estimated via regression modeling historical data. Consider a trial for drug Q. By reviewing completed trials or similar studies of drug Q, physicians assign a severity score to each grade of toxicity and then assign an overall TBS score for each patient, using the severity score as a frame of reference. To improve accuracy, different physicians can assign the scores blinded to other reviewer

TABLE 2.2

Summary of designs with toxicity-scoring approaches.

Method	Authors	Year	Summary
TTB	Bekele and Thall	2004	Sum of severity weights assigned by clinical impressions.
TI	Rogatko et al.	2004	Weighted sum of toxicity grades. The highest grade has the largest weight and gradually reduces weight for lower-grade toxicities.
TAME	Trotti et al.	2007	Three different measures to comprehensively summarize toxicity burden. Assumes equal weights for different types of toxicity. May incorporate long-term AE.
TBS	Lee et al.	2012	Weighted sum of toxicity grade. Weights are estimated by historical data from completed trials.

scores. Once the TBS scores are assigned in the historical data, a regression analysis can be performed, modeling assigned TBS by the grade of each type of toxicity. The estimated coefficients of each grade are the weight of that particular grade of toxicity.

Table 2.2 is a summary of the various approaches of toxicity-scoring methods we introduced and discussed in this section.

2.8 Discussion

For early-phase trial designs, selection of safety endpoints requires careful consideration. It is often not enough to simply quantify the most severe toxicity experienced by each subject as dose-limiting or not. Outcomes should be balanced based on preclinical knowledge of the drugs investigated, the expected toxicity profiles in terms of both quantity and severity, and the timing of an AE (acute versus late onset).

Ordinal models do incorporate more information regarding the severity of an observed toxicity. These are nice extensions to what is already observed and categorized in clinical practice, with reliable guidelines already established such as CTCAE. Options of ordinal models can include proportional odds, CR, or probit models with MLE or Bayesian estimation approaches to obtain parameter estimates. The rule on how to estimate the next dose to test needs to be identified prior to study and can be tailored to traditional DLT approaches, multiple constraints, or EWOC criteria.

There is a need to quantify a more comprehensive picture of a subject's toxicity profile, but this often adds to the complexity of the design. Continuous scales, such as TBS, TI, TTB, and TAME to name a few, do reflect a more comprehensive snapshot of an overall toxicity profile in terms of severity, quantity, and in some cases, timing. However, they require a lot of preclinical knowledge of the drug and assumptions made by clinical investigators over all hypothetical scenarios. This requires much discussion between investigators and statisticians prior to trial activation and extensive simulation work to test various situations, and as such these designs have not been utilized in many trials.

References

J. Babb, A. Rogatko, and S. Zacks. Cancer phase I clinical trials: Efficient dose escalation with overdose control. *Statistics in Medicine*, 17(10):1103–1120, 1998. doi:10.1002/(SICI) 1097-0258(19980530)17:10⟨1103::AID-SIM793⟩3.0.CO;2-9.

B. N. Bekele and P. F. Thall. Dose-finding based on multiple toxicities in a soft tissue sarcoma trial. *Journal of the American Statistical Association*, 99(465):26–35, 2004. doi:10.1198/016214504000000043.

E. V. Dressler and Z. Huang. ordcrm: Likelihood-Based Continual Reassessment (CRM) Dose Finding Designs. R package version 1.0.0, https://cran.r-project.org/package= ordcrm, 2016.

A. Ivanova. Escalation, group and A + B designs for dose-finding trials. *Statistics in Medicine*, 25(21):3668–3678, 2006. doi:10.1002/sim.2470.

S. M. Lee, B. Cheng, and Y. K. Cheung. Continual reassessment method with multiple toxicity constraints. *Biostatistics*, 12(2):386–398, 2011. doi:10.1093/biostatistics/kxq062.

S. M. Lee and Y. K. Cheung. Model calibration in the continual reassessment method. *Clinical Trials*, 6(3):227–238, 2009. doi:10.1177/1740774509105076.

S. M. Lee, D. L. Hershman, P. Martin, J. P. Leonard, and Y. K. Cheung. Toxicity burden score: A novel approach to summarize multiple toxic effects. *Annals of Oncology*, 23(2): 537–541, 2012. doi:10.1093/annonc/mdr146.

Y. Lin and W. J. Shih. Statistical properties of the traditional algorithm-based designs for phase I cancer clinical trials. *Biostatistics*, 2(2):203–215, 2001. doi:10.1093/biostatistics/ 2.2.203.

National Cancer Institute (NCI). Common Terminology Criteria for Adverse Events (CTCAE). Version 4.0, 2009.

E. Reiner, X. Paoletti, and J. O'Quigley. Operating characteristics of the standard phase I clinical trial design. *Computational Statistics and Data Analysis*, 30(3):303–315, 1999. doi:10.1016/S0167-9473(98)00095-4.

A. Rogatko, J. S. Babb, H. Wang, M. J. Slifker, and G. R. Hudes. Patient characteristics compete with dose as predictors of acute treatment toxicity in early phase clinical trials. *Clinical Cancer Research*, 10(14):4645–4651, 2004. doi:10.1158/1078-0432.ccr-03-0535.

J. Ruan, P. Martin, R. R. Furman, S. M. Lee, K. Cheung, J. M. Vose, A. LaCasce, J. Morrison, R. Elstrom, S. Ely, et al. Bortezomib plus CHOP-rituximab for previously untreated diffuse large B-cell lymphoma and mantle cell lymphoma. *Journal of Clinical Oncology*, 29(6):690–697, 2011. doi:10.1200/jco.2010.31.1142.

M. Tighiouart, G. Cook-Wiens, and A. Rogatko. Escalation with overdose control using ordinal toxicity grades for cancer phase I clinical trials. *Journal of Probability and Statistics*, 2012:18, 2012. doi:10.1155/2012/317634.

A. Trotti, T. F. Pajak, C. K. Gwede, R. Paulus, J. Cooper, A. Forastiere, J. A. Ridge, D. Watkins-Bruner, A. S. Garden, K. K. Ang, et al. TAME: Development of a new method for summarising adverse events of cancer treatment by the Radiation Therapy Oncology Group. *Lancet Oncology*, 8(7):613–624, 2007. doi:10.1016/s1470-2045(07)70144-4.

E. M. Van Meter, E. Garrett-Mayer, and D. Bandyopadhyay. Dose-finding clinical trial design for ordinal toxicity grades using the continuation ratio model: An extension of the continual reassessment method. *Clinical Trials*, 9(3):303–313, 2012. doi:10.1177/ 1740774512443593.

E. M. Van Meter, E. Garrett-Mayer, and D. Bandyopadhyay. Proportional odds model for dose-finding clinical trial designs with ordinal toxicity grading. *Statistics in Medicine*, 30 (17):2070–2080, 2011. doi:10.1002/sim.4069.

3

Dose-Finding Methods for Nonbinary Outcomes

Shing M. Lee and Ying Kuen K. Cheung

Columbia University

CONTENTS

3.1 Introduction

The continual reassessment method (CRM) as originally proposed assumes that the outcome is binary. However, in practice, toxicity and adverse event data are captured across all body systems and symptoms on a grade from 0 to 5, with 0 being no toxicity, 1 a mild toxicity, 2 a moderate toxicity, 3 a severe toxicity, 4 a life-threatening toxicity, and 5 being death. To be able to use the CRM, the multidimensional toxicity data are summarized into a single binary endpoint in the presence or absence of a dose-limiting toxicity (DLT), which is generally defined as the presence of a grade 3 or higher nonhematologic toxicity or the presence of a grade 4 or higher hematologic toxicity in the first cycle of therapy. While using this summary measure from the first cycle alone is simple and advantageous for rapid assignment of doses in sequentially treated patients, and for timely study completion when using conventional methods to determine the maximum tolerated dose (MTD), this approach assumes the absence of late-onset toxicities and ignores cumulative toxicity. Moreover, summarizing a wide range of adverse events into a single binary endpoint, though simple, also comes with weaknesses because it does not differentiate between lower grades of toxicity and between types of toxicity. Thus, a lot of information is potentially lost. Several methods have been proposed for summarizing toxicities into a continuous or ordinal outcome and for estimating the MTD associated with such outcomes. Among the proposed methods that work with a continuous or ordinal endpoint directly, several, such as the latent variable approach by Bekele and Thall [1], have already been described in the previous chapter. In this chapter, we will review the CRM with multiple toxicity constraints in more detail [2, 3] and describe the quasi-continual reassessment method (quasi-CRM)

[4, 5] and the unified approach by Ivanova and Kim [6]. While the CRM with multiple constraints defines the MTD as the dose that satisfies various prespecified toxicity thresholds of a continuous or ordinal outcome, the other methods define the MTD as the dose associated with a target level of the continuous or ordinal outcome. Thus, the selection of a target level can be challenging, given that generally little information is known about the summary toxicity measure that would make it possible to specify a relevant target. This is particularly important given that when using these methods, the MTD is defined as the dose associated with the specified target level of the continuous outcome. Each of these methods will be discussed in detail in this chapter. Section 3.2 discusses various methods used for summarizing toxicities into continuous measures and the differences among them. An illustration of a dose-finding clinical trial using the CRM with multiple constraints is presented in Section 3.3. The mathematical framework and the dose-escalation algorithm are presented for the CRM with multiple constraints in Section 3.4, for the quasi-CRM is presented in Section 3.5.1, and for the unified approach by Ivanova and Kim in Section 3.5.2.

The original CRM, like traditional dose-finding methods, also requires complete observations before each dose assignment. To be able to complete trials within a reasonable time frame, in practice, only toxicities in the first cycle of treatment are considered. This practice disregards late-onset and cumulative toxicities, which are particularly important in the context of new anticancer treatments [7]. The time-to-event CRM (TITE-CRM) was proposed to address these shortcomings by allowing for a longer observation window and inclusion of late-onset toxicities [8]. Moreover, by including partial information, the TITE-CRM allows for continuous recruitment, faster accrual, and shorter study duration. Section 3.6 describes the TITE-CRM along with the mathematical framework for the method and the dose-escalation algorithm. An example of a dose-finding trial using the TITE-CRM is presented in Section 3.7.

Several other designs will not be discussed in this chapter. For example, several designs have been proposed to dichotomize the continuous outcome with the objective of identifying the dose associated with a single target percentile of the continuous outcome. Among those methods, we have the stochastic approximation with virtual observations by Cheung and Elkind [9]. Moreover, there are other designs that incorporate information into the toxicity grading but have the same objective as the CRM of estimating the dose associated with a targeted probability of DLT, such as the proportional odds model and the continuation ratio models by Van Meter et al. [10, 11], which are presented in detail in the previous chapter; the design by Wang et al. [12]; and the design by Iasonos et al. [13]. Wang et al. [12] proposed modifications to the CRM that incorporate the information into toxicity grades by including a term for the conditional probability of a grade 4 toxicity given a DLT in the likelihood and also by assigning doses depending on the severity of the DLT observed. The method by Iasonos et al., in contrast, focuses on the information provided by lower-grade toxicities in the context of the two-stage CRM and proposes methods for incorporating information into lower-grade toxicities in the first stage of a two-stage design and for separately modeling the rates of DLT and lower-grade toxicities.

3.2   Summaries of Toxicity Types and Grades

Before diving into the dose-finding methods for nonbinary outcomes, we will first discuss the various methods that have been proposed for summarizing toxicity data into a continuous measure, which can then be used with dose-finding methods for continuous outcomes. Other types of continuous outcomes for dose-finding methods are outcomes that are naturally continuous such as biological biomarkers. Several methods have been proposed for summarizing the individual toxicity data on grades and types. All these methods summarize the individual toxicities into a score using a weighted sum of individual toxicities, even though the severity weight for the toxicities and the toxicities to be included differs among them.

The method proposed by Rogatko et al. [14] summarizes the toxicities into a toxicity index score defined as the weighted sum of toxicity grades where the weights are the product of the reciprocal grades plus 1. The method takes into account all toxicity grades and can accommodate the severity distinction between hematologic and nonhematologic toxicity. However, it does not differentiate the severity of toxicity types within these categorizations. For example, the weight given to a grade 3 nausea would be the same as that given to a grade 3 cardiac toxicity. In addition, the method assumes that the aggregate effect of lower-grade toxicities never amounts to that of higher-grade toxicities.

The method proposed by Bekele and Thall [1] is applied in the context of dose-finding clinical trials. This method defines the total toxicity burden (TTB) as the weighted sum of toxicity grades for a predetermined set of toxicities. The weights are elicited from the physicians based on their impression of the relative impact of the toxicity through a consensus process. The method takes into account the various grades of toxicity and differentiates the severity of various types of toxicity via physician input. However, it only considers a small subset of toxicities. The predetermined set of toxicities differs by therapy, and thus, the method has to be tailored for individual therapies and cannot be generalized easily. Moreover, the elicitation process is very subjective and requires careful planning and collaboration. More details on this method are available in the previous chapter.

Another method proposed in the context of radiotherapy is the TAME method by Trotti et al. [15], which is comprised acute toxicities, late events, and treatment-related mortality. The acute and late events are divided into a fixed number of tissue or organ system categories, which are counted per patient based on the highest grade of any type within the category. They combine grade 3 and 4 toxicities. Thus, the individual toxicity data are the sum of grade 3 and 4 toxicities across categories. Toxicities are then summarized by averaging the individual toxicity data for acute and late events and calculating the cumulative incidence of death due to toxicity separately. This approach dichotomizes toxicities and does not take into account the severity gradation within each category, assumes equal weight for all toxicity categories, and groups toxicities by organ system categories that were selected for head and neck radiotherapy instead of chemotherapy. By assuming equal weight, the method does not differentiate between the severity of hematologic and nonhematologic toxicities, which is essential for chemotherapy agents. In addition, since the approach was proposed for radiotherapy agents, the toxicity categories are specific to radiotherapy.

The method proposed by Lee et al. [16] summarizes adverse events into a numerical score called the toxicity burden score (TBS). The method differentiates between the grades and types of toxicities, and it summarizes toxicities, via a weighted sum of individual toxicities, where the weights are obtained using a regression approach. By using a regression approach and including several raters, the elicitation process is more reliable and reproducible. However, like the method by Bekele and Thall, the toxicities need to be prespecified as they are the toxicities that are most likely thought to be related to treatment. Thus, it has to be tailored to individual therapies, and it is not appropriate for a first-in-human dose-finding trial, where there is little information on the toxicity profiles of an agent.

To use the method to summarize toxicity data, it is necessary to first identify the J toxicities thought to be related to treatment and obtain a historical data on toxicities experienced using the drug of interest. For patient i, let $Y_{i,j} \in \{0, 1, \dots, 5\}$ be the toxicity grade experienced for treatment-related toxicity type j and W_i be an overall measure of toxicity, where $j = 1, \dots, J$. Using the dataset, multiple clinicians are asked to assign severity scores based on the toxicity grades and types experienced for each patient, with the guideline that a score of 1 should amount to a DLT, 0 to no toxicity, and 5 to treatment-related death. Using the assigned severity scores as the dependent variables in a linear mixed effects model and the treatment-related toxicity types and grades and the overall measure of toxicity as covariates, we can estimate the weights using the fixed-effects coefficients obtained from the model. Then, given $(Y_{i,1}, \ldots, Y_{i,J}, W_i)$, we can summarize the severity of multiple toxicities into a TBS defined as

$$T_i = \min\left\{\sum_{j=1}^{J}\sum_{c=1}^{5} a_{jc}I(Y_{i,j} = c) + bW_i, 5\right\},$$

where a_{jc}s and b are the constants pre-estimated by fitting a linear mixed-effects model to the historical data and $a_{j5} \equiv 5$. By definition, $T_i = 5$ when there is a treatment-related death.

This method was illustrated in the context of a bortezomib trial data where the two toxicities thought to be related to treatment were neuropathy and low platelet count, i.e., $J = 2$. The number of grade 3 or higher-grade nonhematological toxicities unrelated to bortezomib is included as variable W because it is believed that excessive toxicities are important in the determination of overall toxicity burden. To obtain the coefficients a_{jc}s and b, three clinicians were asked to assign a severity score based on the toxicity grades and types experienced by 24 patients in a bortezomib trial. Using linear mixed-effects model to fit the data gave the following significant fixed-effects coefficients: $a_{11} = 0.19, a_{12} = 0.64, a_{13} = 1.03$, and $a_{14} = 2.53$ for neuropathy; $a_{21} = a_{22} = 0.17, a_{23} = 0.40$, and $a_{24} = 0.85$ for low platelet count; and $b = 0.17$. Thus, for a patient who is alive or did not die due to treatment,

$$\begin{aligned}T_i = \{&0.19I(Y_{i,1} = 1) + 0.64I(Y_{i,1} = 2) + 1.03I(Y_{i,1} = 3) + 2.53I(Y_{i,1} = 4)\\ &+ 0.17I(Y_{i,2} = 1) + 0.17I(Y_{i,2} = 2) + 0.40I(Y_{i,2} = 3) + 0.85I(Y_{i,2} = 4)\\ &+ bW_i\}.\end{aligned}$$

The severity weights for these toxicities can be applied for a future bortezomib dose-finding trial. For example, if a patient experiences a grade 1 neuropathy, a grade 1 low platelet count, a grade 2 hemoglobin, and a grade 1 nausea, the estimated TBS is 0.19 for the grade 1 neuropathy plus 0.17 for the grade 1 platelet count which equals 0.36. This continuous TBS value can then be used as an outcome along with one of the dose-finding methods for continuous outcomes that will be discussed later in this chapter.

It should be noted that all of the aforementioned methods have been proposed as conceptual ideas and they lack further testing in other disease sites, agents, and applications. As a result, the methods have lacked support from physician and have not been adopted in practice, with the exception of a few applications. This is an area of ongoing research.

3.3   Continual Reassessment Method with Multiple Constraints

The CRM with Multiple Constraints can be applied to any ordinal or continuous outcome where we are interested in controlling the rate at various thresholds of the outcome [3]. Let $D = \{d_1, \ldots, d_K\}$ be the K doses of interest and let Y^* be an ordinal or continuous toxicity outcome such as the National Cancer Institute Common Terminology Criteria for Adverse Events (NCI-CTCAE), or the TBS and the TTB score specified in the previous section. Define Y to an ordinal toxicity outcome that takes on values $0, 1, \ldots, L$ based on the desired constraints, such that L is less than or equal to the number of possible toxicity outcome categories in Y^*. For example, suppose that the raw outcome Y^* is the NCI-CTCAE, which assumes values $0, 1, 2, 3, 4,$ and 5, and we are interested in only two constraints (i.e., $L = 2$): one on $\Pr(Y^* \geq 3)$ and the other on $\Pr(Y^* \geq 4)$. In this case, the variable Y is defined as $Y = 0$ if and only if $Y^* = 0, 1,$ or 2, $Y = 1$ if and only if $Y^* = 3$, and $Y = 2$ if and only if $Y^* \geq 4$. Denote $P(Y \geq l | d_k) = R_l(d_k)$, $k = 1, \ldots, K, l = 1, \ldots, L$. The unknown toxicity probabilities $R_l(d_k)$ satisfy $0 < R_l(d_1) < \cdots < R_l(d_K) < 1$ for $l = 1, \ldots, L$, and $R_{l_1}(d_k) > R_{l_2}(d_k)$ for any $l_1 < l_2$ and fixed k. Thus, it is implicitly assumed that there are L toxicity constraints, where constraint on $\Pr(Y \geq l)$ corresponds to the non-zero value $Y = l, l = 1, \ldots, L$.

Consider a prespecified targeting toxicity vector $\theta = (\theta_1, \ldots, \theta_L)^T$ such that $1 > \theta_1 > \cdots > \theta_L > 0$. For each $l = 1, \ldots, L$, we define the optimal dose associated with the lth toxicity constraint as

$$d_{\nu_l} = \arg\min_{x \in D} |R_l(x) - \theta_l|.$$

In our example, when $l = 1$, $Y \geq 1$ corresponds to the dose-limiting toxicity and d_{ν_1} corresponds to the original definition for the MTD. The MTD under multiple toxicity constraints is defined as follows:

$$d_\nu = \min\{d_{\nu_1}, \ldots, d_{\nu_L}\},$$

which is seen as a generalization of the definition for the MTD.

To estimate the MTD d_ν, consider a generic working model

$$P(Y \geq l) = \psi_l(x, a), \quad l = 1, \ldots, L,$$

where $a = (a_1, \ldots, a_L)^T$ is the unknown parameter. We assume that the above model is rich enough in the sense that for any fixed dose x and any given targeting toxicity θ, there exists a a such that $\psi_l(x, a) = \theta_l, l = 1, \ldots, L$.

Based on the assigned doses and the toxicity outcomes of the first n patients, the likelihood is defined as follows:

$$L_n(a) = \prod_{i=1}^{n} \psi_L\{x(i), a\}^{I(y_i = L)} [1 - \psi_1\{x(i), a\}]^{I(y_i = 0)}$$

$$\times \prod_{l=1}^{L-1} [\psi_l\{x(i), a\} - \psi_{l+1}\{x(i), a\}]^{I(y_i = l)},$$

where $x(i)$ is the dose administered to the ith patient, y_i is the outcome for that patient, and $\psi_l(x, a)$ is the working dose–toxicity model based on the lth threshold. Given the data accrued up to the first n patients, the model parameter a can be estimated using a Bayesian framework or by maximizing the likelihood. The Bayesian approach requires the specification of priors for the model parameters. The choice of prior distributions guarantees that the probability of toxicity is strictly increasing in dose. Using the priors, the joint posterior distribution of model parameters can be obtained using the Markov chain Monte Carlo (MCMC) method, and hence the joint posterior of $(\theta_1, \ldots, \theta_L)$. The next patient is then treated at

$$\hat{x}(n + 1) = \arg\min_{d_k} |d_k - \hat{\theta}_n|,$$

where $\hat{\theta}_n$ is the posterior median of θ. A second potential estimator for θ is $\tilde{\theta}_n = \hat{\theta}_{n, \hat{\lambda}_n}$, where $\hat{\theta}_{n,l}$ denotes the marginal posterior median of θ_l given the first n observations, and $\hat{\lambda}_n = \arg\min_l \hat{\theta}_{n,l}$. The next patient is then given

$$\tilde{x}(n + 1) = \arg\min_{d_k} |d_k - \tilde{\theta}_n|.$$

The likelihood approach does not require the specification of priors, and it is much easier to compute. However, $\hat{a}_n$ may not exist, particularly when n is small, given that it requires heterogeneity of outcomes. That is, the maximum likelihood estimate $\hat{a}_n$ exists when all of the $L + 1$ possible values of Y are observed. Therefore, to make use of all of the L constraints, all of the $L + 1$ possible values of Y must be observed, which we call "full heterogeneity." However, we emphasize that our procedure can be used as long as two or more distinct values are observed, which we call "partial heterogeneity," with the understanding that under "partial heterogeneity," some of the constraints may not be invoked. For example, if the outcome Y can take on values of 0, 1, or 2 and we impose two constraints, "full heteregeneity" requires that 0, 1, and 2 be observed. However, if we have only observed the values of 0 and 1, we have "partial heterogeneity" and we can impose one constraint. Thus, for implementation of the method, we take a multistage approach that depends on the extent of heterogeneity observed. At the start of a trial, we propose an initial dose-escalation sequence. Once partial heterogeneity is achieved, the design switches to the proposed procedure, invoking as many constraints as distinct values of outcomes are observed. Based on partial heterogeneity, $\hat{a}_n$ exists and the recommended dose for the $(n + 1)$th patient is

$$x(n + 1) = \min\{\arg\min_{x \in D} |\psi_l(x, \hat{a}_n) - \theta_l|, l = 1, \dots, L\}.$$

For example, suppose that Y takes on three possible values: 0 (no toxicity), 1 (dose-limiting toxicity), and 2 (life-threatening toxicity), and we are interested in two constraints: $\Pr(Y \geq 1) \leq \theta_1$ and $\Pr(Y \geq 2) \leq \theta_2$. In the first stage, we will specify an initial dose-escalation sequence. If the first toxicity we observe is $Y = 2$, then we proceed by considering only the constraint $\Pr(Y \geq 2) \leq \theta_2$. We invoke the constraint $\Pr(Y \geq 1) \leq \theta_1$ only once $Y = 1$ is observed. This is different from the regular CRM in that the constraint $\Pr(Y \geq 1) \leq \theta_1$ is always used regardless of whether $Y = 1$ or 2 is first observed. In the situation where $Y = 1$ is not observed and all toxicities are $Y = 2$, the CRM will recommend the dose with a toxicity probability of θ_1, while the proposed method will recommend the dose with a toxicity probability of θ_2. This process is continued until a prespecified number of patients N. The recommended dose for the $N + 1$ patient is the estimate of the MTD.

The design parameters that need to be specified when using the CRM with multiple constraints are very similar to the CRM, with the exception of the additional target rates at the various desired thresholds that are selected based on clinical significance. Similarly, the doses to be administered, the starting dose, and the number of patients are all specified with the help of clinicians. The choice of starting dose can be the lowest dose level or solely selecting the prior guess of the MTD based on the primary constraint of interest. Following the CRM convention, the working models can be empiric. While the CRM with multiple constraints has been shown to be consistent, meaning that for large enough sample sizes, the method will select the true MTD [2], it is also important to calibrate the model to yield good operating characteristics in small sample settings. One approach for selecting the initial guesses of the probabilities of toxicity at each dose is to only consider the primary constraint and disregard the other constraints. Another approach is to use the idea of an indifference interval to obtain the initial guesses of the probabilities of DLT based only on the primary constraint, but to select the optimal indifference interval based on calibration scenarios that include various distributions of the probabilities of toxicity based on the thresholds. For example, in the case of two constraints ($L = 2$), the conditional log odds model used for ordinal categorical data can be used to specify the conditional probability of $Y \geq 2$, given $Y \geq 1$ at any dose level, specifically,

$$\text{logit}\{P(Y \geq 2|d_k)/P(Y \geq 1|d_k)\} = \text{logit}(\theta_2/\theta_1) + s(k - k^*),$$

for $k = 1, \dots, K$. A bigger value of s corresponds to a more drastic increase of the probability $\Pr(Y \geq 2|d_k)$ as k increases.

TABLE 3.1
True probabilities of toxicities for the calibration.

	Dose Level				
	1	2	3	4	5
Scenario where $s = 0.30$					
Probability of $Y \geq 1$	0.14	0.14	**0.25**	0.40	0.40
Probability of $Y \geq 2$	0.04	0.05	**0.10**	0.19	0.22
Scenario where $s = 0.70$					
Probability of $Y \geq 1$	0.14	0.14	**0.25**	0.40	0.40
Probability of $Y \geq 2$	0.02	0.04	**0.10**	0.23	0.29

For example, suppose we have five dose levels and $\theta_1 = 0.25$ and $\theta_2 = 0.10$. In order to select the initial guesses of the probabilities of toxicity at each dose, we first start by specifying the calibration set of scenarios based on which the initial guesses will be selected. For $Y \geq 1$, we can select the plateau configuration used by Lee and Cheung [17] and set the true toxicity probability for $Y \geq 1$ as $\Pr(Y \geq 1|d_{k^*}) = 0.25$, $\Pr(Y \geq 1|d_k) = 0.14$ for $k < k^*$, and $\Pr(Y \geq 1|d_k) = 0.40$ for $k > k^*$, where k^*, the true MTD, can take on the values of 1, 2, 3, 4, or 5. Given a fixed value of k^*, we then determine the toxicity probability for $Y \geq 2$ by letting $s = 0.30$ or 0.70 in the following equation:

$$\text{logit}\{P(Y \geq 2|d_k)/P(Y \geq 1|d_k)\} = \text{logit}(0.10/0.25) + s(k - k^*),$$

for $k = 1, \ldots, 5$. To put it more concretely, just looking at $k^* = 3$, i.e., dose level 3 is the true MTD, the true toxicity probabilities for $Y \geq 1$ are $(0.14, 0.14, 0.25, 0.40, 0.40)$. The true probabilities for the calibration scenarios based on the equation above and setting $s = 0.30$ or 0.70 with $k^* = 3$ are provided in Table 3.1.

The likelihood framework for the CRM with multiple constraints also requires the specification of an initial dose-escalation sequence prior to observing "partial" heterogeneity. So far, the choices have been *ad hoc* with the use of either cohorts of three patients at a time or a cohort of one patient at a time. That is, three patients are assigned—or one patient is assigned—to each dose, and if no toxicities are observed, the dose is escalated. Calibration of CRM with multiple constraints has not been fully explored in the literature, and it is an area of ongoing research. Thus, these are just starting points in terms of calibration of the model parameters. Careful simulation studies should be performed when applying the method in practice.

3.4 Example: Application of the Continual Reassessment Method with Multiple Constraints

Consider, for example, a phase I trial in patients with previously untreated diffuse large B-cell or mantle cell non-Hodgkin's lymphoma, where the main objective was to determine the MTD of bortezomib when administered in combination with CHOP + Rituximab (CHOP-R) [18]. The standard dose for CHOP-R was administered every 21 days. There were five dose levels of bortezomib with the third dose level thought to be the best guess of the MTD prior to starting the trial. Being that bortezomib is a potent proteasome inhibitor that could cause neurologic and hematologic toxicities, a DLT was defined as life-threatening or disabling neurologic toxicity, very low platelet count, or symptomatic non-neurologic or nonhematologic toxicity requiring intervention. The MTD was defined as the dose associated with a 25% DLT probability. The original trial was conducted using the CRM with a sample size of 18. Using only the DLT definition, it did not differentiate the gradation and types of severe toxicity. While grade 3 neuropathy is a symptomatic toxicity interfering with activities of daily life, it may be resolved by symptomatic treatment. In contrast, a grade 4 neuropathy is life-threatening or disabling, and hence irreversible. Thus, while 25% grade 3 neuropathy is acceptable in the bortezomib trial, the tolerance for grade 4 neuropathy is much lower. Furthermore, while a grade 4 neuropathy and a very low platelet count are both considered DLT, the tolerance for grade 4 neuropathy is much lower. To account for these differences, the toxicity data can be summarized into a continuous or ordinal outcome such as those previously described in Section 3.2. Let us assume that the TBS approach by Lee et al. is used to summarize the toxicity data into a continuous outcome. We are then interested in imposing two toxicity constraints to differentiate between toxicities that are severe, but reversible and not life-threatening, and those that are life-threatening and irreversible, that is, in terms of TBS: $Y^* < 1$, $1 \leq Y^* < 1.5$, and $Y^* \geq 1.5$. Thus, the outcome Y is defined as $(Y = 0)$ if and only if the patient experiences no toxicity, or a mild or moderate toxicity, $(Y = 1)$ if and only if the patient experiences a severe and reversible toxicity, and $(Y = 2)$ if and only if the patient experiences a life-threatening and irreversible toxicity. The threshold for dose-limiting toxicities (i.e., severe toxicities or worse) is 25% and for life-threatening toxicities is 10%, that is, $\theta_1 = 0.25$ and $\theta_2 = 0.10$. As in the original CRM design, we consider $K = 5$ test doses with a starting dose at level 3 and a sample size of 18. In addition, we do not allow for dose skipping and dose escalation immediately after $Y \geq 1$ is observed. In this illustration, we assume that the dose–toxicity model is empiric and use the multistage likelihood approach with an initial design based on a cohort size of 1. For simplicity, the scaled doses are selected based solely on the primary DLT constraint using the indifference interval approach by Lee and Cheung [17]. With a target of 25%, five dose levels, and dose level 3 being the best guess of the MTD, the optimal indifference interval is 0.09, which yields the following initial guesses or scaled doses (0.02, 0.09, 0.25, 0.44, 0.62).

Figures 3.1 and 3.2 summarize graphically the dose assignments and outcomes for a simulated trial of 18 patients using the CRM with two constraints as specified above and the following two scenarios of true probabilities of toxicities for the three gradations of toxicity in Table 3.2. In the first scenario, the additional constraint is not necessary since the MTDs for both constraints are the same. In the second scenario, the limiting constraint is the second constraint based on life-threatening toxicities, and thus, using only the primary constraint would lead us to an overly toxic dose recommendation.

TABLE 3.2

True probabilities of toxicities for the simulated examples.

	Dose Level				
	1	2	3	4	5
Scenario 1					
Probability of $Y \geq 1$	0.05	0.05	0.10	**0.25**	0.45
Probability of $Y = 2$	0.01	0.01	0.02	**0.10**	0.23
Scenario 2					
Probability of $Y \geq 1$	0.05	0.10	0.16	**0.25**	0.45
Probability of $Y = 2$	0.01	0.03	**0.10**	0.23	0.35

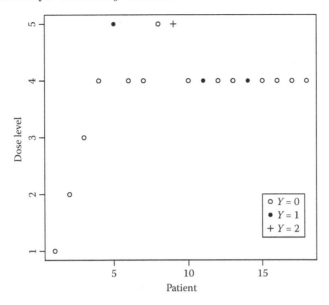

FIGURE 3.1
Simulated trial under scenario 1 using CRM with multiple constraints, where the true MTD is dose level 4 based on both the primary constraint and the secondary constraints. $Y = 0$ is no toxicity, $Y = 1$ is a severe toxicity (grade 3), and $Y = 2$ is a life-threatening toxicity (grade 4).

In the first scenario (Figure 3.1), the dose was escalated after each patient with no toxicities being observed up to the fifth patient, who experienced a severe, but reversible, toxicity ($Y = 1$). At that point, we had partial heterogeneity, and based on the CRM, the sixth and the seventh patients were assigned dose level 4. These patients did not experience toxicities, and thus, the dose was once again escalated to dose level 5 for patients 8 and 9. The ninth patient experienced a life-threatening toxicity ($Y = 2$) at dose level 5. Having observed both severe ($Y = 1$) and life-threatening ($Y = 2$) toxicities, the CRM with multiple constraints is evoked and recommends dose level 4 to the rest of the patients. Two out of nine patients experienced severe toxicities. At the end of the trial, dose level 3, the MTD based on both constraints, was the recommended dose level. Moreover, toxicities were reported in 4 out of the 18 patients (22%), with 1 (6%) patient having a life-threatening toxicity.

In the second scenario (Figure 3.2), the dose was escalated after each patient with no toxicities being observed up to the fifth patient, who experienced a severe toxicity, ($Y = 1$). At that point, we had partial heterogeneity, and based on the CRM, the sixth and the seventh patients were assigned dose level 4. These patients did not experience toxicities, and thus, the dose was once again escalated to dose level 5 for patients 8 and 9. The ninth patient experienced a life-threatening toxicity ($Y = 2$) at dose level 5. With full heterogeneity, the CRM with multiple constraints was initiated at that point and recommended dose level 4 for the next five patients. Two of the five patients experienced life-threatening toxicities ($Y = 2$), and thus, the dose was de-escalated to dose level 3 for the following four patients. None of these patients experienced toxicities. At the end of the trial, dose level 3, the MTD based on the secondary constraint, was the recommended dose level. Furthermore, toxicities were reported in 4 out of the 18 patients (22%), with 3 (17%) patients having a life-threatening toxicity.

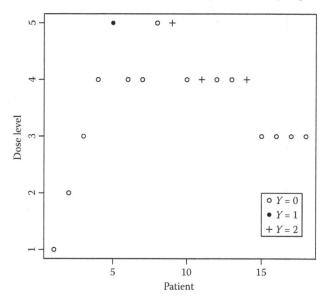

FIGURE 3.2

Simulated trial under scenario 2 using CRM with multiple constraints, where the true MTD is dose level 4 based on the primary constraint and dose level 3 when accounting for both the primary and the secondary constraints. $Y = 0$ is no toxicity, $Y = 1$ is a severe toxicity (grade 3), and $Y = 2$ is a life-threatening toxicity (grade 4).

3.5   Other Methods for Ordinal or Continuous Outcomes

3.5.1   Quasi-continual reassessment method

The quasi-CRM is an approach based on the CRM that differentiates between the various grades of toxicity [4] and targets a level of equivalent toxicity (ET) score. When using this method, the maximal toxicity grades are transformed to ET scores and used as the outcome. Each toxicity grade is assigned an ET score, $w_1, \ldots, w_C$, where C is the number of toxicity grades, and normalized by dividing them by the ET score of the most severe toxicity grade ($w_{\max}$) to obtain fractional events, that is, $w_C^* = w_C/w_{\max}$. The target ET score is obtained by weighting the ET scores by the guess of the probability of each toxicity grade at the MTD and summing them over all grades. Assume that $d_1, \ldots, d_K$ are the K test doses of interest. Let $\psi(x, a)$ be the dose-normalized model. Then, the quasi-Bernoulli likelihood function for the first n patients is

$$L_n(a) = \prod_{i=1}^{n} (\psi(x(i); a))^{w_{[i]}^*} (1 - \psi(x(i); a))^{(1 - w_{[i]}^*)},$$

where $x(i)$ is the dose administered to the ith patient and $w_{[i]}^*$ is the corresponding normalized ET score for that patient. In the Bayesian framework, let $\pi(\cdot)$ be the prior distribution on the model parameter a, the quasi-posterior mean of a can be estimated using the above likelihood. The highest dose level such that its normalized ET score is less than or equal to the normalized target ET score is assigned to the next patient. This process is continued until a prespecified number of patients, N. The recommended dose for the $N + 1$ patient is the estimate of the MTD.

The design parameters that need to be specified when using the quasi-CRM are the doses to be administered, the starting dose, the definition of DLT, the number of patients, the ET scores for each grade of toxicity, the target ET score, the dose-normalized model, the prior distribution of the model parameter, and the initial guesses of the ET scores at each dose. The first four are selected with input from the physicians. The ET scores for each grade are obtained from physicians by assigning the cutoff for the DLT a score of 1 and eliciting the scores for the other grades based on the toxicity relationships. For example, if a DLT is defined as grade 3 or higher toxicity ($w_3 = 1$), two grade 2 toxicities are thought to be equal to a grade 3 toxicity ($2w_2 = w_3 = 1$), two grade 3 toxicities are thought to be equal to a grade 4 toxicity ($2w_3 = w_4 = 2$), and grade 1 is considered nontoxic ($w_1 = 0$), then the ET scores would be 0 for grade 0 or 1, 0.5 for grade 2, 1.0 for grade 3, and 2.0 for grade 4. To obtain the target ET score, it is necessary to provide the guesses of the probability of each toxicity grade at the MTD in addition to the ET scores for each grade of toxicity. Given the importance of the initial guesses and the ET scores at each dose level in defining the target ET score, they should be carefully selected. The same dose–toxicity model and prior distribution of the model parameters used for the CRM can be used. The selection of the initial ET scores at each dose was not discussed and thus should be carefully selected based on detailed simulation studies examining the operating characteristics of the method.

The quasi-CRM approach by Yuan, Chappell, and Bailey was proposed in a Bayesian framework. The work has been further extended to a frequentist framework with a two-stage design by Ezzalfani et al. [5], where an up-and-down design is used before any toxicities are observed. By having the two-stage design, this method avoids the specification of the prior, which is required for the Bayesian quasi-CRM. The method, named the quasi-likelihood CRM, performs similar to its Bayesian counterpart. The quasi-CRM is a simple approach for incorporating the information into a toxicity grade for the estimation of the MTD. It is simpler to apply in practice than the more complicated approaches proposed for incorporating toxicity grade and type information. However, the need to specify a target ET score when little is known about the probability of each toxicity grade at the MTD can be challenging and problematic.

3.5.2 Unified approach with monotone objective function

Ivanova and Kim [6] proposed a unified approach for continuous or ordinal outcomes that are monotone functions of dose, where the aim of the design is to estimate the dose associated with a prespecified value of an outcome. The dose-escalation algorithm is based on a t-statistic. Let $d_1, d_2, \ldots, d_K$ be the K-ordered dose levels. If a patient's response at dose level d_k has distribution function $F(\cdot; \mu_k, \sigma_k^2)$, where μ_k and σ_k^2 are the mean and the variance, respectively, the objective is to find the dose d_m with μ_m closest to the target value of the response μ^*. Let $d_1, d_2, \ldots, d_K$ be the K doses of interest. Patients are assigned starting from the lowest dose. After n patients are enrolled, let $n_1(n), n_2(n), \ldots, n_K(n)$ be the number of patients assigned to each dose level and $Y_{i,k}$ be the outcome for the ith patient assigned to dose d_k, $i = 1, \ldots, n_k(n)$. Define the t-statistic, $T_k(n_k(n))$, to be

$$T_k(n_k(n)) = \frac{\overline{Y}_k(n_k(n)) - \mu^*}{s_k(n_k(n))/\sqrt{n_k(n)}},$$

where $\overline{Y}_k(n_k(n))$ and $s_k(n_k(n))$ are the sample mean and the sample standard deviation from all observations at dose level d_k, respectively. Patient $n + 1$ will be assigned the following:

(1) Dose level d_{k+1} if $T_k(n_k(n)) \leq -\Delta$

(2)   Dose level d_{k-1} if $T_k(n_k(n)) \geq \Delta$

(3)   Dose level d_k if $-\Delta < T_k(n_k(n)) < \Delta$

To estimate the target dose d_m, at the end of the trial, the isotonic estimates of the mean responses are obtained and the dose with the estimated value closest to the target response value μ^* is selected. If there is more than one dose, the highest dose with the estimated value below the target is chosen. The design parameters that need to be specified are the doses to be administered as well as the starting dose, the number of patients, and the parameter Δ. The first three are selected with the input from the clinicians. The optimal Δ depends on the true dose–response relationship and the difference between adjacent doses. Simulation studies should be performed to select a reasonable Δ. For the various examples presented by Ivanova and Kim, a Δ value of 1 was used. Moreover, at least two subjects should be assigned to any untried dose level before escalating to a higher dose.

While the extensions of the CRM (CRM with multiple constraints and quasi-CRM) use available outcome data from all patients up to the current assignment, the unified approach only uses the information for the last dose level assigned. Thus, in cases in which the true MTD is in between doses selected, the design will oscillate between doses and expose a higher number of patients to over-toxic doses. To avoid these scenarios, it is necessary to specify another rule. Moreover, the method is easy to implement, but it also requires the specification of a target level of the outcome of interest.

3.6   Time-to-Event Continual Reassessment Method

The difference between the TITE-CRM and the originally proposed CRM is that TITE-CRM incorporates partial information from patients, in addition to complete observations. In most dose-finding trials, the observation window for DLT is one cycle or 28 days. Thus, only toxicities from the first cycle or 28 days of treatment are considered and included in the definition of DLT. Toxicities occurring beyond that window are disregarded in the dose-escalation decisions and the estimation of the MTD. Protocols using the CRM generally require complete observation, meaning that patients have to be observed for the entire observation window before the next dose is assigned. Thus, for example, if the first patient has only been treated 7 days and the observation window is 28 days, even if the second patient comes on day 10, she cannot be assigned a dose until the first patient completes 28 days. The challenges of requiring complete observations are the need to turn patients away or having patients wait. Moreover, to include late-onset and cumulative toxicities requiring complete observations leads to much longer study duration. The TITE-CRM was developed to address these shortcomings, by including partial information and allowing for continuous recruitment, faster accrual, and shorter study duration compared to methods that required complete observations [8].

Using the same notation as that for the CRM, let $d_1, d_2, \ldots, d_K$ be the K doses of interest, $\psi(x, a)$ be the working dose–toxicity model, and θ be the target probability of DLT. Given the data accrued up to the first n patients, we can estimate a based on a weighted likelihood that weights partially observed information, defined as,

$$L_n(a; \mathbf{w}) \propto \prod_{i=1}^{n} \{\psi(x(i), a)\}^{y_{i,n+1}} \{1 - w_{i,n+1}\psi(x(i), a)\}^{1-y_{i,n+1}},$$

where $x_{(i)}$ is the dose administered to the ith patient, which can take a value from $d_1, d_2, \ldots, d_K$; $y_{i,n+1}$ is the corresponding binary DLT outcome for that patient prior to the enrollment of the $n + 1$ patient; and $w_{i,n+1}$ is the weight assigned to the observation prior to the enrollment of the $n + 1$ patient. Similar to the CRM, the model parameter a can be estimated via the posterior mean in the Bayesian framework or by maximizing the likelihood. The maximum likelihood estimate only exists after heterogeneity of outcomes has been observed. Thus, it requires a two-stage design whereby a dose-escalation sequence is followed before a DLT is observed. Once a DLT has occurred and heterogeneity is observed, the maximum likelihood estimate is used. Regardless of whether Bayesian or maximum likelihood methods are used to obtain the model estimate, $\hat{a}_n^w$, the dose level recommended for the $(n + 1)$th patient is the dose with the model-based DLT probability closest to θ, that is,

$$x(n + 1) = \arg \min_{d_k} |\psi(d_k, \hat{a}_n^w) - \theta|.$$

This process is continued until a prespecified number of patients N. The recommended dose for the $N + 1$ patient is the estimate of the MTD.

The design parameters that need to be specified when using the TITE-CRM are very similar to the CRM with the exception of the weight function and the length of the observation window for DLT. Similar to the CRM, the doses to be administered, the starting dose, the number of patients, and the target probability of DLT are all specified with the help of clinicians. Given that the dose–toxicity modeling and the time-to-toxicity modeling can be performed separately, the calibration of the dose–toxicity model, the prior distribution of the model parameters, and the initial guesses of the toxicity probabilities at each dose are all the same as those for the CRM and can be done using the indifference interval approaches by Lee and Cheung [17, 19]. The impact of the weight function has been evaluated by Cheung and Chappell, and the linear weight, whereby a weight proportional to the total amount of expected follow-up is assigned, is adequate in most scenarios. That is, let T be the maximum length of observation for the DLT:

$$w(t; T, x(i)) = \min(t/T, 1).$$

If a two-stage TITE-CRM is used, then an additional dose-escalation sequence needs to be specified. It is important to check for coherence at the transition point after the first toxcity is observed and the TITE-CRM is used because overconservative dose-escalation sequences can lead to incoherence [20].

3.7 Example: Application of the Time-to-Event Continual Reassessment Method

Consider the same phase I trial in patients with lymphoma that was presented in Section 3.4. The main objective was to determine the MTD of bortezomib when administered in combination with CHOP + Rituximab (CHOP-R) [18]. There were five dose levels of bortezomib, and dose level 3 was the prior guess of the MTD. The MTD was defined as the dose associated with a 25% DLT probability. With a target of 25%, five dose levels and dose level 3 being the best guess of the MTD, the optimal indifference interval is 0.09, which yields the following initial guesses or scaled doses (0.02, 0.09, 0.25, 0.44, 0.62). A linear weight is assumed.

This is a good example for the application of the TITE-CRM, because bortezomib has been associated with late-onset toxicities and defining DLT based only on the first cycle may identify a dose that is not well tolerated over extended administration [7]. Thus, it is of interest to extend the toxicity observation window to three cycles (12 weeks) to account

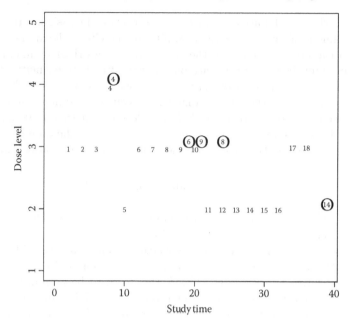

FIGURE 3.3
Simulated trial using TITE-CRM, where the true MTD is dose level 3. The x-axis represents the study time in weeks. The y-axis indicates the dose level assigned to each patient. Each number represents a patient in chronological order. The numbers represent patients enrolled at particular dose level, and the circled numbers indicate the toxicity time (if observed) for a particular patient.

for late-onset toxicities. In this case, even with a sample size of 18, if complete observations are required, the trial would last over 4 years.

We demostrate the TITE-CRM under a simulated scenario where the true probabilities of toxicities at each dose level are 0.05, 0.10, 0.25, 0.45, and 0.55, respectively. Thus, the true MTD is dose level 3. Furthermore, we assume a fixed accrual rate of one patient every 2 weeks. Figure 3.3 displays the dose level assigned to each patient along with their respective outcome for the simulated trial. The x-axis represents the study time in weeks. The y-axis indicates the dose level assigned to each patient. Each number represents a patient in chronological order. The numbers represent patients enrolled at particular dose level, and the circled numbers indicate the toxicity time (if observed) for a particular patient. Patients 1, 2, and 3 were assigned dose level 3 (the initial dose) and showed no toxicity in the first 8 weeks. Patient 4 entered on week 8 and was assigned dose level 4. Within a week, this patient experienced a DLT. Thus, the dose was lowered to dose level 2 for patient 5, who started on week 10. The dose was once again escalated to dose level 3 for patient 6 who started on week 12. The same dose was assigned to patients 7, 8, and 9 who entered on weeks 14, 16, and 18, respectively. By the time patient 10 entered on week 20, patient 6 had experienced a DLT. Given that this was the first DLT out of the seven patients assigned dose level 3, patient 10 was assigned dose level 3. By the time patient 11 entered on week 22, patient 9 had experienced a DLT, and thus, patients 11 and 12 were both assigned dose level 2. Patient 8 experienced a DLT before the arrival of patient 13, and thus, patients 13–16 were all asigned dose level 2. Given that none of these patients expecienced a DLT, the dose was escalated to dose level 3 for patients 17 and 18 who entered on weeks 34 and 36, respectively. By the time all observation windows were closed, one more DLT was observed for patient 14. The recommended MTD for this simulated trial was dose level 3 and 3 out of a total of 10 patients assigned to this dose had a DLT. In contrast, one out of the seven patients assigned to dose level 2 had a DLT.

References

1. B. N. Bekele and P. F. Thall. Dose-finding based on multiple toxicities in a soft tissue sarcoma trial. *Journal of the American Statistical Association*, 99(465):26–35, 2004.

2. B. Cheng and S. M. Lee. On the consistency of the continual reassessment method with multiple toxicity constraints. *Journal of Statistical Planning and Inference*, 164:1–9, 2015.

3. S. M. Lee, B. Cheng, and Y. K. Cheung. Continual reassessment method with multiple toxicity constraints. *Biostatistics*, 12(2):386–398, 2011.

4. Z. Yuan, R. Chappell, and H. Bailey. The continual reassessment method for multiple toxicity grades: A Bayesian quasi-likelihood approach. *Biometrics*, 63(1):173–179, 2007.

5. M. Ezzalfani, S. Zohar, R. Qin, S. J. Mandrekar, and M. C. Deley. Dose-finding designs using a novel quasi-continuous endpoint for multiple toxicities. *Statistics in Medicine*, 32(16):2728–2746, 2013.

6. A. Ivanova and S. H. Kim. Dose finding for continuous and ordinal outcomes with a monotone objective function: A unified approach. *Biometrics*, 65(1):307–315, 2009.

7. S. M. Lee, D. Backenroth, Y. K. Cheung, D. Vulih, B. Anderson, P. Ivy, and L. Minasian. Case example of dose optimization using data from bortezomib dose-finding trials. *Journal of Clinical Oncology*, 34:1395–1401, 2016.

8. Y. K. Cheung and R. Chappell. Sequential designs for phase I clinical trials with late-onset toxicities. *Biometrics*, 56(4):1177–1182, 2000.

9. Y. K. Cheung and M. S. V. Elkind. Stochastic approximation with virtual observations for dose finding on discrete levels. *Biometrika*, 97:109–121, 2010.

10. E. M. Van Meter, E. Garret-Mayer, and D. Bandyopadhyay. Proportional odds model for dose-finding clinical trial desings with ordinal toxicity grading. *Statistics in Medicine*, 30(17):2070–2080, 2011.

11. E. M. Van Meter, E. Garret-Mayer, and D. Bandyopadhyay. Dose-finding clinical trial design for ordinal toxicity grades using the continuation ratio model: An extension of the continual reassessment method. *Clinical Trials*, 9(3):303–313, 2012.

12. C. Wang, T. Chen, and I. Tyan. Designs for phase I cancer clinical trials with differentiation of graded toxicity. *Communications in Statistics: Theory and Method*, 29:975–987, 2000.

13. A. Iasonos, S. Zohar, and J. O'Quigley. Incorporating lower grade toxicity information into dose finding desings. *Clinical Trials*, 8(4):370–379, 2011.

14. A. Rogatko, J. S. Babb, H. Wang, M. J. Slifker, and G. R. Hudes. Patient characteristics compete with dose as predictors of acute treatment toxicity in early phase clinical trials. *Clinical Cancer Research*, 10:4645–4651, 2004.

15. A. Trotti, T. Pajak, C. Gwede, R. Paulus, J. Cooper, A. Forastiere, J. Ridge, D. Watkins-Bruner, A. Garden, K. Ang, and W. Curran. TAME: Development of a new method for summarising adverse events of cancer treatment by the Radiation Therapy Oncology Group. *Lancet Oncology*, 8(7):613–624, 2007.

16. S. M. Lee, D. L. Hershman, P. Martin, J. P. Leonard, and Y. K. Cheung. Toxicity burden score: A novel approach to summarize multiple toxic effects. *Annals of Oncology*, 23(2):537–541, 2012.

17. S. M. Lee and Y. K. Cheung. Model calibration in the continual reassessment method. *Clinical Trials*, 6(3):227–238, 2009.

18. J. P. Leornard, R. R. Furman, and Y. K. Cheung, et al. Phase I/II trial of bortezomib plus CHOP-rituximab in diffuse large B cell and mantle cell lymphoma: Phase I results. *Blood*, 106(11):147A, 2005.

19. S. M. Lee and Y. K. Cheung. Calibration of prior variance in the Bayesian continual reassessment method. *Statistics in Medicine*, 30:2081–2089, 2011.

20. A. Jia, S. M. Lee, and Y. K. Cheung. Characterisation of the likelihood continual reassessment method. *Biometrika*, 101:599–612, 2014.

4

Dose-Finding Trials in Pediatric Oncology

Arzu Onar-Thomas

St. Jude Children's Research Hospital

Fridtjof Thomas

University of Tennessee Health Science Center

CONTENTS

4.1   The Current Landscape for Pediatric Oncology Trials

The popular adage "children are not small adults" represents a double-edged sword when it comes to identifying new medicines to treat childhood cancer: while children are recognized in their own rights and needs, the adage also calls attention to the fact that therapeutic approaches established for adults may not readily extend to children. Even though childhood cancer is a relatively rare diagnosis, it is estimated that 1 in 285 children in the United States will be diagnosed with the disease before the age of 20 years [1]. In contrast, the lifetime risk of developing cancer is approximately one in two for men and one in three for women, where 78% of all cancer diagnoses are in people aged 55 years or older [1]. Pediatric cancers represent 1% of all new cancer diagnoses in the United States [1]. On an annual basis, these rates are estimated to result in 10,450 new cases and 1,350 cancer deaths among U.S. children (aged 0–14 years) and 5,330 new cases and 610 cancer deaths among U.S. adolescents (aged 15–19 years) [1]. The estimated number of annual new diagnoses of cancer in children worldwide is 175,000. In contrast, approximately 1.7 million new adult cancer cases are expected to be diagnosed during 2015 in the United States alone. Nevertheless, cancer is the most common cause of nonviolent death for children in the United States, and it remains a significant area of focus for treatment [2].

    In light of the figures cited above, childhood cancers are typically classified as uncommon, rare, or exceedingly rare. The most common malignant cancer types in children aged 0–14 years are acute lymphocytic leukemia (26%, $n \approx 2670$ new cases annually in the United States), central nervous system (CNS) (21%, $n \approx 2240$), neuroblastoma (7%, $n \approx 710$), and non-Hodgkin's lymphoma (6%, $n \approx 620$), whereas the most common cancers among adolescents aged 15–19 years are Hodgkin's lymphoma (15%, $n \approx 800$), thyroid carcinoma (11%, $n \approx 570$), CNS (10%, $n \approx 540$), and testicular germ cell tumors (8%, $n \approx 430$).

It is important to note that children's cancers are often molecularly quite different from their adult counterparts, and there are certain types of tumors that occur in children but are rarely seen in adults [3–6]. Notable examples are cancers that originate in developing tissues and organ systems such as neuroblastoma, Wilms' tumor, medulloblastoma, rhabdomyosarcomas, and retinoblastoma [1].

The pediatric oncology community as well as regulatory bodies such as the U.S. Food and Drug Administration (FDA) and the European Medicines Agency (EMA) agree that pediatric patients should be treated with medicines that have been properly evaluated in children. In order to ensure timely access to agents that may be beneficial to children, pediatric studies should be incorporated into the product development plans of agents for which there is reasonable expectation of future pediatric use. Note that while pediatric patients do not typically develop breast or prostate cancers, many of the molecular aberrations that are relevant in these and other common adult cancers play a role in pediatric malignancies as well. Therefore, the assessment of reasonable expectation for future pediatric use is not based on the site of cancer but rather on the pathway that is involved or the mechanism of action of the agent (e.g., immunotherapy) that may have efficacy in cancers that are seen in children. While the need to study new agents in children is evident, the economic incentives for pharmaceutical companies to support such trials have been lacking until very recently. The primary reason for the lack of impetus for the pharmaceutical companies to invest in pediatric trials is the rarity of childhood cancers, which makes it unlikely that an agent with an indication in a pediatric cancer would be profitable. According to the Tufts Center for the Study of Drug Development, the average cost of developing a new drug is $2.6 billion [7]. While this figure has been disputed by some [8], it is widely accepted that drug development is a very costly venture with a very high failure rate. It is estimated that only one in thousand new compounds that enter preclinical testing ever reaches the stage of human trials, and only one in five agents that enter human trials receives FDA approval [2]. Given the high risk of failure, the incentive to take that risk is far greater when one considers millions of adult patients with common cancers to whom the agent can be marketed compared to a much smaller pediatric cohort.

Recognizing the discrepancy between financial considerations and the need to study new agents in pediatric populations, both the FDA and the EMA have enacted various regulations to provide incentives to pharmaceutical companies to incorporate pediatric studies into their development plans. In the United States, three key initiatives are at play: the Pediatric Research Equity Act (PREA), the Best Pharmaceuticals for Children Act (BPCA), and the Federal Research and Innovation Safety Act (FDASIA). PREA was passed by Congress in 2003, and under certain conditions, it authorized the FDA to require pediatric assessments from companies that are applying for new indications, new dosing/administration regimens, or new active ingredients. However, this act also incorporated criteria for waivers for which many oncology therapies were eligible, thus limiting PREA's impact. BPCA was passed by Congress in 2002 and among other regulations also incorporated a provision from 1997 that provided financial incentive to companies to voluntarily conduct pediatric studies under a written request from the FDA. The incentive did not require a positive pediatric study but rather simply the conduct of a phase I and II pediatric trial in exchange for a 6-month extension to all existing market exclusivities and patents for the drug moiety. This construction leveraged an economic incentive derived from adult cancers for pediatric cancer drug development. By conducting studies in children, pharmaceutical companies were given 6 additional months of market exclusivity (commonly referred to as "pediatric exclusivity") for all of their drug products using the active moiety in question. While 6 months may not sound like a long period of time, such an extension could in fact be worth in the billions of dollars for highly successful drugs since it delays competing generics from entering the market [9].

This provision was indeed successful in that it led to a notable increase in the number of pediatric trials that were initiated especially for blockbuster drugs (more than $1 billion in revenue annually), where a clear financial incentive was present to prolong market exclusivity. Between 1997 (passage of the FDA Modernization Act) and 2011, the FDA granted pediatric exclusivity to 185 drugs, and the prerequisite trials resulted in 211 associated pediatric label changes [9]. As of November 2015, the number of approved drugs that were granted pediatric exclusivity was 214 for 203 active moieties [10].

Both BPCA and PREA were made permanent laws by the U.S. Congress in 2012 as part of the FDASIA, which also amended PREA to require the submission of a pediatric study plan by the companies, usually by the conclusion of planned phase II studies for adult indications. As part of the same legislation, the FDA also introduced the Pediatric Rare Disease Priority Review Voucher Program, which provided additional incentives for development of medicines for rare pediatric diseases. The FDA's guidance on this defines pediatric rare disease as a condition that affects fewer than 200,000 individuals in the United States who are 18 years old or younger. This program provides a voucher for an expedited "priority review" of any subsequent drug application. Importantly, this voucher can not only be used outside pediatric or orphan disease settings, but it can also be transferred or sold to other companies, potentially leading to large revenues. It is the hope of the pediatric healthcare community as well as patients and families that this new regulatory environment with its "carrots and sticks" will increase the number of clinical trials that are conducted in pediatric populations leading to new, safe, and effective treatments for pediatric diseases.

4.2 Phase I Trial Considerations in Children

With a few exceptions, most new oncology agents enter the pediatric arena with a phase I trial. The aim is to identify a pediatric recommended dose and to establish safety of this dose in children. It is well accepted that for many therapeutic agents, the pharmacokinetic (PK) characteristics in children might be different from those in adults. This is typically due to developmental and physiological changes that occur throughout childhood, including changes in intestinal pH and motility as well as in enzyme activity that can affect drug absorption. Changes in body composition as a child matures, such as the total body water and the amount of fatty tissue, as well as alterations in circulating plasma proteins, can modify the degree, as well as the location, of the distribution of a medication. Furthermore, the developmental stage of various organs such as the liver and the kidneys can affect the safety profile of the agent and can lead to toxicities not reported in adults [11, 12]. Examples of differing safety profiles of various agents between pediatric and adult populations include *trans* retinoic acid where children are notably more susceptible to CNS toxicities compared to adults [13], acetaminophen hepatotoxicity where young children are more resistant, and valporic acid-induced hepatotoxicity to which children are more susceptible [14]. These differences necessitate studies in pediatric populations before a drug can be safely administered to children.

For most pediatric trials, "children" have traditionally been defined as subjects who are aged less than 21 years, though more recently this definition has been restricted to individuals who are aged 18 years and younger, especially for phase I trials. More often than not, when a phase I trial is initiated in a pediatric population, an adult maximum tolerated dose (MTD) and/or recommended phase II dose (RP2D) is available along with information about toxicity as well as PK data from adult cohorts. This information is of course quite helpful in designing a phase I trial in children with respect to dose levels that may be studied as well as PK parameters that could be targeted for maximal efficacy, etc. Since most adult trials enroll patients aged 18 years and older, restricting pediatric trials to subjects aged 18 years and younger allows the toxicity and PK data to be complementary to the data generated by the adult trials.

Most pediatric trials in children are initiated at 80% of the adult MTD and/or recommended phase II dose. This is done for pragmatic reasons and seems to be a good compromise between the need for ensuring safety and the desire to complete the phase I trial as quickly as possible. With a very few exceptions, pediatric phase I trials are conducted in patients with relapsed or refractory disease for whom no curative therapy is available. Given that over 80% of pediatric cancer patients are expected to be cured [1], the number of children with recurrent cancer who are eligible to participate in phase I trials is small. Therefore, minimizing the number of patients needed to identify a pediatric MTD/RP2D is very important.

In an influential paper, Lee et al. [15] reviewed 69 (53 cytotoxic and 16 biologic) pediatric phase I oncology trials that enrolled 1,973 patients during 1990 and 2004. The authors noted that for a vast majority of the trials, the pediatric MTD was within two dose levels of the adult MTD and recommended that no more than four dose levels be studied in a pediatric phase I trial of an agent when an adult MTD/RP2D is available. Furthermore, pharmaceutical companies sponsoring these studies are often against studying doses that far exceed the adult MTD. Hence, it is not unusual to conduct a pediatric phase I trial with only two to three dose levels. In many pediatric trials, the starting dose is designated as 80% of the adult MTD, and dose escalation is stopped at the adult MTD or one dose level above that.

While the small number of patients needed to complete these studies is a desirable aspect of this approach, determining the MTD is not the only reason one conducts a phase I trial in pediatrics. In addition, defining the agent's PK properties in children is of great interest. When a pediatric MTD/RP2D is identified, it is common practice to expand the cohort at the MTD to 10 or 12 patients and to stratify accrual in such a way that half of the patients at the MTD are aged less than 12 years at enrollment in an effort to obtain specific safety and PK information in younger patients. The other "soft" aim of pediatric phase I trials is detecting an early signal of efficacy, which is a conflicting goal with the one that tries to minimize sample size. While efficient algorithms are desirable in conducting these trials, this efficiency needs to be balanced against the objective to generate adequate PK/PD data as well as the aim to understand the relationship between dose and response and dose and toxicity, especially when only a few dose levels are proposed. Note that the safety and PK/PD information obtained from doses lower than the single-agent MTD may be relevant for future combination trials or for single-agent dosing in more heavily pretreated populations.

With the heightened recent emphasis on therapeutic intent in phase I trials by the recently released ASCO phase I policy [16], there may be a shift in how phase I trials are conducted. The presence of therapeutic intent in the context of pediatric phase I trials predates the ASCO guidelines by at least two decades. This long-standing intention, coupled with the fact that the starting doses in pediatric trials are often quite close to the adult MTD, substantially reduces the likelihood that the doses studied in a pediatric trial will be biologically inactive. This helps justify enrolling larger cohorts of subjects at each dose level. In practice, these considerations often translate to studying cohorts of 3–6 patients at each dose level. Algorithms such as the 3 + 3 design as well as the Rolling-6 design remain popular in pediatric settings for these reasons as well as due to their simplicity and ease of implementation [17]. While the more efficient algorithms such as the continual reassessment method (CRM) [18] are also used, they are not as popular even among groups that have the operational and statistical capabilities to implement them since some of the primary advantages offered by such approaches are somewhat muted in pediatric settings. One of the main advantages of model-based designs is the fact that they facilitate reaching the biologically active doses quickly and identifying the MTD accurately. In pediatric trials, since the starting dose is often one dose level lower than the adult MTD, or sometimes the adult MTD itself, the goal of reaching therapeutic doses quickly is often not relevant. Similarly, while the rarity of the pediatric patients invariably restricts the sample size, since only two or three dose levels are typically studied, the sample size is not a major constraint in pediatric trials. Often, the intent is to determine the safety of the adult MTD in pediatrics and understand its PK characteristics in children rather than identifying the pediatric MTD, though exceptions certainly exist. Nevertheless, there are other more nuanced advantages that model-based designs offer in pediatric trials, which could help motivate their use. Those advantages mainly relate to unique dosing considerations in pediatrics, which will be discussed in Section 4.3.

4.3 Dosing in Pediatric Phase I Trials

As noted above, pediatric phase I trials often enroll patients from birth up to the age of 21 years. This frequently leads to a very heterogeneous cohort with respect to organ function as well as body size and composition, which could affect the toxicity and response rate to the agent being studied. Given this heterogeneity in subjects enrolled on early-phase trials, some extra provisions are needed in adjusting doses. This is most typically done in a relatively simplistic fashion by adjusting the dose to the patient's size as measured by weight or body surface area (BSA). The former is often used in very young patients (typically less than 1 year of age) and the latter in patients who are older. Thus, dose levels in a pediatric phase I trial are often defined not in mg units but in mg/m^2 or in mg/m units. The median BSA in the Pediatric Brain Tumor Consortium (PBTC) database based on patients treated during the past 10 years was $1.15\,m^2$ with a range of 0.36–$2.78\,m^2$. The 25th and 75th percentiles of the observed BSAs were 0.82 and $1.51m^2$, respectively. In contrast, a "typical" adult BSA is considered to be $1.7\,m^2$. In order to illustrate the impact of BSA-based dosing an agent whose MTD was determined to be $50\,mg$ in adult trials is considered. The equivalent pediatric BSA-adjusted MTD would be calculated based on the "typical adult" BSA of $1.7\,m^2$ and thus would be given as approximately $30\,mg/m^2$, i.e., 50 divided by 1.7. Hence, a patient with a BSA of $0.6\,m^2$ who is assigned to this dose level would ideally receive $18\,mg$ of drug whereas another patient whose BSA is $1.9\,m^2$ would receive $57\,mg$ of drug. The BSA-based adjustments described above are mathematically simple, and they are often incorporated into protocols via BSA-specific dosing tables in order to assure accuracy in dosing, etc. Note, however, that this approach to dosing is very different from how dosing is handled in adult trials, where all subjects receive a flat mg dose regardless of their body size.

Oral drugs are generally preferred both in the adult and pediatric oncology settings since their administration does not require hospitalizations, unlike IV agents. This could potentially provide better quality of life for patients and their families by reducing the number of trips to the hospital, disruptions in daily routines, etc. Administering oral drugs to pediatric patients also comes with some significant challenges, however, since in many cases the agents are in capsule form that cannot be opened or in tablet form that cannot be crushed or cut. Many young children cannot swallow conventionally sized capsules or tablets whole, which could result in their exclusion from trials. There are also specific obstacles for children with regard to taste of medicines, including the ones that are available in liquid formulation, which can significantly affect adherence. Lack of adherence would clearly result in suboptimal data from clinical trials but also, more importantly, reduced efficacy in the treatment of the disease in question. Another important consideration in the use of medicines formulated for adults in pediatric populations is the safety of excipients, very few of which have any safety data for children. An excellent review article by Ivanovska et al. [12] provides a comprehensive discussion regarding the considerations and the complexity associated with pediatric drug formulations.

An additional concern for dose-finding trials in children arises in the cases of oral agents that come in fixed pill sizes that cannot be opened, crushed, or cut. This is a very common occurrence in early-phase pediatric trials since the timing of these trials generally coincides with a premarket period for the adult indication(s) being pursued. Most studies that involve new routes of administration or new dosage strengths for an agent are done in the postmarket environment. Even in cases where the agent already has FDA approval for an adult indication, there is little incentive to create a new formulation more suitable for children during the early stages of studying the agent due to the relatively high cost associated with the necessary studies [7].

The lack of pediatric formulations that allow dosage flexibility can lead to large differences between targeted and deliverable doses due to the BSA-adjusted dosing employed in children (see, e.g., Refs [19–22]). For example, if the available pill sizes are in multiples of 25 mg for a given agent with 25 mg being the smallest pill size, as in the example introduced earlier in this section, then the closest deliverable dose for a patient with a BSA of $0.6\,\mathrm{m}^2$ is 25 mg; whereas this patient should ideally receive 18 mg of drug. Therefore, this patient will effectively receive $41.7\,\mathrm{mg/m}^2$ (i.e., 25 mg divided by $0.6\,\mathrm{m}^2$), which is substantially higher than the desired $30\,\mathrm{mg/m}^2$. Similarly, the deliverable drug dose that is closest to the ideal dose of 56 mg for a patient with a BSA of $1.9\,\mathrm{m}^2$ is 50 mg, which is equivalent to $26.3\,\mathrm{mg/m}^2$ when adjusted for BSA and, thus, lower than the desired $30\,\mathrm{mg/m}^2$.

Figure 4.1 illustrates the BSA-adjusted deliverable total daily doses for dasatinib (Sprycel, BMS-354825, Bristol-Myers Squibb, Princeton, NJ) used in an institutional combination phase I trial in children with newly diagnosed diffuse intrinsic pontine glioma (SJBG09 NCT00996723) [23].

In this trial, two doses of dasatinib were to be studied in combination with vandetanib (Caprelsa, AstraZeneca, Macclesfield, UK). The proposed doses for dasatinib were $65\,\mathrm{mg/m}^2$ BID ($130\,\mathrm{mg/m}^2$ per day) and $85\,\mathrm{mg/m}^2$ BID ($170\,\mathrm{mg/m}^2$ per day). These dose levels were equivalent to one dose level below the single-agent MTD in children and the single-agent MTD in children, respectively. The smallest available tablet size for dasatinib at the time the trial was conducted was 20 mg and the BSA-based dosages were rounded to the nearest deliverable dose, i.e., up or down to the nearest 20. This approach results in the jagged appearance of the plot where each arc corresponds to fixed mg doses in increments of 20, i.e., the first arc represents 20 mg, the second arc 40 mg, third arc 60 mg etc. Within each arc, as the BSA increases (left to right on the x-axis), the administered BSA-adjusted dose decreases due to the constant mg dose represented by the arc, until one more pill is added. Addition of another pill results in a BSA-adjusted dose higher than the target dose but closer than what it would have been if another pill were not added. Then, again, the BSA-adjusted dose falls below this target dose as BSA increases further until the next pill is added to the administered dosage. The relative effect of adding another pill on the BSA-adjusted dosage diminishes as BSA increases, which gives rise to the funnel-shaped appearance of the deliverable dosage as a function of BSA. As is apparent from Figure 4.1, while some variation from the target dose is present for both 130 and $170\,\mathrm{mg/m}^2$ BSA-adjusted actual daily doses, the proposed dose levels are sufficiently far apart (the two "funnels" are clearly separated) to enable the study of this agent in pediatric populations even when some variations from targeted doses are preset.

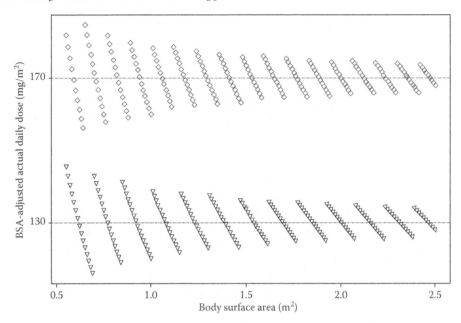

FIGURE 4.1
Deviations from target doses for dasatinib based on 20 mg tablets due to BSA-based dosing.

To illustrate this further, we will use a vignette from a recently published PBTC trial [19] of GDC-0449 (PBTC-025, NCT00822458). GDC-0449 (Vismodegib, Genentech, San Francisco, CA) was a first-in-class SHH pathway inhibitor via the inhibition of *SMO*. *SMO* is a membrane-associated protein that functions downstream of the *PTCH1* gene in the SHH pathway [19]. Initial phase I trial of GDC-0449 was conducted for a population of patients with advanced, metastatic solid tumors [24]. An impressive response rate of 60% was observed in patients with basal cell carcinoma on this trial. There was one additional response that was noted which occurred in a patient with metastatic medulloblastoma [24]. Medulloblastoma is a malignant brain tumor that occurs predominantly in children, though it can also occur in adults. The SHH pathway is known to be aberrant in a subset of these patients. Responses are exceedingly rare in patients with recurrent/progressive medulloblastoma, and thus, a phase I trial was initiated by the PBTC to study the safety and tolerability of this agent in pediatric patients with recurrent medulloblastoma based on an abundance of preclinical data and rationale [26, 27] as well as the response noted above. The trial also aimed to study the PK characteristics of this agent in children and even more importantly, to determine whether developmental toxicities specific to children such as growth defects in bones and teeth in skeletally immature patients were associated with the use of this agent as suggested by preclinical experiments conducted in young mice [28, 29]. GDC-0449 was supplied by Genentech and was distributed by the National Cancer Institute's (NCI) Cancer Therapy Evaluation Program (CTEP).

The pediatric trial was designed to use safety and PK data to select between two dose levels, namely 85 and $170 \, \text{mg/m}^2$, to recommend for the subsequent phase II trial. The adult recommended dose was 150 mg/day, which was equivalent to the $85 \, \text{mg/m}^2$ dose level. Enrollment was initiated at $85 \, \text{mg/m}^2$, and barring excessive toxicity, treatment of six patients per dose level was planned where patients were to be enrolled in cohorts of three. The safety observation period was defined as the first 28 days of treatment, and a lower dose, $60 \, \text{mg/m}^2$, was provided in the event that $85 \, \text{mg/m}^2$ turned out to be unsafe. Similar to the escalation rules used in the $3 + 3$ design, if no more than one patient in a cohort of six patients experienced a dose-limiting toxicity (DLT), then the dose would be escalated to 170 mg/m^2 and a similar approach would be used to study its safety. If both dose levels proved to be safe (i.e., no more than one DLT in six patients), then the PK parameters would be used to choose the dose to be carried forward to the phase II trial. Thus, PK studies were mandatory for this study and were part of the primary objectives.

At the beginning of the trial, GDC-0449 was available in 25 and 150 mg capsules, so the dosing strategy incorporated into the trial was to round BSA-adjusted doses to the nearest 25 mg. Initially, a suggestion was made by the company in the interest of safety to round down the BSA-adjusted dose to the nearest 25 mg rather than rounding up or down to the nearest 25 mg dose, but this was not pursued for reasons illustrated in Figure 4.2.

The two panels in Figure 4.2 compare the BSA-adjusted daily doses with BSA for the two strategies. The plot on the left is based on rounding down to the nearest 25 mg and the plot on the right is rounding to the nearest 25 mg. Note that with the round-down strategy, almost every patient would receive a dose that is below the target level. In fact, with this approach, some of the patients who are assigned to 85 mg/m^2 would receive less than 60 mg/m^2 (the overlapping crosses and triangles in the lower part of Figure 4.2). There is some overlap in the graph on the right as well (based on the "round to the nearest 25 mg" approach), but this occurs in the region between 60 and 85 mg/m^2. Furthermore, the average variation from the target dose is larger in the "round-down" approach compared to the "round to the nearest multiple of 25 mg" approach.

While it is clear from the discussion above and from Figure 4.2 that rounding up or down to the nearest deliverable dose level is preferable, the overlapping regions in the BSA-adjusted doses pose challenges in clinical and operational aspects of phase I trials. In the absence of additional safeguards, these regions represent BSAs for which patients assigned to 60 mg/m^2 or 85 mg/m^2 would actually receive the same amount of drug. For example, in the case of GDC-0449, a patient with a BSA of 0.65 m^2 assigned to 85 mg/m^2 dose level would ideally receive 55.25 mg of drug. This is not possible, however, since the smallest pill size is 25 mg; thus, the closest deliverable amount is 50 mg. If the same patient is assigned to 60 mg/m^2 following a de-escalation, the ideal dose would have been 39 mg, which is also not deliverable and for which the closest deliverable dose is still 50 mg. Thus, based on the, "rounding to the nearest 25 mg" strategy, this patient would receive 50 mg of drug

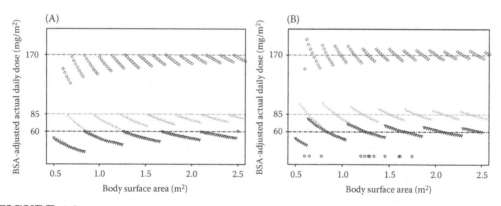

FIGURE 4.2

Deviations from target doses for GDC-0449 based on 25 mg capsules due to BSA-based dosing. (A) Using "round-down" strategy and (B) using "round up or down to the nearest multiple of 25 mg" strategy. The horizontal indications above BSA axis in (B) mark actual BSAs of patients enrolled in the phase I trial.

whether he/she is assigned to dose level 0 ($60\,\mathrm{mg/m^2}$) or 1 ($85\,\mathrm{mg/m^2}$). In a setting of dose finding, it is clearly not acceptable that patients with different assigned doses receive the same amount of drug in practice; what is more, in the event of a de-escalation from dose level 1 to dose level 0 due to excessive toxicities, practically applying an unchanged dose poses ethical questions.

When limited pill sizes are present, such overlaps are common when BSA-adjusted doses are used no matter the rounding strategy. In fact, in designing a phase I pediatric trial with an oral agent, one of the first questions that the study team needs to answer is whether pediatric dosing is feasible with the current formulation. The pill size limitations almost always affect lower dose levels and lower BSA ranges because higher doses and/or higher BSAs allow for a relatively closer match of desired dose with the deliverable dose. For an intuitive rationale for this, note that "the arcs that comprise the funnels" in Figures 4.1 and 4.2 are wider for lower dose levels and for smaller BSAs within a dose level. The wider these "arcs," the more likely that the overlaps will occur.

There are several approaches one could use to accommodate these overlaps; one option would be to choose the dose levels in such a way that these overlaps are avoided. If the dose levels are far apart enough, then these overlapping regions do not manifest or can be minimized. Separating dose levels adequately so as to avoid the overlaps is not always a viable strategy, however, since this could result in very large increments between dose levels and could compromise safety. This is an important consideration since these overlaps almost always affect lower dose levels and thus are relevant to phases of the trial during which little safety information is available. A trial is typically initiated at lower dose levels, and dose is escalated one level at a time as more safety information is accumulated from the patient cohorts treated. Thus, large increments between initial dose levels are often impractical especially given the fact that the starting doses for pediatric trials are already high. A common increment used in pediatric trials between dose levels is 30%.

A second approach to dealing with these overlaps in the setting of a phase I trial is to exclude patients with BSAs that correspond to these regions. While this is not ideal as it often leads to excluding some of the smaller patients from enrollment at the lower dose levels, it can be a pragmatic way to proceed with the trial. In practice, a combination of these two approaches is often used in an effort to operationally optimize the trial conduct.

The PBTC-025 study was conducted as described above, and after treating six patients at each dose level, it was determined that both dose levels were safe, and $170\,\mathrm{mg/m^2}$ was chosen as the RP2D based on its more favorable PK properties. Shortly thereafter, the company informed CTEP and the PBTC that they were discontinuing the production of the 25 mg capsules and recommended that, given the established safety of $170\,\mathrm{mg/m^2}$ in children, the pediatric patients enrolled on the phase II trial be treated with 150 mg flat dose per day, similar to their adult counterparts. The PBTC study team felt that this recommendation was not acceptable due to the wide range of BSAs inherent in pediatric patients and the resulting differences in BSA-adjusted doses. Figure 4.3 illustrates the effect of flat 150 mg/day dosing on BSA-adjusted doses in pediatric patients.

This concern was heightened as the study team had already demonstrated in the first part of the trial that PK exposure parameters were dependent on dosage (as measured by $\mathrm{mg/m^2}$). The study team countered this proposal with a different strategy where the patients would be dosed at $170\,\mathrm{mg/m^2}$ by rounding to the nearest 150 mg capsules. While this strategy would also lead to large variations from the targeted doses, the study team felt that it was preferable under the current pill size constraints. After extensive discussions, the study teams proposal was approved and the second stage of the trial commenced testing the safety and PK characteristics of this approach in pediatric patients. Given the single large pill size, the smallest/youngest patients had to be excluded from the second portion of the study and BSA of eligible patients were limited to $>0.67\mathrm{m^2}$. Table 4.1

TABLE 4.1

Dosing strategy based on 150 mg capsules targeting 170 mg/m^2.

BSA Range	Dose (mg)	BSA-Adjusted Dose (mg/m^2)	Deviation (%)
0.67–1.32	150	113.64–223.88	−34 to +32
1.33–2.20	300	136.36–225.56	−20 to +33
2.21–2.50	450	180.00–203.62	+6 to +20

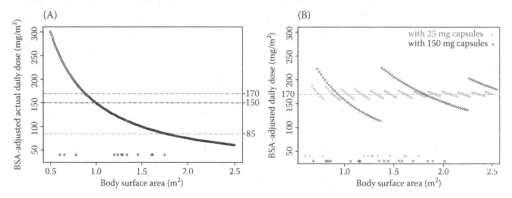

FIGURE 4.3

BSA adjusted dosages with capsule sizes limited to 150 mg. (A) Flat dosing based on 150 mg/day. (B) BSA-adjusted doses based on rounding to the nearest multiple of 25 mg versus 150 mg. The horizontal indications above BSA axes mark actual BSAs of patients enrolled in the phase I trial, where for (B) "∘" indicates patients receiving 25 mg capsules and "×" indicates patients receiving 150 mg capsules.

demonstrates the dosing nomogram based on this approach that was used in the second part of the trial and the anticipated percent deviation from the target dose.

Figure 4.3 (B) illustrates the BSA-adjusted doses proposed for the second part of the trial as compared to the approach used during the first part, when the 25 mg capsules were available. The circles ("∘") in the plot represent the dosing variation associated with the first portion of the trial, and the crosses ("×") represent the same in the second portion. The symbols at the lower part of the plot just above the x-axis mark the BSAs of the patients who enrolled on the first portion ("∘") and the second portion ("×") of the trial. The trial was completed successfully after establishing the safety of the revised approach used in part 2 of the study and demonstrated favorable PK characteristics [19]. The two phase II trials, one in adults and the other in pediatric patients, were subsequently conducted, which showed notable efficacy, though transient, in SHH-driven medulloblastoma [30].

4.4 Use of Model-Based Designs in Pediatric Trials

As noted previously in this chapter, and also similar to adult trials, algorithmic approaches such as 3 + 3 and the Rolling-6 dominate the dose-finding designs used in pediatric settings. The use of the Rolling-6 design has gained popularity since its introduction due to the promise that it may reduce downtime during toxicity evaluation and hence lead to shorter overall trial duration. Simulation studies in Ref. [31] as well as in [32] demonstrate that the 3 + 3 and the Rolling-6 designs are comparable with respect to patient safety and the likelihood of recommending a reasonable dose as the MTD. With respect to trial duration and the number of patients enrolled, the same studies showed that on average, the Rolling-6 design requires more patients but does lead to shorter overall trial duration. Note, however, that the reduction in the length of the trial may be very modest if the trial has very high per patient costs. In such cases, the reduction in duration may not justify the increase in cost due to the larger sample size often required by the Rolling-6 design [32]. Furthermore, while the toxicity rate is similar between the Rolling-6 and the 3 + 3 designs, the fact that the Rolling-6 design requires a larger number of patients implies that the number of toxicities is likely to be larger as well. For agents where severe and potentially irreversible toxicities are likely, the use of the Rolling-6 design may be inadvisable. On the other hand, a scenario where only two dose levels are proposed around the adult MTD as a brief safety trial prior to proceeding to a phase II study where no or little toxicity is expected based on the adult experience may be ideally suited for the Rolling-6 design. Additionally, phase I trials with longer dose-finding periods where accrual rate is expected to be high may also be suitable for the use of the Rolling-6 design, as a way of shortening the trial duration and allowing more patients to participate in the trial. For example, trials where radiotherapy and chemotherapy are administered concurrently and the dose-finding period spans the entire radiotherapy treatment (usually 6–8 weeks), plus 2–4 weeks of additional observation period for delayed toxicities, may represent a scenario where the Rolling-6 design may be preferable. In these settings, the extended suspension of accrual is often a source of frustration for clinicians as well as patients and families. Thus, such trials may create a favorable setting for the use of the Rolling-6 design, especially if the expected toxicity incidence is low. Note, however, that if the accrual rate is not fast enough, extended DLT observation periods in a Rolling-6 design may lead to longer accrual suspensions compared to the 3 + 3 or the CRM design since one would have to wait for the fourth, fifth, and sixth patients to complete the observation period. It is worth mentioning that model-based designs, such as the TITE-CRM [33, 34], that could be effectively used in a setting with long DLT observation periods are available.

While empirical designs are simpler to implement, model-based dose-finding approaches such as the CRM [18] have been shown to be more efficient and effective in identifying the MTD without sacrificing safety [35–37]. Furthermore, trial durations associated with the CRM-type designs are comparable or shorter than those of the Rolling-6 designs [31]. The use of BSA-adjusted doses provides an additional motivation for implementing model-based designs in pediatric dose-finding trials. Notably, however, most available CRM-type algorithms treat dose levels as ordinal and do not utilize information from the actual dose level other than its order among the proposed dose levels. As demonstrated above, in a pediatric setting, there is additional information available that results from the variation generated from BSA-based dosing that could be used in determining the RP2D. More specifically, in a pediatric trial, the assumption that all patients in a cohort are treated at the same dose level is no longer true, as each patient within a cohort will likely receive a slightly different dose. While there are CRM-type designs that use dose as a continuous variable, such as the one introduced in Ref. [38] in an HIV setting, these approaches are not commonly used in oncology trials. Part of the reason for this may be the fact that in most adult trials, the ordinal dose levels may adequately capture the information needed for these models and the fact that using designs that rely on continuous dosing inherently requires stronger assumptions between dose and toxicity. In pediatric trials, however, where BSA-based dosing may introduce a lot of variability in the delivered dose within a dose level, the former may not be true and the latter may be justified.

In a limited simulation study, it has been shown that taking this information into account can lead to a different MTD estimate compared to cases where one assumes that all patients in a cohort are treated at the same dose level [31]. Based on six dose–toxicity probability scenarios studied in that manuscript and 1,000 simulated trials using the same patient cohort and toxicity outcomes for each trial with the exception of BSA-adjusted doses vs.

not adjusted doses (denoted as CRM-BSA vs. CRM, respectively), the percentage of simulated trials where the MTD estimate was different between CRM and CRM-BSA approaches ranged between 6.4% and 13.8%. Similarly, the estimated rank correlations of the MTD estimates obtained for the CRM and CRM-BSA approaches were quite high (0.835 − 0.955) but not perfect. This difference was notable as it was caused by the BSA-based dosing variations alone since the patient cohort and the toxicity outcomes were kept the same. Furthermore, based on the same simulation study, it was estimated that the dose-escalation/de-escalation decisions were not identical between the CRM and the CRM-BSA in 10.7–28.3% of trials, which is nonignorable. In addition to the latent dose–toxicity relationship, the likelihood that one would determine a different MTD when incorporating BSA-adjusted doses compared to the case where this information is not taken into account depends on the variability in BSA-adjusted doses as determined by preset dose levels and pill size limitations as well as the range of BSAs associated with patients that enroll on the trial. Nevertheless, ignoring this information by only using the ordinal dose information can be suboptimal in a setting where information is already scarce and could, in some cases, justify the stronger assumptions needed to implement a model with a continuous dose–toxicity relationship.

In addition to incorporating variations within cohorts as a potential source of variability, model-based designs have another distinct advantage in the pediatric setting in that they can formalize the use of already available information from previous adult trials. A notable example of this approach is introduced in Ref. [39], where the authors describe bridging studies in the context of heterogeneity. In this approach, the authors illustrate how model-based designs can be used to study two cohorts simultaneously or in a staggered setting. They also describe how data from a previous trial can be formally incorporated into the design of a subsequent study via a parameter in the model in order to improve the efficiency of the trial with respect to duration as well as sample size.

4.5   Conclusions

As noted numerous times in this chapter, pediatric cancer is a rare disease in a heterogeneous and vulnerable population. These factors as well as several others discussed above, pose significant challenges in conducting early-phase trials in children. There are, however, a number of factors that can significantly aid in accomplishing this goal. One of the most notable is the fact that there are several NCI-funded consortia that focus on pediatric cancer. The most comprehensive is the Childrens Oncology Group (COG), which is the largest pediatric clinical trials consortium in the world. Its membership includes approximately 220 participating hospitals, a vast majority of which are in the United States. According to the COG website, 60% of patients under the age of 29 years diagnosed with cancer in the United States are enrolled on trials. In contrast, only 3% of adult cancer patients in the United States participate in clinical trials [40]. St. Baldrick's Foundation estimates that 90% of children with cancer are treated at a COG institution. Thus, a vast majority of children receive cancer care at specialized centers with expert pediatric oncology teams who are aware of and have access to ongoing clinical trials. In addition, the NCI sponsors smaller, more specialized pediatric consortia such as the PBTC (www.PBTC.org), the COG phase I and Pilot Consortium (https://childrensoncologygroup.org/index.php/phase-1-home), and New Approaches to Neuroblastoma Therapy Consortium (NANT, www.nant.org), which are focused on identifying and developing new treatments for pediatric cancers with the worst outcomes. A variety of other consortia funded by philanthropic or industry support are also available, including Pediatric Oncology Experimental Therapeutics Investigators'

Consortium (POETC, http://www.poeticphase1.org/) and Pacific Pediatric Neuro-Oncology Consortium (PNOC, http://www.pnoc.us/).

Due to the aforementioned lack of incentive in conducting pediatric trials by pharmaceutical companies in the past, there have been relatively few phase I trials conducted in children. As a result, despite the limited number of pediatric patients eligible for phase I trials, when a promising trial is open for a pediatric population, accrual has almost never been an issue [41, 42]. In fact, the lack of suitable studies for patients with recurrent or refractory cancers is a common lament of pediatric oncologists and families of patients. It is the expectation and hope of the pediatric oncology community that with the new regulatory environment, the number and the variety of trials available for children with cancer will increase dramatically in the coming years. If this materializes, the successful completion of these studies will require a collaborative effort and the pediatric oncology community is well positioned to respond to this need with the existing NCI-funded consortia as well as various other collaborative groups that have been formed by expert pediatric oncology centers nationally and internationally using other funding mechanisms. There are a variety of philanthropic and advocacy organizations focused on childhood cancer that have done a tremendous job in raising awareness of the issues specific to pediatric cancer and regarding the need for new regulations. They have also been very effective in generating the funds to support research efforts in pediatric cancers at all phases, starting from preclinical studies, continuing with clinical trials, and following up with late-effect studies in childhood cancer survivors.

The long-standing partnerships between government, academic centers, and philanthropic and advocacy organizations that have recently been supplemented with increasing collaborations with industry have created an environment where the pediatric oncology trials can be conducted via an expanded portfolio with the objective of developing new, safe, and effective therapies for children paving the way for achieving the ultimate goal of ending pediatric cancer. Clinical trial biostatisticians have an important role to play in these efforts by ensuring that the state-of-the-art statistical approaches often developed in adult settings are properly translated to pediatric trials. Doing so could facilitate improving both efficiency and the quality of information that can be derived from small early-phase trials in an effort to inform and guide later-phase studies, which can change how the children with cancer are treated for the better.

Acknowledgments

Grant Support: A. Onar-Thomas's contribution to this work was supported, in part, by the National Institutes of Health (grant no. U01 CA081457 to the PBTC), the St. Jude Cancer Center CORE (grant no. CA 21765), and the American Lebanese Syrian Associated Charities (ALSAC).

References

1. American Cancer Society. Cancer facts & figures 2014—special section: Childhood & adolescent cancers. http://www.cancer.org/acs/groups/content/@research/documents/webcontent/acspc-042151.pdf, 2014. Accessed: November 24, 2015.

2. J. Boklan. Little patients, losing patience: Pediatric cancer drug development. *Molecular Cancer Therapeutics*, 5(8):1905–1908, 2006.

3. K. E. Deffenbacher, J. Iqbal, W. Sanger, Y. Shen, C. Lachel, Z. Liu, Y. Liu, M. S. Lim, S. L. Perkins, K. Fu, et al. Molecular distinctions between pediatric and adult mature B-cell non-Hodgkin lymphomas identified through genomic profiling. *Blood*, 119(16):3757–3766, 2012.

4. J. R. Downing, R. K. Wilson, J. Zhang, E. R. Mardis, C.-H. Pui, L. Ding, T. J. Ley, and W. E. Evans. The pediatric cancer genome project. *Nature Genetics*, 44(6):619–622, 2012. doi: 10.1038/ng.2287.

5. C. Jones, L. Perryman, and D. Hargrave. Paediatric and adult malignant glioma: Close relatives or distant cousins? *Nature Reviews Clinical Oncolgy*, 9(7):400–413, 2012. doi: 10.1038/nrclinonc.2012.87.

6. D. W. Parsons, M. Li, X. Zhang, S. Jones, R. J. Leary, J. C.-H. Lin, S. M. Boca, H. Carter, J. Samayoa, C. Bettegowda, et al. The genetic landscape of the childhood cancer medulloblastoma. *Science* 331(6016):435–439, 2011.

7. Tufts Center for the Study of Drug Development. How the Tufts Center for the Study of Drug Development pegged the cost of a new drug at $2.6 billion. http://csdd.tufts.edu/files/uploads/cost_study_backgrounder.pdf, November 18, 2014. Accessed: November 24, 2015.

8. J. Avorn. The $2.6 billion pill—Methodologic and policy considerations. *New England Journal of Medicine*, 372(20):1877–1879, 2015.

9. N. Aumock, J. Smith, and S. Townsend. Do incentives drive pediatric research? McKinsey Center for Government, October 2013.

10. Federal Drug Administration (FDA). Pediatric exclusivity granted: Drugs to which FDA has granted pediatric exclusivity for pediatric studies under Section 505A of the Federal Food, Drug, and Cosmetic Act. http://www.fda.gov/Drugs/DevelopmentApproval-Process/DevelopmentResources/ucm050005.htm, October 2015. Accessed: November 19, 2015.

11. M. E. Ceja, A. M. Christensen, and S. P. Yang. Dosing considerations in pediatric oncology. *U.S. Pharmacist*, 38(Oncology suppl):8–11, 2013.

12. V. Ivanovska, C. M. A. Rademaker, L. van Dijk, and A. K. Mantel-Teeuwisse. Pediatric drug formulations: A review of challenges and progress. *Pediatrics*, 134(2):361–372, 2014.

13. M. Smith, M. Bernstein, W. A. Bleyer, J. D. Borsi, P. Ho, I. J. Lewis, A. Pearson, F. Pein, C. Pratt, G. Reaman, et al. Conduct of phase I trials in children with cancer. *Journal of Clinical Oncology*, 16(3):966–978, 1998.

14. V. M. Piñeiro-Carrero and E. O. Piñeiro. Liver. *Pediatrics*, 113(4 Suppl):1097–1106, 2004.

15. D. P. Lee, J. M. Skolnik, and P. C. Adamson. Pediatric phase I trials in oncology: An analysis of study conduct efficiency. *Journal of Clinical Oncology*, 23(33):8431–8441, 2005.

16. J. S. Weber, L. A. Levit, P. C. Adamson, S. Bruinooge, H. A. Burris, M. A. Carducci, A. P. Dicker, M. Gönen, S. M. Keefe, M. A. Postow, et al. American society of clinical oncology policy statement update: The critical role of phase I trials in cancer research and treatment. *Journal of Clinical Oncology*, 33(3):278–284, 2015.

17. J. M. Skolnik, J. S. Barrett, B. Jayaraman, D. Patel, and P. C. Adamson. Shortening the timeline of pediatric phase I trials: The rolling six design. *Journal of Clinical Oncology*, 26(2):190–195, 2008.

18. J. O'Quigley, M. Pepe, and L. Fisher. Continual reassessment method: A practical design for phase I clinical trials in cancer. *Biometrics*, 46(1):33–48, 1990.

19. A. Gajjar, C. F. Stewart, D. W. Ellison, S. Kaste, L. E. Kun, R. J. Packer, S. Goldman, M. Chintagumpala, D. Wallace, N. Takebe, et al. Phase I study of vismodegib in children with recurrent or refractory medulloblastoma: A pediatric brain tumor consortium study. *Clinical Cancer Research*, 19(22):6305–6312, 2013.

20. M. W. Kieran, R. J. Packer, A. Onar, S. M. Blaney, P. Phillips, I. F. Pollack, J. R. Geyer, S. Gururangan, A. Banerjee, S. Goldman, et al. Phase I and pharmacokinetic study of the oral farnesyltransferase inhibitor lonafarnib administered twice daily to pediatric patients with advanced central nervous system tumors using a modified continuous reassessment method: A pediatric brain tumor consortium study. *Journal of Clinical Oncology*, 25(21):3137–3143, 2007.

21. J. G. Villablanca, M. D. Krailo, M. M. Ames, J. M. Reid, G. H. Reaman, and C. P. Reynolds. Phase I trial of oral fenretinide in children with high-risk solid tumors: A report from the Children's Oncology Group (CCG 09709). *Journal of Clinical Oncology*, 24(21):3423–3430, 2006.

22. B. C. Widemann, W. L. Salzer, R. J. Arceci, S. M. Blaney, E. Fox, D. End, A. Gillespie, P. Whitcomb, J. S. Palumbo, A. Pitney, et al. Phase I trial and pharmacokinetic study of the farnesyltransferase inhibitor tipifarnib in children with refractory solid tumors or neurofibromatosis type I and plexiform neurofibromas. *Journal of Clinical Oncology*, 24(3):507–516, 2006.

23. A. Broniscer, S. D. Baker, C. Wetmore, A. S. Pai Panandiker, J. Huang, A. M. Davidoff, A. Onar-Thomas, J. C. Panetta, T. K. Chin, T. E. Merchant, et al. Phase I trial, pharmacokinetics, and pharmacodynamics of vandetanib and dasatinib in children with newly diagnosed diffuse intrinsic pontine glioma. *Clinical Cancer Research*, 19(11):3050–3058, 2013.

24. D. D. Von Hoff, P. M. LoRusso, C. M. Rudin, J. C. Reddy, R. L. Yauch, R. Tibes, G. J. Weiss, M. J. Borad, C. L. Hann, J. R. Brahmer, et al. Inhibition of the hedgehog pathway in advanced basal-cell carcinoma. *New England Journal of Medicine*, 361(12):1164–1172, 2009.

25. C. M. Rudin, C. L. Hann, J. Laterra, R. L. Yauch, C. A. Callahan, L. Fu, T. Holcomb, J. Stinson, S. E. Gould, B. Coleman, et al. Treatment of medulloblastoma with hedgehog pathway inhibitor GDC-0449. *New England Journal of Medicine*, 361(12):1173–1178, 2009.

26. K. D. Robarge, S. A. Brunton, G. M. Castanedo, Y. Cui, M. S. Dina, R. Goldsmith, S. E. Gould, O. Guichert, J. L. Gunzner, J. Halladay, et al. GDC-0449—A potent inhibitor of the hedgehog pathway. *Bioorganic & Medicinal Chemistry Letters*, 19(19):5576–5581, 2009.

27. J. T. Romer, H. Kimura, S. Magdaleno, K. Sasai, C. Fuller, H. Baines, M. Connelly, C. F. Stewart, S. Gould, L. L. Rubin et al. Suppression of the Shh pathway using a small molecule inhibitor eliminates medulloblastoma in $Ptc1^{+/-}p53^{-/-}$ mice. *Cancer Cell*, 6(3):229–240, 2004.

28. H. Kimura, J. M. Y. Ng, and T. Curran. Transient inhibition of the hedgehog pathway in young mice causes permanent defects in bone structure. *Cancer Cell*, 13(3):249–260, 2008.

29. K. Seidel, C. P. Ahn, D. Lyons, A. Nee, K. Ting, I. Brownell, T. Cao, R. A. D. Carano, T. Curran, M. Schober, et al. Hedgehog signaling regulates the generation of ameloblast progenitors in the continuously growing mouse incisor. *Development*, 137(22):3753–3761, 2010.

30. G. W. Robinson, B. A. Orr, G. Wu, S. Gururangan, T. Lin, I. Qaddoumi, R. J. Packer, S. Goldman, M. D. Prados, A. Desjardins, et al. Vismodegib exerts targeted efficacy against recurrent sonic hedgehog-subgroup medulloblastoma: Results from phase II pediatric brain tumor consortium studies PBTC-025b and PBTC-032. *Journal of Clinical Oncology*, 33(24):2646–2654, 2015.

31. A. Onar-Thomas and Z. Xiong. A simulation-based comparison of the traditional method, Rolling-6 design and a frequentist version of the continual reassessment method with special attention to trial duration in pediatric phase I oncology trials. *Contemporary Clinical Trials*, 31(3):259–270, 2010.

32. R. Sposto and S. Groshen. A wide-spectrum paired comparison of the properties of the Rolling 6 and 3 + 3 phase I study designs. *Contemporary Clinical Trials*, 32(5):694–703, 2011.

33. Y. K. Cheung and R. Chappell. Sequential designs for phase I clinical trials with late-onset toxicities. *Biometrics*, 56(4):1177–1182, 2000.

34. T. M. Braun. Generalizing the TITE-CRM to adapt for early- and late-onset toxicities. *Statistics in Medicine*, 25(12):2071–2083, 2006.

35. A. Iasonos, A. S. Wilton, E. R. Riedel, V. E. Seshan, and D. R. Spriggs. A comprehensive comparison of the continual reassessment method to the standard 3 + 3 dose escalation scheme in phase I dose-finding studies. *Clinical Trials*, 5(5):465–477, 2008.

36. A. Onar, M. Kocak, and J. M. Boyett. Continual reassessment method vs. traditional empirically-based design: Modifications motivated by phase I trials in pediatric oncology by the pediatric brain tumor consortium. *Journal of Biopharmaceutical Statistics*, 19(3):437–455, 2009.

37. N. A. Wages, M. R. Conaway, and J. O'Quigley. Performance of two-stage continual reassessment method relative to an optimal benchmark. *Clinical Trials*, 10(6):862–875, 2013.

38. J. O'Quigley, M. D. Hughes, and T. Fenton. Dose-finding designs for HIV studies. *Biometrics*, 57(4):1018–1029, 2001.

39. J. O'Quigley and A. Iasonos. Bridging solutions in dose finding problems. *Statistics in Biopharmaceutical Research*, 6(2):185–197, 2014.

40. Institute of Medicine (US). Clinical trials in cancer. *Forum on Drug Discovery, Development, and Translation. Transforming Clinical Research in the United States: Challenges and Opportunities*, Chapter 6. Workshop Summary. Washington, DC: National Academies Press. http://www.ncbi.nlm.nih.gov/books/NBK50895/, 2010. Accessed: November 30, 2015.

41. S. B. Bavdekar. Pediatric clinical trials. *Perspectives in Clinical Research*, 4(1):89–99, 2013.

42. National Cancer Institute (NCI). An analysis of the National Cancer institute's investment in pediatric cancer research. http://www.cancer.gov/types/childhood-cancers/research/pediatric-analy sis. pdf, September 2013. Accessed: August 22, 2016.

Part II

More Advanced Phase I and Phase I/II Methodology

5

Phase I/II Dose-Finding Designs with Efficacy and Safety Endpoints

Oleksandr Sverdlov

Novartis Institutes for Biomedical Research

Lei Gao

Sanofi US

CONTENTS

5.1 Introduction

The primary objective of a conventional phase I oncology trial of a cytotoxic agent is to identify the maximum tolerated dose (MTD) for testing in subsequent studies. The major assumption is that both the probability of toxicity and the probability of therapeutic response are monotonically increasing with dose; therefore, by determining the MTD, one indirectly determines a dose with maximum potential for therapeutic effect. Many phase I trial designs for determining the MTD with a prespecified level of toxicity rate have been proposed in the literature [53].

With recent developments in personalized medicine, there has been an increasing interest in clinical trials of cytostatic agents—the therapies that act on specific molecular targets expressed in cancer cells and, due to their specific mechanism of action, can inhibit tumor growth or prevent proliferation of cancer cells at doses that are not necessarily very toxic. Clinical trial designs of cytostatic agents generally require special considerations, different from those of cytotoxic agents [31, 71]. In particular, for a cytostatic agent, the risk of toxicity may not necessarily increase with increased doses. In addition, the dose–efficacy curve may have a peak or may reach a plateau at some dose levels below the MTD, and therefore, higher doses may at best result in only marginal improvements in clinical benefit. Hence, a simultaneous assessment of early signals of efficacy along with toxicity can be of great importance for a successful development of a cytostatic therapy. Recently, there has been significant methodological research on statistical designs for phase I clinical trials that incorporate both efficacy and toxicity outcomes in dose-finding objectives (see Refs [10, 52, 54, 76] for recent reviews). Such designs are also referred to as *seamless phase I/II designs* [10] because they integrate the objectives of traditional phases I and II—namely, identifying a dose or doses that exhibit promising signals of efficacy (phase II goal) with acceptable levels of toxicity (phase I goal)—in a single study.

An advantage of pursuing a seamless phase I/II trial is that doses with desirable benefit–risk ratio can be identified faster and more efficiently than in a conventional sequence of separate phase I and II trials. Clinical development programs can be potentially accelerated because a phase I/II trial avoids an administrative wait between phase I and II protocol activation. Gains in statistical efficiency can be achieved because a phase I/II trial would typically be larger and collect more data than would a single phase I trial. Since therapeutic response and toxicity are frequently correlated, one can perform joint modeling of the dose–efficacy–toxicity relationship—this can yield many insightful findings on the benefit–risk ratio of the compound.

The goal of this chapter is to provide an overview of state-of-the-art seamless phase I/II dose escalation oncology designs that utilize both efficacy and toxicity outcomes in dose assignment decisions. In Section 5.2, we present statistical background, define experimental objectives of a phase I/II trial, and discuss adaptive designs to achieve these objectives in practice. In Section 5.3, we discuss several important types of phase I/II designs for trials where efficacy and toxicity are correlated binary random variables. In Section 5.4, we describe phase I/II designs for more complex settings, namely when the toxicity is binary and efficacy is continuous, when efficacy (and toxicity) outcomes are delayed, and when study patients have heterogeneous prognostic profiles. Section 5.5 provides a discussion.

Note that in this chapter, we exclude phase I/II "cohort expansion" designs where phase I toxicity-based dose escalation is followed by a phase II single-arm or multiarm randomized selection design using efficacy response. Examples of "cohort expansion" designs can be found elsewhere [29, 32]. Also, our review is focused on phase I/II dose-escalation studies of a single compound. More complex phase I/II drug combination and dose-schedule-finding studies are discussed in Chapters 6 and 7 of the present volume. For a recent book-length discussion on Bayesian phase I/II trial designs, refer to [69].

5.2   Statistical Background

5.2.1   Basic concepts

Let $D = \{d_1 < d_2 < \cdots < d_K\}$ denote the set of prespecified doses of the selected agent to be investigated in the study. We first consider with the simplest case, when both toxicity and efficacy are binary random variables, that is,

$$Y_T = \begin{cases} 1, & \text{if toxicity;} \\ 0, & \text{otherwise.} \end{cases} \qquad Y_E = \begin{cases} 1, & \text{if efficacy;} \\ 0, & \text{otherwise.} \end{cases}$$

The definitions of toxicity and efficacy will depend on a particular medical setting. In oncology, toxicity commonly refers to any severe (requiring hospitalization) or life-threatening adverse event, whereas efficacy can refer to objective response according to RECIST criteria, progression-free survival status at a given time point, or some other indication of therapeutic benefit. Let X denote the dose assignment ($X \in D$), and let $p(d) = \Pr(Y_T = 1 | X = d)$ and $q(d) = \Pr(Y_E = 1 | X = d)$ denote, respectively, marginal probabilities of toxicity and efficacy for a patient treated at dose $d \in D$. Frequently, it is sensible to assume that both $p(d)$ and $q(d)$ are monotone increasing in dose, that is, $0 < p_1(d) < \cdots < p_K(d) < 1$ and $0 < q_1(d) < \cdots < q_K(d) < 1$. However, $q(d)$ can be also nonmonotone [31].

Let $0 < \overline{p}_T < 1$ and $0 < \underline{q}_E < 1$ denote two thresholds for the maximum acceptable toxicity probability ($\overline{p}_T$) and the minimum acceptable efficacy probability ($\underline{q}_E$), prespecified by the clinical investigator, respectively. Then, one can define the MTD as

$$MTD = \max\{d \in D : p(d) \leq \overline{p}_T\},$$

and the *minimum effective dose (MED)* as

$$MED = \min\{d \in D : q(d) \geq \underline{q}_E\}.$$

In situations when $MED < MTD$, the interval $[MED, MTD]$ is referred to as the *therapeutic window (TW)* [63]. Doses within the TW are suitable for clinical investigation. If $MED > MTD$, then the TW is an empty set (the investigational drug has no practical value).

If one looks at (Y_T, Y_E) jointly, several types of outcomes can be considered. The simplest approach is to suppress the pair of outcomes to a single dichotomous variable: $U = 1$, if $(Y_E, Y_T) = (1, 0)$ (efficacy without toxicity) and $U = 0$ otherwise. However, such dichotomization results in loss of important information.

Another approach is a three-category model that defines an ordinal variable Z as follows:

$$Z = \begin{cases} 0, & \text{if } (Y_E, Y_T) = (0, 0) \text{ (no efficacy and no toxicity);} \\ 1, & \text{if } (Y_E, Y_T) = (1, 0) \text{ (efficacy without toxicity);} \\ 2, & \text{if } Y_T = 1 \text{ (toxicity).} \end{cases} \qquad (5.1)$$

The grading in model (5.1) is appropriate, for instance, in trials where toxicity causes irreversible organ damage or regimen-related death, and if it occurs, then efficacy is simply not applicable. Throughout this chapter, we shall also use the following notations: $\overline{E} \cap \overline{T}$ for $Z = 0$, $E \cap \overline{T}$ for $Z = 1$, and T for $Z = 2$.

Finally, the most informative approach is a four-category model for which all four efficacy–toxicity combinations $(Y_E, Y_T) = \{(0, 0), (0, 1), (1, 0), (1, 1)\}$ can be observed.

With any approach, the desirable outcome for any patient is efficacy without toxicity. Throughout the chapter, the outcome $(Y_E, Y_T) = (1, 0)$ is referred to as *success*.

Let $\widetilde{q}(d) = \Pr(Y_E = 1 | Y_T = 0, X = d)$ denote the conditional probability of efficacy given no toxicity at dose d. Then, the probability of success, $s(d)$, is given by the product

$$s(d) = \widetilde{q}(d)(1 - p(d)). \qquad (5.2)$$

If $s(d)$ in (5.2) is unimodal, then one can define the *most successful dose (MSD)* as

$$MSD = \arg\max_{d \in D} s(d).$$

Durham et al. [13] (see also Ref. [42]) give conditions for the existence and uniqueness of MSD (which they refer to as *optimal dose*). In general, the MSD may fall outside the TW if its associated risk of toxicity is higher than maximally acceptable, i.e., if $p(MSD) > \overline{p}_T$.

One can also define the *safe MSD* (*sMSD*) as one that maximizes $s(d)$ in (5.2), with an additional restriction that the marginal probability of toxicity at this dose must not exceed $\bar{p}_T$ [34, 45]:

$$sMSD = \arg \max_{d \in D:p(d) \leq \bar{p}_T} s(d).$$

The *sMSD* (if it exists) can be thought of as the dose with the most desirable efficacy–toxicity profile, which merits to be moved forward within the clinical development program.

5.2.2   A Bayesian formulation

Concepts similar to the ones in Section 5.2.1 can be developed from a Bayesian perspective [54]. This requires postulation of a parametric model to describe the dose–toxicity–efficacy relationship and a prior distribution for the parameters of interest. Note that due to very limited information on the properties of an investigational product at the trial outset, the chosen model is likely to be misspecified, and it should be viewed only as a *working model* to calibrate study design and facilitate adaptive dose assignments. As such, Bayesian adaptive design in this case should be viewed as a working approach, but not as a formal statistical inference tool. Parsimonious models should be preferred because complex models may be difficult to estimate given small sample sizes in phase I/II trials [9].

Let $\boldsymbol{\theta}$ denote the vector of model parameters. Assume that marginal dose–toxicity and dose–efficacy probability relationships are modeled using some given nonlinear functions $\pi_T(x, \boldsymbol{\theta})$ and $\pi_E(x, \boldsymbol{\theta})$ such that $0 \leq \pi_T(x, \boldsymbol{\theta}) \leq 1$ and $0 \leq \pi_E(x, \boldsymbol{\theta}) \leq 1$ for $x \in [d_1, d_K]$. Here, we use notation x, not d, for the dose (or its logarithmic or some other transformation) to indicate that it is a continuous predictor in a regression model. Furthermore, assume that the joint probabilities are modeled as

$$\pi_{a,b}(x, \boldsymbol{\theta}) = \Pr\left(Y_E = a, Y_T = b | x, \boldsymbol{\theta}\right), \quad a, b \in \{0, 1\} \tag{5.3}$$

for some nonlinear functions $\pi_{a,b} = \pi_{a,b}(x, \boldsymbol{\theta})$, where $0 \leq \pi_{a,b} \leq 1$ and $\sum_{a=0}^{1}\sum_{b=0}^{1} \pi_{a,b} = 1$. The likelihood for a single observation at dose x using model (5.3) is

$$\mathcal{L}(\boldsymbol{\theta}; x, a, b) = \pi_{1,1}^{ab}\pi_{1,0}^{a(1-b)}\pi_{0,1}^{(1-a)b}\pi_{0,0}^{(1-a)(1-b)}.$$

Suppose that we have efficacy–toxicity data from m patients; the jth patient's observation is $(x_j, y_{E,j}, y_{T,j})$, where $x_j \in D$ (dose assignment), $y_{E,j} \in \{0, 1\}$ (efficacy outcome), and $y_{T,j} \in \{0, 1\}$ (toxicity outcome). Given data from m patients, the full likelihood is $\mathcal{L}_m(\boldsymbol{\theta}) = \prod_{j=1}^{m} \mathcal{L}(\boldsymbol{\theta}; x_j, y_{E,j}, y_{T,j})$.

In a Bayesian framework, $\boldsymbol{\theta}$ is assumed to be random. Let $g(\boldsymbol{\theta})$ denote the prior density of $\boldsymbol{\theta}$. Using Bayes' theorem, the posterior of $\boldsymbol{\theta}$ is $g(\boldsymbol{\theta}|data) \propto \mathcal{L}_m(\boldsymbol{\theta})g(\boldsymbol{\theta})$, and for every $d \in D$, one can obtain posterior distributions of the marginal probabilities $\pi_T(d, \boldsymbol{\theta})$ and $\pi_E(d, \boldsymbol{\theta})$.

A dose $d \in D$ is said to be *acceptable* if it satisfies

$$\Pr\left(\pi_T(d, \boldsymbol{\theta}) < \bar{\pi}_T | data\right) > c_T \quad \text{and} \quad \Pr\left(\pi_E(d, \boldsymbol{\theta}) > \underline{\pi}_E | data\right) > c_E, \tag{5.4}$$

where $\bar{\pi}_T$ and $\underline{\pi}_E$ are some clinically acceptable thresholds for toxicity and efficacy probabilities, prespecified by the clinical investigator, respectively, and c_T and c_E are some predefined probability cutoffs that determine stringency of the acceptability criteria. Commonly, c_T and c_E are set in the range of 0.05–0.20; one possibility is $c_T = c_E = 0.10$. To get a better insight into why the latter choice is sensible, it is instructive to think about acceptability criteria in terms of complementary events that render a dose *unacceptable* if either $\Pr\left(\pi_T(d, \boldsymbol{\theta}) > \bar{\pi}_T | data\right) > 1 - c_T = 0.90$ (the dose is likely to be too toxic) or $\Pr\left(\pi_E(d, \boldsymbol{\theta}) < \bar{\pi}_E | data\right) > 1 - c_E = 0.90$ (the dose is likely to be inefficacious).

Let $\mathscr{A}$ denote the set of acceptable doses. Provided that $\mathscr{A} \neq \emptyset$, the *most desirable dose* is one that maximizes posterior mean probability of success:

$$d^* = \arg \max_{d \in D \cap \mathscr{A}} E_{\boldsymbol{\theta}}\{\pi_{1,0}(d, \boldsymbol{\theta})|data\}.$$

The described Bayesian framework forms the basis for many phase I/II adaptive designs, which will be discussed in Sections 5.3 and 5.4.

5.2.3 Phase I/II trial objectives

Broadly speaking, the objectives of a phase I/II trial can be classified into three types: statistical, clinical, and operational. More specifically,

Statistical Objectives:

- To identify the $sMSD$ when it exists or terminate the trial early if no dose satisfies safety and efficacy requirements.
- To estimate $p(d)$, $q(d)$, and $s(d)$ at $sMSD$.
- To estimate $sMSD$ and possibly other parameters from the dose–response curve at the end of the study.

Clinical Objectives:

- To cluster dose assignments at and around $sMSD$.
- To ensure that the majority of trial patients are treated at doses in TW.

Operational Objective:

- To achieve the primary trial objective(s) with the smallest sample size in a timely manner.

Note that even seemingly similar statistical objectives (e.g., identification or estimation of $sMSD$) can require different design considerations. It goes without saying that clinical objectives should be prime in any cancer trial due to ethical obligations to research participants.

5.2.4 Adaptive designs

At the time when a trial is designed, knowledge about the dose–toxicity–efficacy relationship is scant, so adaptive designs are a scientifically sound approach. Due to ethical obligations to study participants, most of the phase I/II oncology trials are cast as dose-escalation designs, which start at low dose levels and escalate to higher doses, provided that previously tested doses are acceptably safe. A phase I/II clinical trial protocol should specify the trial objectives, the dose space D, the starting dose, the criteria for assessment of efficacy and toxicity outcomes, the rules for dose escalation/de-escalation, the working model for dose–response (which should capture the general shape of the true relationships in the range of doses to be investigated), the maximum sample size for the study, the stopping rules (e.g., for excess toxicity), and the statistical methodology for estimating various quantities of interest throughout the trial and at the end of the study.

Eligible patients are enrolled in the trial in cohorts of size M. If $M = 1$, we have *sequential* enrollment. For the mth cohort of patients, the triple $(x_m, \boldsymbol{Y}_{E,m}, \boldsymbol{Y}_{T,m})$ contains the dose assignment ($x_m \in D$), the efficacy outcomes from individual patients in the mth cohort $\boldsymbol{Y}_{E,m} = (y_{E,m1}, \dots, y_{E,mM})$ ($y_{E,mk} \in \{0,1\}$, $k = 1, \dots, M$), and the toxicity outcomes

$\boldsymbol{Y}_{T,m} = (y_{T,m1}, \dots, y_{T,mM})$ $(y_{T,mk} \in \{0,1\}, k = 1, \dots, M)$. It is assumed that efficacy and toxicity are both observed within a comparable time frame and can efficiently be utilized in design adaptations. Let $\mathscr{F}_m = \{(x_1, \boldsymbol{Y}_{E,1}, \boldsymbol{Y}_{T,1}), \dots, (x_m, \boldsymbol{Y}_{E,m}, \boldsymbol{Y}_{T,m})\}$ denote cumulative data from cohorts $1, \dots, m$. In general, the dose assignment for the $(m + 1)$th cohort of patients is determined as

$$X_{m+1} = \mathscr{D}(\mathscr{F}_m), \tag{5.5}$$

where $\mathscr{D}$ is some prospectively defined dose-escalation/de-escalation rule. The rule $\mathscr{D}$ in Equation 5.5 is the core element of the trial design. It must be chosen judiciously and calibrated via computer simulations under a variety of standard to worst-case experimental scenarios. The design should achieve selected experimental objectives (cf. Section 5.2.3) with high probability, and it should be robust to deviations from model assumptions.

Adaptive phase I/II designs can be *nonparametric* or *parametric model based*. The non-parametric designs (cf. Section 5.3.1) make no specific parametric assumptions about the shape of dose–response curves. Many of these designs utilize data only from the most recent cohort of patients, in which case the rule (5.5) is $X_{m+1} = \mathscr{D}(\{x_m, \boldsymbol{Y}_{E,m}, \boldsymbol{Y}_{T,m}\})$ ("short-memory" designs). In contrast, parametric model-based adaptive designs (cf. Section 5.3.2) utilize the entire history $\mathscr{F}_m = \{(x_1, \boldsymbol{Y}_{E,1}, \boldsymbol{Y}_{T,1}), \dots, (x_m, \boldsymbol{Y}_{E,m}, \boldsymbol{Y}_{T,m})\}$ to estimate underlying dose–response by borrowing information across different dose levels ("long-memory" designs).

In the next section, we discuss in detail various phase I/II adaptive designs for bivariate binary efficacy–toxicity outcomes.

5.3   Phase I/II Designs with Bivariate Binary Outcomes

5.3.1   Nonparametric designs

Gooley et al.'s [22] paper was perhaps the first that considered phase I/II dose-finding designs with efficacy–toxicity outcomes. Their motivating example was a phase I trial in bone marrow transplantation where the objective was to determine an optimum dose of T cells to enable nonrejection of the donor marrow (efficacy) without graft-versus-host disease (GVHD) (toxicity). The key assumption was that an increase in the dose of T cells would decrease the risk of rejection of the donor marrow, but at the same time, it would increase the risk of GVHD. The desired dose d^* would satisfy $\Pr(\text{rejection}|d^*) \leq 0.05$ and $\Pr(\text{GVHD}|d^*) < 0.15$. Three different algorithms (Designs *A*, *B*, and *C*) were proposed and evaluated via simulation under three experimental scenarios. The design adaptation rules were heuristic, based on the observed numbers of efficacy and toxicity events among the patients at a given dose. The authors found that the originally proposed Design *A* had too stringent dose-modification rules and higher frequency of incorrect dose selection compared to Designs *B* and *C*. The authors emphasized the importance of simulations for evaluating statistical properties of candidate designs.

Several papers developed nonparametric designs for trials where the outcome is suppressed to a dichotomous variable, i.e., $U = 1$ if success (efficacy without toxicity), and $U = 0$ otherwise [13, 26, 25, 40, 41].

In particular, Durham et al. [13] proposed a response–adaptive randomized Pólya urn design to skew treatment allocation to the most successful dose(s). The design makes no assumption of a functional relationship between success probabilities and the dose. In this design, the urn initially contains at least one ball to represent each dose and exactly one control ball to introduce the stopping rule for the experiment. The treatment assignment for a new patient is determined as follows. A ball is drawn from the urn at random with replacement. The patient is allocated to the corresponding dose, and if the treatment outcome is a "success," then a ball representing the same dose is added to the urn; if the outcome is a "failure," no new ball is added. If a control ball is drawn, then one new control ball is added. This algorithm is repeated sequentially for new patients until a control ball is drawn ν times ($\nu \geq 1$ is prespecified). The theoretical operating characteristics of this design (including the expected numbers of assignments per dose and the expected total sample size) are available in Ref. [13].

Kpamegan and Flournoy [40, 41] proposed an *optimizing up-and-down design*, assuming that $\Pr(U = 1|d)$ is unimodal. The design makes dose assignments to pairs of subjects at adjacent doses depending on the outcome of the previous pair of subjects. It induces a nonhomogeneous random walk on the lattice of doses and converges to a unimodal stationary distribution with a mode very close to the optimum dose.

Another notable nonparametric design that can be used in a unimodal response setting is the *stochastic approximation* method, which is aimed at finding the local maximum of a regression function [38].

Hardwick and Stout [26] compared via simulation four designs, including the Pólya urn design [13], the optimizing up-and-down design [40], the stochastic approximation method [38], and a *univariate bandit* design (Hardwick and Stout's [26] proposal). The latter design updates the unimodal dose–response curve using posterior beta distributions for response rates at individual doses and allocates a new patient according to the values of the Gittins index for each dose and the outcome of the current patient. The four designs were compared with respect to the percentage of correct dose recommendations (decision efficiency) and the expected number of successes in the trial (sampling efficiency) under four different dose–response scenarios and with sample sizes in the range of 25–200. The authors found that the bandit design performed best, the up-and-down design [40] was generally coming in second, and the Pólya urn design [13] and the stochastic approximation method [38] were generally less efficient than the other designs. The loss of efficiency of the Pólya urn in small samples can be explained by extra variability in allocation induced by response–adaptive randomization [30].

For a three-category outcome model (5.1), Ivanova [34] proposed a simple intuitive dose allocation rule: based on z_j, the outcome of the jth subject at dose d_k, the $(j+1)$th subject is assigned to dose d_{k+1}, if $z_j = 0$ (no efficacy and no toxicity); to dose d_k, if $z_j = 1$ (efficacy without toxicity); or to dose d_{k-1}, if $z_j = 2$ (toxicity). Appropriate modifications are made at d_1 and d_K. This design induces a Markov chain on the lattice of doses and has a stationary distribution that can easily be computed for a given set of toxicity–efficacy probabilities. Simulations in Ref. [34] showed that the proposed design is competitive in terms of decision and sampling efficiency to designs of O'Quigley et al. [45] and Kpamegan and Flournoy [40]. However, Dragalin and Fedorov [11] and Pronzato [50] found that Ivanova's [34] design has lower estimation efficiency than model-based penalized adaptive optimal designs.

By combining nonparametric rules with modeling, one can create more flexible designs with enhanced statistical properties. For instance, Hardwick et al. [25] proposed a *directed walk algorithm* (DWA) for trials with independent efficacy and toxicity outcomes and unimodal dose–success probability curve $s(d) = \tilde{q}(d)(1 - p(d))$. The DWA involves sequential estimation of $p(d)$, $\tilde{q}(d)$, and $s(d)$ based on cumulative outcome data in the trial (i.e., non-Markovian design). Seven different estimation methods, both parametric and nonparametric, were considered in Ref. [25]. At each step, the DWA moved at most one dose in the direction of the updated optimum. The authors found through simulations that the DWA with either parametric or smoothed shape-constrained method for estimating probability curves performed best in terms of decision and sampling efficiency, whereas the up-and-down design [40] performed less well than the other designs.

In another recent paper, Zang et al. [71] proposed three different designs for trials of molecularly targeted agents where a dose–efficacy curve can possibly be unimodal or reach a plateau at some dose below the MTD. The first design assumed a logistic dose–efficacy probability with linear and quadratic dose effects. The second design was nonparametric, using a double-sided isotonic regression for the dose–efficacy curve. The third design was semiparametric, using logistic model only locally around the current dose. Toxicity was monitored during the trial using a beta-binomial model. Within the set of admissible safe doses, the algorithm could move one level up, one level down, or stay at a current dose according to posterior estimates from dose–efficacy relationships. The three designs were compared through simulation with a traditional $3 + 3$ design, followed by a randomized two-arm selection design [28] and the *slope-sign* design [31]. The slope-sign design aims to identify a biologically adequate dose [either a dose that yields a specific (high) response rate or a dose in the plateau], while using few patients. The design escalation rule is based on the estimated slope of the dose–efficacy curve using data from a certain number of adjacent dose levels. If the estimated slope is > 0, the dose level is escalated; otherwise, the trial is terminated, and the dose with the highest response rate is recommended as biologically adequate. The authors of Ref. [71] reported that the nonparametric design and the semiparametric design significantly outperformed the slope-sign design and the traditional design both in terms of percentage of optimal dose recommendation and the percentage of efficacy, toxicity, and promising dose allocations. The parametric logistic design had reasonably good performance in some but not all scenarios.

5.3.2   Parametric model-based designs

Model-based designs have been proposed as alternatives to nonparametric designs. These designs utilize some (parsimonious) parametric working model for dose–efficacy–toxicity relationship and perform dose assignments adaptively, according to updated knowledge of the dose–response curve.

One can distinguish three classes of model-based adaptive designs (although there may be some overlap between the classes). The first class is "best intention" (BI) designs [17, 19]. A BI design allocates each new patient a cohort of patients to the dose currently viewed as the best, (for instance, the seemingly most efficacious). Two types of BI designs for phase I/II trials will be discussed momentarily: extensions of the continual reassessment method (CRM) [46] (Section 5.3.2.1), and designs based on efficacy–toxicity trade-off (Section 5.3.2.2).

The second class is Bayesian decision-theoretic designs [63, 64]. These designs make dose assignments to maximize the posterior expected utility function which is chosen for the given study objectives (Section 5.3.2.3).

The third class is penalized optimal adaptive designs [11]. These designs have been proposed to provide a scientifically sound trade-off between estimation and treatment goals in the study (Section 5.3.2.4).

5.3.2.1   Extensions of the CRM

O'Quigley et al. [45] proposed an extension of the CRM [46] in a setting of a phase I/II clinical trial of new antiretroviral treatments for HIV-infected children. The objective was to identify a dose level (among four doses) which is both safe and biologically active, or, if no dose appears to be promising, to stop the trial early and conclude that treatment is inefficacious. The marginal toxicity probability $\pi_T(x, \beta_1)$ and the conditional probability of viral reduction given no toxicity $\pi_{E|\overline{T}}(x, \beta_2)$ were one-parameter models, and the probability of success was defined as $S(x) = \pi_{E|\overline{T}}(x, \beta_2)(1 - \pi_T(x, \beta_1))$. The dose-finding algorithm had two components. Initially, a likelihood-based CRM was used to target a dose with some acceptable toxicity rate ($\widetilde{\pi}_T = 0.10$ in the paper). As experimental data accrued, a sequential probability ratio test was applied to test $H_0 : S(d_k) = s_0$ versus $H_1 : S(d_k) = s_1$ for some prespecified $s_0 < s_1$. A conclusion in favor of H_0 would lead to removal of d_k and all other lower levels from the study and increase in the target toxicity rate (to at most $\widetilde{\pi}_T = 0.3$ in the paper). A conclusion in favor of H_1 would lead to completion of the trial with the recommendation of the current dose. An indeterminate decision would lead to further experimentation at a dose level guided by the toxicity criterion. Simulations under four experimental scenarios with different target doses showed promising performance of the proposed design in terms of the percentage of correct dose recommendation, the expected number of patients treated at the optimum dose, and overall sample size distribution. In Ref. [78], the designs described in Refs [34, 45] were compared against the nonparametric optimum benchmark that provides the upper bound on decision efficiency (rate of correct *sMSD* identification). Both of these designs were found to be very close to the optimum, and it was concluded that "...any rewards for trying to construct alternative designs with yet better performance are most likely going to be small."

Subsequently, Zohar and O'Quigley [77] explored applications of the method described in Ref. [45] in a cancer trial setting. Four competing designs were studied [46]. The first one was the original proposal, also called "dose escalation guided by a compromise structure" (CS). The second one was a "design guided by undepraparameterized models" (UM). This design uses a simple up-and-down allocation rule until the first instance of toxicity and efficacy, at which point $\pi_T(x, \beta_1)$ and $\pi_{E|\overline{T}}(x, \beta_2)$ can be estimated. Given estimates $(\widehat{\beta}_{1j}, \widehat{\beta}_{2j})$ after j patients, the $(j + 1)$th patient's dose is chosen to maximize the probability of success:

$$X_{j+1} = \arg\max_{d \in D} \left\{ \pi_{E|\overline{T}}(d, \widehat{\beta}_{2j}) \left(1 - \pi_T(d, \widehat{\beta}_{1j})\right) \right\}.$$

In addition, two modifications of the CS and UM designs (*mUM* and *mCS*) were explored. These designs had extra constraints relevant to oncology trials, such as control for excess toxicity. The authors reported a simulation study under 6 different dose–efficacy–toxicity scenarios with the sample size (n) of 50. They found that CS had a higher percentage of correct dose selection than UM in five of the six scenarios (most likely due to that UM had lower sample size than CS at stopping). The authors also reported that mCS and mUM designs had more robust performance than CS and UM.

Braun [6] proposed a *bivariate CRM* (bCRM) in the context of a trial of allogenic cell transplantation for high-risk leukemia patients. The marginal probabilities $\pi_T(x, \beta_1)$ and $\pi_E(x, \beta_2)$ were one-parameter logistic models with fixed intercepts, which were combined into a joint model with correlation ρ between efficacy and toxicity. Noninformative priors were assumed for the components of $\theta = (\beta_1, \beta_2, \rho)$. The optimal dose was defined as one which, in the efficacy–toxicity probability space, has the closest weighted Euclidean distance to the "desirable" prespecified pair of efficacy and toxicity rates (π_E^*, π_T^*). Based on data from j patients in the trial, compute posterior mean $\widehat{\theta}_j$ and update marginal probabilities at study dose levels as $\pi_T(d_k, \widehat{\theta}_j)$ and $\pi_E(d_k, \widehat{\theta}_j)$, $k = 1, ..., K$. The $(j + 1)$th patient's dose assignment is then chosen as

$$X_{j+1} = \arg\min_{d \in D} \left\{ w(\pi_T(d, \widehat{\theta}_j) - \pi_T^*)^2 + (1 - w)(\pi_E(d, \widehat{\theta}_j) - \pi_E^*)^2 \right\}, \quad (5.6)$$

where $w \in [0, 1]$ is user defined ($w = 0.5$ is one practical choice). Early stopping rules for excess toxicity and/or or lack of efficacy were added as well. Simulations in Ref. [6] showed that the bCRM was more likely to correctly identify the optimum dose when the dose–response curves were steeper around that dose. The starting dose had an impact on the design performance. The bCRM was also compared to nonparametric Designs B and C of Gooley et al. [22] (see Table 1 of Ref. [22] for the description of these algorithms) for an allogenic bone marrow transplantation trial with 18 dose levels, under three hypothetical scenarios: (1) 5 of the 18 doses are acceptable, (2) Two of the 18 doses are acceptable, and (3) no doses are acceptable. It was found via simulation that Design C outperformed bCRM in the first two scenarios; yet, bCRM was more likely to correctly stop the trial early in the third scenario when the target dose did not exist. While the 18 dose levels are not typical in a phase I study, it is important to highlight that a specific design for a specific study (Design C in this case) can have better operating characteristics under certain experimental conditions than the other designs (e.g., bCRM).

Asakawa et al. [2] combined the bCRM [6] with the Bayesian model averaging (BMA) method [67] in a new design *BMA-bCRM*. This method uses multiple prespecified working models (skeletons) for $\pi_T(x, \beta_1)$ and $\pi_E(x, \beta_2)$, to mitigate the risk of model misspecification. At each dose, BMA estimation is performed, with a weight for each working model adjusted adaptively according to the quality of fit to the observed data. Bayesian criteria are introduced to focus the search on the doses that satisfy minimum efficacy and maximum toxicity constraints, and the trial is terminated if the set of acceptable doses is empty. The dose assignment for the next cohort is made as in Equation 5.6. BMA-bCRM was assessed via simulation in a trial with five doses, eight dose–response scenarios, and four sets of working models (in four of the eight scenarios, one of the working models coincided with the true dose–response curve), with the maximum sample size (n) of 45. BMA-bCRM had the second best performance among the five examined designs. Not surprisingly, the best design in each scenario was one whose skeleton was correctly specified.

Zhang et al. [72] proposed a modification of the CRM for the trinary-outcome case (5.1) (*TriCRM*). Their approach is conceptually similar to the methods of Thall and Russell [59] (cf. Section 5.3.2.2) and O'Quigley et al. [45], but it uses a more flexible continuation-ratio model (5.9) and some special utility functions. For the dose-finding algorithm, a Bayesian CRM-type design was used. Independent uniform prior distributions were assumed for the components of $\boldsymbol{\theta}$. The design specified two decision functions: $\delta_1(x; \boldsymbol{\theta}) = 1_{\{\pi_T(x, \boldsymbol{\theta}) < \overline{\pi}_T\}}$ and $\delta_2(x; \boldsymbol{\theta}) = \pi_{E \cap \overline{T}}(x, \boldsymbol{\theta}) - \lambda \pi_T(x, \boldsymbol{\theta})$, where $1_{\{\cdot\}}$ is an indicator function and $\lambda \in [0, 1]$ is a user-specified constant ($\lambda = 0$ and $\lambda = 1$ were explored in the paper). The doses that satisfy the toxicity constraint $\delta_1(x; \boldsymbol{\theta}) = 1$ are said to be acceptable. The *biologically optimal dose* (BOD) is defined as the one that maximizes $\delta_2(d; \boldsymbol{\theta})$ subject to $\delta_1(d; \boldsymbol{\theta}) = 1$. The experiment starts with the lowest dose, and no dose can be skipped when escalating. After m cohorts, a posterior estimate $\widehat{\boldsymbol{\theta}}_m$ of $\boldsymbol{\theta}$ is obtained, and the decision criteria $\delta_1(d; \widehat{\boldsymbol{\theta}}_m)$ and $\delta_2(d; \widehat{\boldsymbol{\theta}}_m)$ are evaluated for each $d \in D$. Suppose $\delta_1(d; \widehat{\boldsymbol{\theta}}_m) = 0$ for all $d \in D$. Then, if $X_m = d_1$, the trial is stopped and no dose is recommended; if $X_m > d_1$, set $X_{m+1} = d_1$. If $\delta_1(d; \widehat{\boldsymbol{\theta}}_m) = 1$ for some $d \in D$, then select

$$X_{m+1} = \arg \max_{d \in D: \delta_1(d; \widehat{\boldsymbol{\theta}}_m) = 1} \{\delta_2(d; \widehat{\boldsymbol{\theta}}_m)\}. \tag{5.7}$$

In other words, the new cohort is treated at the dose that satisfies the toxicity constraint and maximizes utility $\delta_2(d; \boldsymbol{\theta})$, given data accrued so far. The TriCRM was studied via simulation under nine different dose–success probability curves (including monotone increasing, decreasing, and unimodal), when data followed a continuation-ratio model, a proportional odds model, and model-free pattern. It was found to have favorable operating characteristics including high percentages of correct dose selection (when BOD existed) or early stopping when no dose was acceptable.

In some settings, such as oncohematology trials, efficacy without toxicity is viewed as too stringent an outcome. Instead, investigators are interested in maximizing efficacy acknowledging that some acceptable level of toxicity is mandatory. Seegers et al. [51] proposed a

CRM-type phase I/II design [*marginal approach* (MA)] that attempts to find a dose with the highest marginal probability of efficacy response, subject to a constraint on the marginal probability of toxicity. Assume that the marginal probabilities $\pi_T(x, \beta_1)$ and $\pi_E(x, \beta_2)$ are monotone one parameter power models, which are combined into a bivariate Gumbel model to account for correlation between the outcomes. Given $\widehat{\beta}_{1j}$ and $\widehat{\beta}_{2j}$ after j patients, the $(j+1)$th patient is assigned to the dose $d_\ell = \arg\max_{d \in D}\{\pi_E(d, \widehat{\beta}_{2j})\}$, which must also satisfy $\pi_T(d_\ell, \widehat{\beta}_{1j}) \leq \tau$ for some prespecified toxicity threshold $\tau \in (0,1)$. Simulation studies compared four competing designs: (1) *MA* with maximum likelihood estimation, *MA(F)* in Ref. [51]; (2) *MA* with Bayesian estimation, *MF(B)*; (3) design guided by undepraprameterized models, *UM* [77]; and (4) EffTox method [55]. No stopping rules were used for the first three designs. Six dose–efficacy–toxicity scenarios and two choices of correlation between efficacy and toxicity were investigated. In four of the six scenarios, all methods successfully found their own target dose (however, there were some differences in the percentage of correct selection), and in one scenario, all methods failed to identify their target dose. In terms of quality of estimation of toxicity and efficacy probabilities, the *MA(B)* and *MA(F)* designs performed better than the *UM* design.

An important question is the choice of a copula working model to account for correlation between efficacy and toxicity. In a recent study, Cunanan and Koopmeiners [9] found that there is a lack of benefit when trying to use a correctly specified copula model in the design, and a simple model that assumes independence between the outcomes performs quite stably even in the presence of strong correlation. This may be due to the fact that correlation is difficult to estimate given small sample sizes in phase I/II trials. This observation is also in line with the other recent findings of Iasonos et al. [33] that increasing the number of parameters is counterproductive in terms of operating characteristics.

5.3.2.2 Designs based on efficacy–toxicity tradeoff

Thall and Russell [59] proposed a Bayesian dose-finding procedure (*TR design*) for the trinary-outcome case (5.1). They used a proportional odds model for the probabilities $\gamma_j(x) = \Pr(Z \geq j|x)$, $j = 0, 1, 2$ as follows:

$$\text{logit}\{\gamma_1(x)\} = \mu + \alpha + \beta x \quad \text{and} \quad \text{logit}\{\gamma_2(x)\} = \mu + \beta x, \tag{5.8}$$

where $\text{logit}(p) = \log\{p/(1-p)\}$. For model (5.8), one has $\alpha > 0$, $\beta > 0$, $\boldsymbol{\theta} = (\mu, \alpha, \beta)$, $\pi_T(x, \boldsymbol{\theta}) = (1 + e^{-(\mu+\beta x)})^{-1}$, and $\pi_{E \cap \overline{T}}(x, \boldsymbol{\theta}) + \pi_T(x, \boldsymbol{\theta}) = (1 + e^{-(\mu+\alpha+\beta x)})^{-1}$. Clearly, $\pi_T(x, \boldsymbol{\theta})$ is monotone increasing in dose, whereas $\pi_{E \cap \overline{T}}(x, \boldsymbol{\theta})$ can be nonmonotone. Uniform prior distributions are assumed for the components of $\boldsymbol{\theta}$. The Bayesian criteria as in Equation 5.4 are introduced to define acceptable doses. The TR algorithm prescribes treating patients in cohorts of size $c = 1, 2$, or 3, up to a maximum of n patients. Skipping dose levels when escalating or de-escalating is not allowed unless all intermediate doses have been sampled previously. After m cohorts, the algorithm evaluates conditions (5.4) to determine a set of acceptable doses $\mathscr{A}$, and the next cohort is assigned to the dose $d_\ell \in D \cap \mathscr{A}$, which has the maximum value of the efficacy criterion $\pi_{E \cap \overline{T}}(d, \widehat{\boldsymbol{\theta}}_m)$. If $\mathscr{A} = \emptyset$, the trial is terminated.

In Ref. [59], the TR design was evaluated via simulation for two clinical trial examples: a bone marrow transplantation trial to stimulate moderate GVHD without severe toxicity and a trial of biologic agent IL-12 in malignant melanoma. The results varied across scenarios, but overall they were quite promising. Subsequently, Thall et al. [56] compared the TR design with the 3 + 3 design and a CRM [46], which were based on toxicity only. The TR was reported to have more stable performance in terms of correct decision probabilities and the average number of patients treated at safe and efficacious doses. However, one may argue that a comparison of TR design with the 3 + 3 and CRM designs is not quite relevant because TR uses both efficacy and toxicity, whereas the two other designs are based only on toxicity.

Thall and Cook [55] proposed the efficacy–toxicity tradeoff method (*EffTox*) by improving the TR design [59] in a number of ways. First, for trinary outcomes (Equation 5.1), they proposed a more flexible, four-parameter continuation-ratio model:

$$\log \frac{\pi_{E \cap \overline{T}}(x, \boldsymbol{\theta})}{\pi_{\overline{E} \cap \overline{T}}(x, \boldsymbol{\theta})} = \mu + \alpha + \beta_2 x \quad \text{and} \quad \log \frac{\pi_T(x, \boldsymbol{\theta})}{1 - \pi_T(x, \boldsymbol{\theta})} = \mu + \beta_1 x, \tag{5.9}$$

where $\alpha \geq 0$ and $\beta_1 > 0$, $\beta_2 > 0$. For model (5.9), the dose for which $\pi_{E \cap \overline{T}}(x, \boldsymbol{\theta})$ is maximized exists and is unique [15, 14].

Second, EffTox can be applied with four-category bivariate binary outcomes. The authors considered a bivariate Gumbel model. The marginal probabilities of efficacy and toxicity are modeled using the logistic distribution function $F(x) = (1 + e^{-x})^{-1}$; that is, $\pi_E = \pi_E(x, \boldsymbol{\theta}) = F(\mu_E + \beta_E x + \gamma_E x^2)$ and $\pi_T = \pi_T(x, \boldsymbol{\theta}) = F(\mu_T + \beta_T x)$, where $\beta_T > 0$ to ensure toxicity is monotone increasing. Let ρ be a parameter to characterize the correlation between efficacy and toxicity ($|\rho| < 1$). The joint probabilities are

$$\begin{aligned} \pi_{a,b}(x, \boldsymbol{\theta}) &= \{\pi_E\}^a \{\pi_T\}^b \{1 - \pi_E\}^{1-a} \{1 - \pi_T\}^{1-b} \\ &\quad + (-1)^{a+b} \pi_E \pi_T \{1 - \pi_E\} \{1 - \pi_T\} \{e^\rho - 1\} / \{e^\rho + 1\}. \end{aligned} \tag{5.10}$$

The described model (5.10) is a six-parameter model with $\boldsymbol{\theta} = (\mu_E, \beta_E, \gamma_E, \mu_T, \beta_T, \rho)$. Independent normal priors are assumed for the components of $\boldsymbol{\theta}$ (although *a posteriori* these parameters are not independent).

Third, the EffTox design uses an investigator-elicited efficacy–toxicity contour to quantify desirability of the dose levels and facilitate dose assignments. The design starts with the dose specified by the physician. For each subsequent cohort, no untried dose may be skipped either when escalating or de-escalating. At any step, a set of acceptable doses that satisfy the constraints of Equation 5.4 is determined. If this set is empty, then the trial is terminated early and no dose is selected; otherwise, the patients in the given cohort are treated at the dose $d_\ell = \arg\max_{d \in D} \{\delta(d, \mathscr{F})\}$, where $\delta(d, \mathscr{F})$ is the desirability of dose d given data $\mathscr{F}$. At the end of the trial (if it has not stopped early and there is at least one acceptable dose), the dose with maximum desirability is selected as the winner.

The EffTox method was evaluated in Ref. [55] via simulation in a trial for rapid treatment of acute ischemic stroke (trinary-outcome case) and in a trial for treatment of GVHD (four-category outcome case). For each trial, six different experimental scenarios were considered. The design-operating characteristics included correct dose selection probability, probability of early stopping when no dose was acceptable, and the average number of patients treated at the desirable doses. In the trinary-outcome case, the EffTox with a continuation-ratio model had overall a more robust performance than the EffTox with a proportional odds model and the TR design. In the four-category outcome case, the EffTox was reported to have a good performance across all considered scenarios. The authors concluded that EffTox provides a substantial improvement over the TR method [59], and despite the fact that its methodology is complex and requires significant collaboration between a statistician and a clinician, such extra effort is justified.

It should be also noted that the performance of EffTox method is sensitive to specification of target contours and the informativeness of the prior [69]. As such, careful calibration of EffTox for a specific trial is essential.

Yin et al. [66] proposed a Bayesian dose-finding design for trials where the joint probabilities of efficacy and toxicity are modeled nonparametrically, while incorporating the requirement of monotone increasing dose–toxicity curve. A multivariate normal prior distribution is assumed for the logits of marginal probabilities of efficacy and toxicity among different dose levels. The Bayesian criteria, similar to the ones in Equation 5.4, are used to define acceptable doses. The efficacy–toxicity odds ratio equivalence contour is constructed to quantify desirability of the doses. The design assigns the next cohort of patients to the acceptable dose with the highest desirability provided that the set of acceptable doses is nonempty. Appropriate stopping rules are introduced as well. Simulations in Ref. [66] explored operating characteristics of three versions of the new design and the EffTox design [55] in an exemplary trial with 5 dose levels and 13 different dose–efficacy–toxicity scenarios, and in the context of a real trial in breast cancer. The maximum sample size was 60, and the patients were accrued in cohorts of size 3. The new design exhibited quite satisfactory and robust performance. No design was uniformly best in terms of correct dose selection. One advantage of the design [66] is its nonparametric nature. However, in terms of operating characteristics and computational complexity, the design [66] is reasonably similar to the EffTox [55].

5.3.2.3 Bayesian decision-theoretic designs

A Bayesian decision-theoretic framework for phase I dose-finding designs was developed by Whitehead and Brunier [61] and Whitehead and Williamson [62] in the context of toxicity outcomes. Whitehead et al. [63, 64] generalized these ideas to bivariate binary efficacy–toxicity outcomes. The framework is very general as it can encompass many model-based methods under one paradigm. For instance, BI designs can be cast as decision-theoretic designs by specifying a utility function that reflects individual treatment goal.

A Bayesian decision-theoretic approach requires specification of a dose–outcome model, a prior distribution for the parameters, a set of possible decisions (dose-level assignments), and a utility function $U(d, \boldsymbol{\theta})$ that measures the gain from assigning dose d when parameter $\boldsymbol{\theta}$ is valid. Let $\mathscr{F}_m$ denote data from m patients in the trial. A *Bayes action* is to choose a dose for the $(m+1)$th patient that maximizes the posterior expected utility:

$$X_{m+1} = \arg\max_{d \in D} \mathrm{E}_{\boldsymbol{\theta}}\{U(d, \boldsymbol{\theta})|\mathscr{F}_m\}.$$

If the model, prior, and utility are all chosen judiciously, the resulting clinical trial design should be both scientifically sound and ethical. However, a key challenge is specification of the utility function.

Whitehead et al. [63, 64] considered the trinary-outcome case (5.1), for which $\pi_{E \cap \overline{T}}(x, \boldsymbol{\theta})$ and $\pi_T(x, \boldsymbol{\theta})$ are modeled using two-parameter logistic regressions. The study goal is to determine the TW $[d_L, d_U]$, where $d_L = d_L(\boldsymbol{\theta}) = MED$ and $d_U = d_U(\boldsymbol{\theta}) = MTD$. The following utility function is proposed:

$$U(d, \boldsymbol{\theta}) = \{w\mathrm{Var}(\widehat{d}_L|\mathscr{F}_m) + (1-w)\mathrm{Var}(\widehat{d}_U|\mathscr{F}_m)\}^{-1}, \tag{5.11}$$

where $\mathrm{Var}(\widehat{d}_L|\mathscr{F}_m)$ and $\mathrm{Var}(\widehat{d}_U|\mathscr{F}_m)$ are variances of the estimates of d_L and d_U, respectively, assuming that m patients have been treated at doses $x_1, \ldots, x_m$ and the $(m+1)$th patient is treated at dose d. These variances can be calculated using delta method. The weight $w \in [0, 1]$ represents the relative importance of estimation of d_L and d_U. For instance, if $w = 0$, the objective is to estimate the MTD only. The choice of $w = 0.5$ corresponds to equal interest in estimation of d_L and d_U. The dose assignment for the $(m+1)$th patient is made to maximize the posterior expected utility in Equation 5.11, or alternatively a more convenient measure with a plug-in estimate $X_{m+1} = \arg\max_{d \in D}\{U(d, \widehat{\boldsymbol{\theta}}_m)\}$, where $\widehat{\boldsymbol{\theta}}_m$ is either a mean or mode of the posterior distribution of $\boldsymbol{\theta}$. The design also imposes a safety constraint that prevents administration of any dose with an estimated probability of toxicity greater than some clinically meaningful threshold, and a stopping rule for situations when all doses are excessively toxic and/or terminating the study once d_L and d_U have been estimated with a reasonable level of accuracy.

One can argue that utility for parameter estimation (i.e., optimality in estimation), as a goal, would violate basic ethical constraints because an experimenter would put patients at high and low levels deliberately to gain information. In cancer trials, ethical issues are at stake and "patient gain" is the only useable utility. Whitehead et al. [64] suggested using $U(d, \boldsymbol{\theta}) = \pi_{E \cap \overline{T}}(d, \boldsymbol{\theta})(1 - \pi_T(d, \boldsymbol{\theta}))$ to prioritize patient benefit over the estimation objective.

In Ref. [63], the design with utility (Equation 5.11) was assessed through simulation in a context of a trial in inflammatory lung disease with two choices of prior (a pessimistic prior that assumes there was no TW, and a more optimistic prior), two stopping policies (for safety only and for safety and estimation accuracy), and two choices of the weight ($w = 0$ and 0.5). Four different scenarios for the TW (narrow, wide, safe, and unsafe) and two different sets of dose levels (five and nine doses) were explored. Two versions of the proposed design (both based on the pessimistic prior) came out best in terms of the average number of toxicities and successful outcomes and accuracy of estimation. The design performance was sensitive to the choice of prior. Overall, based on the considered scenarios, the authors recommended using a pessimistic prior, including a larger number of doses (nine is better than five), and assessing competing designs through simulation under different plausible experimental settings. They also emphasized that the proposed dose recommendation rules should aid in decision making but not replace real clinical judgment.

Loke et al. [44] proposed a *Bayesian utility design* (*BUD*) that assigns a utility value to each possible combination of decisions (de-escalate the dose, stay at the current dose, or escalate to the next higher level) and observed the efficacy–toxicity outcome (four combinations of bivariate binary-outcome values were assumed to be possible). At each step, the optimal action was taken to maximize the expected utility under the posterior distribution of efficacy–toxicity probabilities that are modeled using conjugate Dirichlet priors at different dose levels. The goal was to locate an optimal safe dose with a prespecified target probability for efficacy without toxicity. When the outcome probability estimate was very close to the target probability, the decision to escalate or de-escalate would share the same utility. A stopping rule was triggered once a firm decision on the optimal safe dose could be made. The proposed design was compared with the method of O'Quigley et al. [45] via simulation under the same experimental scenarios as in Ref. [45]. The two designs had very comparable operating characteristics. A sensitivity analysis suggested that BUD is quite robust to prior distribution assumptions, choice of the utility, and choice of the stopping criterion.

Wang and Day [60] proposed another phase I/II Bayesian decision-theoretic design. Unlike other methods that model probabilities of efficacy and toxicity directly, Wang and Day's method considers a joint model for the continuous thresholds θ_T and θ_E for doses that cause toxicity and efficacy. It is assumed that $(\log \theta_T, \log \theta_E)$ follow *a priori* a bivariate normal distribution, with hyperparameters elicited from the investigator. The authors proposed four different utility functions to quantify the relative merit of efficacy–toxicity outcomes ("simple," "additive," "aggressive," and "cautious" utility functions). The proposed Bayesian design with additive utility function, a fixed sample size (n) of 30, and no early stopping was compared through simulations with the standard MTD design. The Bayesian design was more efficient in identifying the right dose and led on average to more patients in the trial experiencing efficacy without toxicity than the standard MTD design. While these simulations were not comprehensive, they did provide additional evidence that incorporating efficacy data can bring extra value and lead to more efficient designs than dose escalation designs driven by toxicity alone.

5.3.2.4   Penalized optimal adaptive designs

Dragalin and Fedorov [11] proposed optimal and penalized optimal adaptive designs for phase I/II clinical trials with bivariate binary efficacy–toxicity outcomes. Their methodology is based on optimal design theory for convex objective functions with convex constraints [8, 16]. Unlike BI designs that assign a current cohort of patients to a dose that is viewed as most successful given data collected so far, penalized optimal adaptive designs attempt to maximize at each step an incremental increase in information while penalizing doses that are overly toxic and/or have a low probability of success.

It is worth pointing out that there are challenges to implementation of optimal adaptive designs in real clinical oncology dose-finding trials. It may be very difficult to justify optimization of some statistical criterion without risking Institutional Review Board ethical issues related to experimentation with human subjects. In real dose-finding cancer trials, ideas about future patient benefit rather than current patient benefit are outlawed by the World Medical Association (WMA) Declaration of Helsinki [65], and therefore, BI designs have been regarded as the only appropriate option. Despite these challenges, optimal designs do provide useful tools in phase I/II trials. For instance, they provide theoretical measures of statistical estimation precision against which other designs can be compared. Also, these designs can be more readily applied in animal experiments where a frequent goal is to estimate the whole dose–response curve and where ethical issues are at a lower stake compared to experiments on humans.

The development of optimal adaptive designs starts with postulating a statistical model for the dose–response relationship. Dragalin and Fedorov [11] considered two parametric models. One is a five-parameter bivariate Gumbel model, for which the marginal probabilities of efficacy and toxicity are modeled using the logistic distribution function $F(x) = (1 + e^{-x})^{-1}$ (i.e., $\pi_E(x, \boldsymbol{\theta}) = F(\mu_E + \beta_E x)$ and $\pi_T(x, \boldsymbol{\theta}) = F(\mu_T + \beta_T x)$, $\beta_T > 0$), and the correlation ρ between efficacy and toxicity is introduced via the Gumbel copula $G(y, z) = F(y) \cdot F(z) \cdot \{1 + \rho(1 - F(y))(1 - F(z))\}$, $-\infty < y, z < +\infty$, $|\rho| < 1$. The second model is a six-parameter Cox bivariate binary model, for which the marginal probabilities of efficacy and toxicity are, in general, neither logistic nor necessarily monotone in dose; yet, the conditional probability of efficacy given no toxicity is logistic in dose (see Ref. [11] for details).

Let $\boldsymbol{\xi}_n = \{(d_k, \lambda_{k,n}), k = 1, \dots, K\}$ denote the design measure over the dose space D for a trial with n patients, where $\lambda_{k,n} = n_k/n \in [0, 1]$ is the allocation proportion for d_k with an obvious constraint $\sum_{k=1}^{K} \lambda_{k,n} = 1$. The design $\boldsymbol{\xi}_n$ assigns n_1 patients to d_1, n_2 patients to d_2, etc. For mathematical convenience, one can also consider the limiting design measure $\boldsymbol{\xi}$ (without regard to n), characterized by allocation λ_k to d_k with $\sum_{k=1}^{K} \lambda_k = 1$.

A measure of estimation precision of the design $\boldsymbol{\xi}$ is the Fisher information matrix, defined as

$$\mathbf{M}(\boldsymbol{\xi}, \boldsymbol{\theta}) = \sum_{k=1}^{K} \lambda_k \boldsymbol{\mu}(d_k, \boldsymbol{\theta}),$$

where $\boldsymbol{\mu}(d_k, \boldsymbol{\theta}) = -\mathrm{E}\left\{ \frac{\partial^2}{\partial \boldsymbol{\theta} \partial \boldsymbol{\theta}'} \log \mathcal{L}(\boldsymbol{\theta}; d_k, a, b) \right\}$ is the information of a single observation at d_k. Importantly, $\mathbf{M}^{-1}(\boldsymbol{\xi}, \boldsymbol{\theta})$ provides the lower bound on the variance–covariance matrix of an efficient estimator of $\boldsymbol{\theta}$, and by choosing a $\boldsymbol{\xi}$ that minimizes $\mathbf{M}^{-1}(\boldsymbol{\xi}, \boldsymbol{\theta})$ (in some sense), one can have an experiment that delivers most precise estimates of the parameters of interest. Depending on the trial objectives, different design criteria can be optimized [3]. A popular choice is the D-optimal criterion $\log |\mathbf{M}^{-1}(\boldsymbol{\xi}, \boldsymbol{\theta})|$. The *D-optimal design* minimizes the volume of the confidence ellipsoid for $\boldsymbol{\theta}$, and it can be thought of as the design that results in the most accurate estimation of the entire dose–outcome relationship.

On the other hand, investigators may be more interested in accurate estimation of some target dose rather than the entire model. Let $X^* = X^*(\boldsymbol{\theta})$ denote the estimand of interest (say, the dose with the most desirable risk–benefit ratio, according to some predefined criteria). The asymptotic variance of $\widehat{X}^*$, an efficient estimator of X^*, can be obtained using a delta-method: $\mathrm{Var}(\widehat{X}^*(\boldsymbol{\theta})) = \boldsymbol{c}^{\mathrm{T}}(\boldsymbol{\theta})\mathbf{M}^{-1}(\boldsymbol{\xi}, \boldsymbol{\theta})\boldsymbol{c}(\boldsymbol{\theta})$, where $\boldsymbol{c}(\boldsymbol{\theta}) = \partial X^*(\boldsymbol{\theta})/\partial \boldsymbol{\theta}$. The *c-optimal design* is found as $\boldsymbol{\xi}(\boldsymbol{\theta}) = \arg \min_{\boldsymbol{\xi}} \{\text{Var}(\widehat{X}^*(\boldsymbol{\theta}))\}$. Here, we assume that $\mathbf{M}^{-1}(\boldsymbol{\xi}, \boldsymbol{\theta})$ exists. In some circumstances, the design information matrix may be singular, in which case a *regularized* c-optimal design can be constructed [18].

In general, the *D*- and *c*-optimal designs are quite different. The *D*-optimal design may be suboptimal in terms of *c*-optimality and vice versa [15, 14]. Moreover, the *D*-optimal design can result in a high proportion of study subjects assigned to overly toxic and/or inefficacious doses, which is inappropriate from the individual ethical perspective.

In an effort to provide a scientifically sound trade-off between estimation and treatment goals, Dragalin and Fedorov [11] proposed *penalized optimal designs*. They introduced a cost function

$$\phi(x, \boldsymbol{\theta}; C_E, C_T) = \{\pi_{1,0}(x, \boldsymbol{\theta})\}^{-C_E} \{1 - \pi_T(x, \boldsymbol{\theta})\}^{-C_T},$$

where $C_E \geq 0$ and $C_T \geq 0$ are user-defined parameters that control penalties for doses with low success rate and high toxicity rate. The total cost of the design $\boldsymbol{\xi}$ is expressed as $\Phi(\boldsymbol{\xi}, \boldsymbol{\theta}) = \sum_{k=1}^{K} \lambda_k \phi(d_k, \boldsymbol{\theta}; C_E, C_T)$. The penalized *D*-optimal design is found as a solution to the following optimization problem:

$$\boldsymbol{\xi}(\boldsymbol{\theta}) = \arg \min_{\boldsymbol{\xi}} \left\{ \log \frac{|\mathbf{M}^{-1}(\boldsymbol{\xi}, \boldsymbol{\theta})|}{\Phi(\boldsymbol{\xi}, \boldsymbol{\theta})} \right\}, \tag{5.12}$$

which can be solved by application of the Kiefer–Wolfowitz equivalence theorem [37]. The penalized *D*-optimal design provides maximum information per cost unit, and the cost in this case is the penalty for treating patients at doses with low success rate and/or high toxicity rate. If $C_E = C_T = 0$, then the problem is simplified to finding the *D*-optimal design.

All optimal designs discussed here are important theoretical benchmarks. However, they cannot be implemented directly because they depend on the underlying dose–toxicity–efficacy relationship (through $\boldsymbol{\theta}$), which is unknown at the outset. One solution is to estimate $\boldsymbol{\theta}$ and amend the design adaptively as the trial progresses. At initial points in the trial, estimates of $\boldsymbol{\theta}$ can be highly variable; therefore, initial dose allocations should be made using some nonparametric rule, such as Ivanova's design [34], until a sufficient amount of data are available to reliably estimate $\boldsymbol{\theta}$. Simulations may be useful to determine the length of the start-up phase.

Consider a point when m patients have been treated and their outcome data have been observed. Let $\widehat{\boldsymbol{\theta}}_m$ denote the maximum likelihood estimate of $\boldsymbol{\theta}$ and $\boldsymbol{\xi}_m$ denote the design based on allocation of the m subjects. For an adaptive penalized *D*-optimal design, the dose assignment for the $(m + 1)$th subject is chosen according to the first-order algorithm [18] to maximize an incremental increase of information per cost unit as follows:

$$X_{m+1} = \arg \max_{d \in D} \{\Delta(d, \boldsymbol{\xi}_m, \widehat{\boldsymbol{\theta}}_m)\}, \tag{5.13}$$

where $\Delta(d, \boldsymbol{\xi}, \boldsymbol{\theta}) = \phi^{-1}(d, \boldsymbol{\theta}; C_E, C_T) \text{tr}\{\boldsymbol{\mu}(d, \boldsymbol{\theta}) \mathbf{M}^{-1}(\boldsymbol{\xi}, \boldsymbol{\theta})\}$ is the sensitivity function of the penalized *D*-optimal criterion. The algorithm is continued until the maximum sample size is reached or until a stopping rule for excess toxicity is triggered.

Dragalin and Fedorov [11] reported a simulation study to compare the penalized adaptive *D*-optimal design with Ivanova's up-and-down design [34]. The outcomes were simulated from the Cox correlated bivariate binary distribution under four experimental scenarios. The design used a fixed sample size (n) of 36 without stopping rules. In three of the four scenarios, the penalized adaptive optimal design was more efficient, and in one scenario, it had the same efficiency (in terms of information per cost ratio) as Ivanova's procedure [34].

Following Ref. [11], Dragalin et al. [12] proposed two-stage penalized *D*-optimal and penalized *c*-optimal designs. In Stage 1, a locally optimal design based on historical data or some other start-up procedure such as that described in Ref. [34] is implemented. In Stage 2, a locally optimal design using an estimate of $\boldsymbol{\theta}$ obtained from Stage 1 is implemented. In Ref. [12], two-stage penalized D-optimal and c-optimal designs were compared with the equal allocation design through simulation for a trial with $n = 200$ patients (90 patients for Stage 1 and 110 patients for Stage 2). The performance metrics included D-information, D-information per penalty unit, c-information, and c-information per penalty unit. The adaptive penalized optimal designs provided substantial improvements over equal allocation design on all four metrics and provide some improvement over single-stage penalized D-optimal and c-optimal designs. In terms of accuracy of estimation of the target dose, the two-stage penalized c-optimal design was the best, the two-stage penalized D-optimal design came in second, and the equal allocation design was the least efficient. Additional simulations were performed to investigate the merit of fully sequential adaptive designs compared to two-stage adaptive designs—no major difference between the two approaches was found.

Pronzato [50] performed a theoretical study of penalized optimal designs. He found that for suitable penalty functions with judiciously chosen penalty coefficients, an investigator can construct a small-cost design that concentrates dose assignments around the optimal dose when it is unique. The paper reported a simulation study comparing Ivanova's [34] up-and-down design, an adaptive D-optimal design, and penalized adaptive D-optimal designs with different values of penalty coefficients when data were generated from a six-parameter Cox model. It was found that Ivanova's [34] procedure had low cost but also low estimation accuracy of the optimal safe dose, the adaptive D-optimal design had high quality of estimation but at the same time a high cost, and the adaptive penalized D-optimal designs provided a very reasonable compromise between the two strategies—the cost was close to Ivanova's [34] design, while estimation precision was close to the adaptive D-optimal design. Pronzato [48, 49] established some important asymptotic properties of adaptive penalized D-optimal designs. Under widely satisfied conditions, the maximum likelihood estimator of the model parameters is strongly consistent and asymptotically normal, and the adaptive designs converge weakly to the locally optimal designs. In practice, simulations should be used to validate asymptotic behavior of adaptive designs.

It should be noted that adaptive penalized optimal designs [11, 12] are likelihood-based procedures. Gao and Rosenberger [21] proposed Bayesian adaptive penalized optimal designs using a bivariate Gumbel model. The Bayesian penalized D-optimal design minimizes the criterion $\mathrm{E}_{\boldsymbol{\theta}}\{-\log|\mathbf{M}(\boldsymbol{\xi}, \boldsymbol{\theta})| - \log\Phi(\boldsymbol{\xi}, \boldsymbol{\theta}_\pi)\}$, where $\boldsymbol{\theta}_\pi$, the mean of the posterior distribution of $\boldsymbol{\theta}$, is substituted into the penalty function. A Bayesian adaptive penalized D-optimal design is constructed using similar ideas, as in Ref. [24]. The Bayesian penalized procedure was compared with the EffTox method [55] through simulation under two scenarios of the Gumbel response model. The two competing designs appeared to be similar in terms of ethical criteria (expected number of toxicity, efficacy, and efficacy without toxicity); yet, the Bayesian penalized method had larger information per cost in both scenarios, and it was competitive with the EffTox in terms of average efficacy–toxicity tradeoff desirability (cf. Section 5.3.2.2). The merits of the Bayesian penalized method were more pronounced when efficacy increased faster than toxicity.

5.4 More Complex Settings

5.4.1 Binary toxicity and continuous efficacy

In many clinical settings, efficacy is continuous, while toxicity is binary. Joint modeling of a mixed type of outcomes may not be straightforward. Of course, a continuous variable can be dichotomized with respect to some clinically relevant thresholds. However, this may induce loss of information, and it may reduce the quality of a dose-finding algorithm [20].

Bekele and Shen [5] suggested the use of a latent variable to jointly model a continuous biomarker expression (an indicator of the compound's biological activity) and binary toxicity. For the dose-finding algorithm, they used toxicity-constrained dose escalation with response–adaptive randomization such that doses with higher posterior means of the biomarker expression are more likely to be assigned. Simulations in Ref. [5] showed stable performance of the proposed design over a range of experimental scenarios. Hirakawa [27] proposed another joint model for which a continuous efficacy endpoint follows a normal distribution with mean four-parameter logistic model and multiplicative heteroscedastic variance, and binary toxicity is modeled with a two-parameter logistic regression. The dose-escalation algorithm is based on minimizing a weighted Mahalanobis distance of the posterior mean of the outcomes to the "most desirable" point. Simulations comparing Hirakawa's [27] method with Bekele and Shen's [5] method showed that the former had a lower average number of dose assignments to unacceptably toxic or futile doses, and the two methods had comparable statistical characteristics for a range of considered scenarios.

Zhou et al. [75] extended an earlier work on Bayesian decision-theoretic designs with bivariate binary outcomes [63, 64] to the case of binary safety modeled using a two-parameter logistic regression and continuous efficacy modeled using normal linear mixed-effects model. The design assigns a new cohort of patients to a dose with the highest posterior mean of the continuous outcome provided that the adverse event probability at this dose is less than a prespecified clinical threshold. Such a design yields meaningful dose-escalation decisions, as shown in Refs. [75, 76].

Padmanabhan et al. [47] considered penalized adaptive D-optimal designs for bivariate normal efficacy and safety outcomes, with a four-parameter sigmoid $E_{\max}$ model for the mean dose–efficacy curve, a two-parameter exponential for the mean dose–safety curve, and a known correlation between efficacy and safety. When the penalty function was appropriately specified, penalized adaptive designs provided a substantial improvement over equal randomization designs in terms of frequency of correct identification of MED, MTD, and $sMSD$, and in terms of frequency of dose assignments within TW.

5.4.2   Handling late-onset outcomes

The designs discussed so far are based on the assumption that efficacy and toxicity outcomes are observed within a comparable time frame. In practice, there may be a non-negligible time lag between treatment administration and observing the outcome. One solution is to enroll a new cohort of patients only after all data from the previous cohort are available. However, this can substantially prolong the trial, and it is also not a practical solution if patient enrollment is fast. Several approaches for handling late-onset efficacy (and toxicity) outcomes will be discussed in Sections 5.4.2.1–5.4.2.3.

5.4.2.1   Using surrogate efficacy outcomes

In some situations, a quickly available surrogate efficacy outcome can be used to partially compensate for missing true efficacy outcome. Zhong et al. [74] extended the bCRM of Braun [6] to a trivariate model for toxicity, surrogate efficacy, and true efficacy (all binary variables). The trivariate model included fixed-intercept logistic regressions for marginal probabilities and copula models for the joint probabilities. Weakly informative priors were used to facilitate Bayesian modeling. A simulation study was run for a trial with five dose levels, three scenarios for efficacy–toxicity curves, and two types of surrogate efficacy ("good" and "bad"). Four designs were examined: two new designs based on trivariate models with different copulas (*exB*, *exG*), and two designs based on bivariate models (i.e., only surrogate efficacy and toxicity) (*Braun*, *Gumbel*). It was found that under "good" surrogacy, all designs performed better than under "bad" surrogacy, and also the trivariate models had somewhat higher percentage of correct dose selection than the bivariate ones. In a follow-up paper, Zhong et al. [73] explored different monotone semiparametric and nonparametric link functions for modeling marginal dose–efficacy and dose–toxicity probabilities in the trivariate CRM [74]. They found that some semiparametric and nonparametric link functions can robustify the performance of the trivariate method [74] under model misspecification.

In a similar vein to Ref. [74], Asakawa and Hamada [1] extended bCRM to phase I/II trials with short-term surrogate efficacy outcomes that are assumed to be moderately positively correlated with the main efficacy outcomes. A surrogate efficacy outcome is used in the likelihood provisionally, and it is replaced by a confirmed efficacy outcome once the latter becomes available. In the simulation study [1], five designs were compared: the original bCRM using true efficacy outcome (*Standard*), three variants of the new proposal (*Proposed L*, *Proposed QL*, and *Proposed WL*), and the original bCRM using surrogate efficacy outcome (*Surrogate*). A total of 12 experimental scenarios were considered: 4 different dose–toxicity–efficacy probability curves, and variations of the surrogate efficacy probability across the dose range: (1) constant surrogate efficacy probability of 20%; (2) monotone nondecreasing surrogate efficacy probability, lower than the one for the confirmed efficacy; and (3) identical to the one for the confirmed efficacy. The designs were compared for a study with five dose levels and the maximum sample size (n) of 30. The operating characteristics included correct dose selection probability (and probability of no dose recommendation), average number of patients treated at each dose, average probability of patients experiencing efficacy based on the confirmed response, average probability of toxicity, average total sample size, and average study duration. In the four scenarios where surrogate efficacy probability was constant at 20%, the three new designs had sufficiently similar statistical characteristics to the *Standard* approach. In the four scenarios with moderate association between surrogate and confirmed efficacy outcomes, the statistical criteria of three new designs improved, and in the four scenarios when surrogate efficacy and true efficacy probabilities were identical, the results were most promising.

5.4.2.2 Bayesian data augmentation

Jin et al. [36] proposed a very general approach to impute delayed outcomes in phase I/II trials. At the time when a new treatment decision is to be made, any unobserved outcomes are viewed as missing data. A Bayesian data augmentation (DA) algorithm based on predictive distributions from partial follow-up times and complete outcome data is applied, and decision rules are constructed using the augmented dataset. For the dose-escalation algorithm, Jin et al. [36] considered piecewise exponential marginal models for time-to-efficacy and time-to-toxicity (combined in a joint model via the Clayton copula), weakly informative priors for Bayesian modeling, and the EffTox design [55] to direct dose assignments. In Ref. [36], the new algorithm (*Late-Onset EffTox*) was studied along with three other competing designs through simulation over a range of experimental scenarios. The new design outperformed other methods in terms of correct dose selection rate and measures of clinical benefit.

Another interesting application of Bayesian DA can be found in Chen et al. [7] who extended the Escalation with Overdose Control (EWOC) method [4] to a phase I/II setting. The new design (*EWOUC*) attempts to find the dose with best efficacy–toxicity utility index while handling delayed efficacy data via Bayesian DA to support continuous enrollment. EWOUC uses two-parameter logistic regression models for marginal probabilities of toxicity and efficacy and a Gumbel copula model for the joint outcome. The authors of Ref. [7]

compared four designs via simulation: (1) the original *EWOC* [4], (2) EWOUC with DA to handle missing efficacy data (*EWOUC-DA*), (3) EWOUC that requires complete efficacy observations (*EWOUC-Comp*), and (4) EWOUC that discards all incomplete efficacy data at the moment of new dose decision (*EWOUC-NW*). The designs were compared in terms of dose recommendation accuracy, therapeutic effect (DLT rate and utility value), and trial duration. Five experimental scenarios representing "extremely good," "good," "moderate," "bad," and "extremely bad" agents were investigated. Efficacy was assumed to be evaluated after 3 months, and the maximum sample size was 30. The performance of *EWOUC-DA* was in between *EWOUC-Comp* (which represents the ideal case of no missing efficacy data and is the most efficient) and *EWOUC-NW* (the least efficient method).

5.4.2.3   Efficacy as a time-to-event outcome

Several papers proposed adaptive phase I/II designs that handle delayed efficacy (and possibly delayed toxicity) data by modeling them as time-to-event variables [23, 35, 39, 43, 57, 68, 70]. Due to a limited space here, we shall only discuss three of the aforementioned references.

Ji and Bekele [35] considered a leukemia trial with three treatment arms to be compared with respect to 52-week efficacy and toxicity rates. The study objective is to treat more patients at the doses with high efficacy and low toxicity and select the most favorable treatment at the end of the trial. Data from patients who have not yet completed 52 weeks of follow-up are utilized through a model that uses a weight function to link joint probabilities of outcomes at interim times with the same probabilities at the end of a follow-up period. A Bayesian criterion is used to quantify desirability of treatment arms with respect to efficacy–toxicity tradeoff. Response–adaptive randomization is used to increase allocation frequency of treatments with higher week-52 success rate. Simulations under six different experimental scenarios for a leukemia trial showed that the proposed design performs quite stably and has reasonably high probabilities of correct treatment selection and allocation to superior treatment arms. Variability of allocation was quite high, and therefore, it is important to investigate not only the average performance of the design in terms of correct treatment selection but also the whole distribution of treatment allocation numbers.

Lei et al. [43] proposed a phase I/II response–adaptive randomization design for time-to-event efficacy and binary toxicity. The design objective is to randomize more study patients to better treatment arms based on both efficacy and toxicity and select the best treatment arm at the end of the trial. The efficacy and toxicity outcomes are combined into a model with shared random effects and selected prognostic covariates. At the points of decision making, any unobserved efficacy data are naturally censored by the time of analysis. A Bayesian response–adaptive randomization is cast using a novel efficacy–toxicity tradeoff index (a ratio of the quality-adjusted probability of efficacy to the probability of toxicity). Stopping rules for excess toxicity and futility are introduced to possibly terminate unsafe or inefficacious dose arms. Operating characteristics of the proposed design were assessed by simulation under seven different efficacy–toxicity scenarios and some additional scenarios when the model or prior was misspecified. In the considered scenarios, the design assigned, on average, more patients to treatment arms with better riskbenefit ratio while accounting for the patients' prognostic covariates. It also had higher correct selection probabilities compared to efficacy-only driven design and was likely to shorten the trial duration since it required no suspension of accrual of patients.

Guo and Yuan [23] considered a setting where toxicity is binary, efficacy is time-to-event, and subjects who do not experience efficacy are likely to drop out from the study. Their motivating example was a dose-finding trial in acute myeloid leukemia where toxicity is likely to occur during the first 30 days from the start of treatment, while efficacy is evaluated up to 90 days post-treatment. The goal was to adaptively assign patients to desirable doses and select the target dose satisfying both efficacy and toxicity requirements. The authors used a logistic model for the marginal toxicity probability, a bivariate Cox proportional hazards model for efficacy, and dropout times with a shared frailty term to induce correlation to account for informative dropouts. A Bayesian adaptive dose-escalation design was assessed via simulations under 10 experimental scenarios, with the maximum sample size of 51 patients. Patient accrual followed a Poisson process with a rate of three per month. The new design was compared with two variants of the EffTox method [55] that modeled efficacy and toxicity as binary outcomes and used different strategies for handling dropouts. Two choices of dropout rate—30% and 50%—were explored. While the results varied across scenarios, the new method had competitive performance. It was particularly advantageous over the EffTox method in two scenarios common to the biological agents—when efficacy probability curve is unimodal and toxicity curve is fairly flat. The design was also found to be robust to violations of the proportional hazards assumption, misspecification of the baseline hazard, and the presence of dose–toxicity interactions.

5.4.3 Incorporating covariates

In some settings, it is known at the outset that patients may respond to treatment differentially depending on their covariate profiles. In this case, a dose-finding algorithm should account for selected important covariates.

Thall et al. [58] extended the EffTox design [55] to a procedure that aims at finding a dose with the best efficacy–toxicity trade-off for a patient's covariate profile. The marginal probabilities of efficacy and toxicity include the effects of dose, selected covariates, and dose-by-covariate interactions. The joint probabilities are obtained from the marginal ones via a copula model. Informative priors are elicited for covariate effects based on historical data, and noninformative priors are used for dose-related effects. Consider a point when $m-1$ patients have already been treated and the mth patient with covariate profile Z_m is enrolled. Based on available data, determine the set $\mathscr{A}(Z_m)$ of doses that are acceptable for the given covariate profile using constraints similar to those in Equation 5.4 and construct a target contour [55] to quantify desirability of each dose for the covariate Z_m, i.e., $\delta(d_k, Z_m)$, $k = 1, \ldots, K$. If $\mathscr{A}(Z_m) \neq \emptyset$, then the mth patient is treated at the dose with the maximum value of $\delta(d_k, Z_m)$; otherwise, the mth patient does not receive treatment under protocol. The trial may also be stopped early if for any observed covariate profile Z, $\mathscr{A}(Z) = \emptyset$. At the end of the trial, the acceptability and desirability criteria are used to select doses for future patients. Applicability of the design was demonstrated for a trial in AML patients with two prognostic covariates: age (14–41, 43–52, 53–59) and cytogenetic status ("good," "intermediate," "poor"), and five dose levels. The maximum sample size in the study was set at 60. Simulations were reported for four experimental scenarios for toxicity and efficacy probabilities. Three designs were compared: (1) the new method based on a full model with the effects of dose, covariates, and dose–covariate interactions, (2) the new method based on a reduced model (without dose–covariate interactions), and (3) a simplified version of the new method that ignores covariates completely. The design based on the full model outperformed two other designs in terms of percentage of correct covariate-specific dose selection, especially when non-negligible dose–covariate interactions were present. Therefore, the authors concluded that the proposed method could be attractive in phase I/II trials with heterogeneous patient populations.

One should be mindful of the possibility of model and prior misspecification in complex dose–response settings. As was already mentioned, the EffTox design (and its extensions) are sensitive to specification of target contours and the informativeness of the prior [69], which warrants careful calibration of the design for a specific trial.

5.5   Discussion

In this chapter, we have reviewed seamless phase I/II adaptive designs for dose-finding oncology trials where efficacy and toxicity outcomes are considered simultaneously. These designs make dose assignments adaptively, based on outcomes from patients in the trial, with the goal to identify a dose with the most desirable efficacy–toxicity trade-off and to achieve possibly other experimental goals.

Various phase I/II designs, including nonparametric and parametric model-based approaches, have been proposed in the literature over the past two decades. The nonparametric designs make minimum assumptions about underlying dose–response relationships, and they use simple and intuitive dose-escalation/de-escalation rules to cluster dose assignments at and around the target dose, such as the $sMSD$. By contrast, parametric model-based designs utilize statistical models to estimate dose–response and facilitate design adaptations. Frequently, Bayesian methods are applied to update statistical models and direct dose assignments. Model-based approaches are subject to certain assumptions, including the form of the model and the prior. Simulations must be run to evaluate design operating characteristics under a variety of plausible experimental scenarios before the design is implemented in practice.

Within the class of model-based phase I/II adaptive designs, it is particularly important to contrast "BI" designs and penalized optimal adaptive designs. These approaches address study objectives differently. For instance, BI designs attempt to achieve individual ethical goal by assigning a current cohort of patients to a dose that is viewed as the most successful in light of collected data. By contrast, penalized optimal adaptive designs attempt to balance gain in information about dose–response (learning goal) with the individual ethical (treatment goal) via maximization of some statistical criterion while penalizing excessively toxic and inefficacious dose levels. Many clinical investigators would argue that only the individual ethics goal is acceptable in dose-finding cancer trials, and this has to be considered in the design of such experiments.

Overall, it is difficult to recommend any particular design as the "best" for use in practice. Our current review shows that many innovative methods exist in the literature, and the body of knowledge is increasingly growing. The designs based on bivariate binary efficacy–toxicity outcomes have recently been extended to more complex situations of mixed (continuous and binary) outcomes, dose-finding trials with delayed outcomes, and dose-finding trials incorporating important patient covariates.

Some desirable properties of a phase I/II design include, but are not limited to, the following:

- The design reliably achieves selected study objectives (cf. Section 5.2.3) for a range of selected dose–toxicity–efficacy scenarios.

- The design has robust performance, even in situations when main assumptions are violated, e.g., when model and/or prior are misspecified.

- The design has supportive statistical software to perform simulations and validated information technology infrastructure to perform adaptations quickly and efficiently.

In summary, while planning of a seamless phase I/II trial is a long and complex process requiring collaborative efforts from clinical investigator and statistician, such an investment of effort is often justified, as the resulting designs are more efficient and more ethical than separate phase I and phase II trials.

References

1. Asakawa, T., Hamada, C. (2013). A pragmatic dose-finding approach using short-term surrogate efficacy outcomes to evaluate binary efficacy and toxicity outcomes in phase I cancer clinical trials. *Pharmaceutical Statistics* 12(5), 315–327.

2. Asakawa, T., Hirakawa, A., Hamada, C. (2013). Bayesian model averaging continual reassessment method for bivariate binary efficacy and toxicity outcomes in phase I oncology trials. *Journal of Biopharmaceutical Statistics* 24(2), 310–325.

3. Atkinson, A. C., Donev, A. N., Tobias, R. (2007). *Optimum Experimental Designs, with SAS*. Oxford University Press, Oxford, UK.

4. Babb, J., Rogatko, A., Zacks, S. (1998). Cancer phase I clinical trials: Efficient dose escalation with overdose control. *Statistics in Medicine* 17, 1103–1120.

5. Bekele, B. N., Shen, Y. (2005). A Bayesian approach to jointly modeling toxicity and biomarker expression in a phase I/II dose-finding trial. *Biometrics* 61, 344–354.

6. Braun, T. M. (2002). The bivariate continual reassessment method: extending the CRM to phase I trials of two competing outcomes. *Controlled Clinical Trials* 23, 240–256.

7. Chen, Z., Yuan, Y., Li, Z., Kutner, M., Owonikoko, T., Curran, W. J., Khuri, F., Kowalski, J. (2015). Dose escalation with over-dose and under-dose controls in phase I/II clinical trials. *Contemporary Clinical Trials* 43, 133–141.

8. Cook, R. D., Fedorov, V. V. (1995). Constrained optimization of experimental design. *Statistics* 26, 129–178.

9. Cunanan, K., Koopmeiners, J. S. (2014). Evaluating the performance of copula models in phase I–II clinical trials under model misspecification. *BMC Medical Research Methodology* 14, 51. doi:10.1186/1471-2288-14-51.

10. Dragalin, V. (2010). Seamless phase I/II designs. In A. Pong and S.-C. Chow (eds.), *Handbook of Adaptive Designs in Pharmaceutical and Clinical Development*, pp. 12.1–12.23, Chapman & Hall, Boca Raton, FL.

11. Dragalin, V., Fedorov, V. V. (2006). Adaptive designs for dose-finding based on efficacy-toxicity response. *Journal of Statistical Planning and Inference* 136, 1800–1823.

12. Dragalin, V., Fedorov, V. V., Wu, Y. (2008). Two-stage design for dose-finding that accounts for both efficacy and safety. *Statistics in Medicine* 27, 5156–5176.

13. Durham, S. D., Flournoy, N., Li, W. (1998). A sequential design for maximizing the probability of a favourable response. *Canadian Journal of Statistics* 26(3), 479–495.

14. Fan, S. K., Chaloner, K. (2004). Optimal designs and limiting optimal designs for a trinomial response. *Journal of Statistical Planning and Inference* 126, 347–360.

15. Fan, S. K, Chaloner, K. (2001). Optimal designs for a continuation-ratio model. In A. Atkinson, P. Hackl, W. G. Müller (eds.), *mODa 6—Advances in Model-Oriented Design and Analysis*, pp. 77–85, Springer-Verlag, Berlin and Heidelberg GmbH.

16. Fedorov, V. V. (1972). *Theory of Optimal Experiments*. Academic Press, New York and London.

17. Fedorov, V. V., Flournoy, N., Wu, Y., Zhang, R. (2011). *Best Intention Designs in Dose Finding Studies*. Isaac Newton Institute for Mathematical Sciences, Cambridge, UK.

18. Fedorov, V. V., Hackl, P. (1997). *Model-Oriented Design of Experiments*. Springer Science + Business Media, New York.

19. Fedorov, V. V., Leonov, S. L. (2014). *Optimal Design for Nonlinear Response Models*. CRC Press, Boca Raton, FL.

20. Fedorov, V. V., Wu, Y. (2007). Dose finding designs for continuous responses and binary utility. *Journal of Biopharmaceutical Statistics* 17(6), 1085–1096.

21. Gao, L., Rosenberger, W. F. (2013). Adaptive Bayesian design with penalty based on toxicity-efficacy response. In D. Uciński, A. C. Atkinson, M. Patan (eds.), *mODa 10— Advances in Model-Oriented Design and Analysis*, pp. 91–98, Springer International Publishing, Basel, Switzerland.

22. Gooley, T. A., Martin, P. J., Fisher, L. D., Pettinger, M. (1994). Simulation as a design tool for phase I/II clinical trials: An example from bone marrow transplantation. *Controlled Clinical Trials* 15, 450–462.

23. Guo, B., Yuan, Y. (2015). A Bayesian dose-finding design for phase I/II clinical trials with nonignorable dropouts. *Statistics in Medicine* 34(10), 1721–1732.

24. Haines, L., Perevozskaya, I., Rosenberger, W. F. (2003). Bayesian optimal designs for phase I clinical trials. *Biometrics* 59, 591–600.

25. Hardwick, J., Mayer, M. C., Stout, V. (2003). Directed walk designs for dose-response problems with competing failure modes. *Biometrics* 59, 229–236.

26. Hardwick, J., Stout, V. (2001). Optimizing a unimodal response function for binary variables. In A. Atkinson, B. Bogacka, A. Zhigljavsky (eds.), *Optimum Design 2000*, pp. 195–208, Springer-Verlag, US.

27. Hirakawa, A. (2012). An adaptive dose finding approach for correlated bivariate binary and continuous outcomes in phase I oncology trials. *Statistics in Medicine* 31, 516–532.

28. Hoering, A., LeBlanc, M., Crowley, J. (2011). Seamless phase I/II trial design for assessing toxicity and efficacy for targeted agents. *Clinical Cancer Research* 17(4), 640–646.

29. Hoering, A., Mitchell, A., LeBlanc, M., Crowley, J. (2013). Early phase trial design for assessing several dose levels for toxicity and efficacy for targeted agents. *Clinical Trials* 10(2), 422–429.

30. Hu, F., Rosenberger, W. F. (2006). *The Theory of Response-Adaptive Randomization in Clinical Trials*. John Wiley & Sons, New York.

31. Hunsberger, S., Rubinstein, L. V., Dancey, J., Korn, E. L. (2005). Dose escalation trial designs based on molecularly targeted endpoint. *Statistics in Medicine* 24, 2171–2181.

32. Iasonos, A., O'Quigley, J. (2016). Dose expansion cohorts in phase I trials. *Statistics in Biopharmaceutical Research* 8(2), 161–170.

33. Iasonos, A., Wages, N. A., Conaway, M. R., Cheung, K., Yuan, Y., O'Quigley, J. (2016). Dimension of model parameter space and operating characteristics in adaptive dose-finding studies. *Statistics in Medicine* 35, 3760–3775.

34. Ivanova, A. V. (2003). A new dose-finding design for bivariate outcomes. *Biometrics* 59, 1001–1007.

35. Ji, Y., Bekele, N. (2009). Adaptive randomization for multiarm comparative clinical trials based on joint efficacy/toxicity outcomes. *Biometrics* 65, 876–884.

36. Jin, I. H., Liu, S., Thall, P. F., Yuan, Y. (2014). Using data augmentation to facilitate conduct of phase I–II clinical trials with delayed outcomes. *Journal of the American Statistical Association* 109, 525–536.

37. Kiefer, J., Wolfowitz, J. (1960). The equivalence of two extremum problems. *Canadian Journal of Mathematics* 12, 363–366.

38. Kiefer, J., Wolfowitz, J. (1952). Stochastic estimation of the maximum of regression function. *Annals of Mathematical Statistics* 25, 529–532.

39. Koopmeiners, J. S., Modiano, J. (2014). A Bayesian adaptive phase I-II clinical trial for evaluating efficacy and toxicity with delayed outcomes. *Clinical Trials* 11, 38–48.

40. Kpamegan, E. E., Flournoy, N. (2001). An optimizing up-and-down design. In A. Atkinson, B. Bogacka, A. Zhigljavsky (eds), *Optimum Design 2000*, pp. 211–223, Springer-Verlag, US.

41. Kpamegan, E. E., Flournoy, N. (2008). Up-and-down designs for selecting the dose with maximum success probability. *Sequential Analysis* 27, 78–96.

42. Li, W., Durham, S. D., Flournoy, N. (1995). An adaptive design for maximization of a contingent binary response. In N. Flournoy, W. F. Rosenberger (eds.), *Adaptive Designs*, pp. 179–196, IMS Lecture Notes Monograph Series 25, Hayward, CA.

43. Lei, X., Yuan, Y., Yin, G. (2011). Bayesian phase II adaptive randomization by jointly modeling time-to-event efficacy and binary toxicity. *Lifetime Data Analysis* 17(1), 156–174.

44. Loke, Y. C., Tan, S. B., Cai, Y. Y., Machin, D. (2006). A Bayesian dose finding design for dual endpoint phase I trials. *Statistics in Medicine* 25, 3–22.

45. O'Quigley, J., Hughes, M. D., Fenton, T. (2001). Dose-finding designs for HIV studies. *Biometrics* 57, 1018–1029.

46. O'Quigley, J., Pepe, M., Fisher, L. (1990). Continual reassessment method: A practical design for phase I clinical studies in cancer. *Biometrics* 46, 33–48.

47. Padmanabhan, S. K., Hsuan, F., Dragalin, V. (2010). Adaptive penalized D-optimal designs for dose finding based on continuous efficacy and toxicity. *Statistics in Biopharmaceutical Research* 2(2), 182–198.

48. Pronzato, L. (2008). Asymptotic properties of adaptive penalized optimal designs with application to dose finding. Technical Report ISRN I3S/RR-2008-19-FR, University Nice Sophia Antipolis, 33 pp.

49. Pronzato, L. (2010). Asymptotic properties of adaptive penalized optimal designs over a finite space. In A. Giovagnoli, A. C. Atkinson, B. Torsney (eds) and C. May (co-ed.) *mODa 9—Advances in Model-Oriented Design and Analysis*, pp. 165–172, Springer-Verlag, Berlin and Heidelberg.

50. Pronzato, L. (2010). Penalized optimal adaptive designs for dose finding. *Journal of Statistical Planning and Inference* 140, 283–296.

51. Seegers, V., Chevret, S., Resche-Rigon, M. (2011). Dose-finding design driven by efficacy in onco-hematology phase I/II trials. *Statistics in Medicine* 30, 1574–1583.

52. Sverdlov, O., Wong, W. K. (2014). Novel statistical designs for phase I/II and phase II clinical trials with dose-finding objectives. *Therapeutic Innovation and Regulatory Science* 48(5), 601–615.

53. Sverdlov, O., Wong, W. K., Ryeznik, Y. (2014). Adaptive clinical trial designs for phase I cancer studies. *Statistics Surveys* 8, 2–44.

54. Thall, P. F. (2010). Bayesian models and decision algorithms for complex early phase clinical trials. *Statistical Science* 25(2), 227–244.

55. Thall, P. F., Cook, J. D. (2004). Dose-finding based on efficacy-toxicity trade-offs. *Biometrics* 60, 684–693.

56. Thall, P. F., Estey, E. H., Sung, H. G. (1999). A new statistical method for dose-finding based on efficacy and toxicity in early phase clinical trials. *Investigational New Drugs* 17, 155–167.

57. Thall, P. F., Inoue, L. Y. T., Martin, T. G. (2002). Adaptive decision making in a lymphocyte infusion trial. *Biometrics* 58, 560–568.

58. Thall, P. F., Nguyen, H. Q., Estey, E. H. (2008). Patient-specific dose finding based on bivariate outcomes and covariates. *Biometrics* 64, 1126–1136.

59. Thall, P. F., Russell, K. T. (1998). A strategy for dose finding and safety monitoring based on efficacy and adverse outcomes in phase I/II clinical trials. *Biometrics* 54, 532–540.

60. Wang, M., Day, R. (2010). Adaptive Bayesian design for phase I dose-finding trials using a joint model of response and toxicity. *Journal of Biopharmaceutical Statistics* 20(1), 125–144.

61. Whitehead, J., Brunier, H. (1995). Bayesian decision procedures for dose determining experiments. *Statistics in Medicine* 14, 885–893.

62. Whitehead, J., Williamson, D. (1998). Bayesian decision procedures based on logistic regression models for dose-finding studies. *Journal of Biopharmaceutical Statistics* 8(3), 445–467.

63. Whitehead, J., Zhou, Y., Stevens, J., Blakey, G. (2004). An evaluation of a Bayesian method of dose escalation based on bivariate binary responses. *Journal of Biopharmaceutical Statistics* 14(4), 969–983.

64. Whitehead, J., Zhou, Y., Stevens, J., Blakey, G., Price, J., Leadbetter, J. (2006). Bayesian decision procedures for dose-escalation based on evidence of undesirable events and therapeutic benefit. *Statistics in Medicine* 25, 37–53.

65. World Medical Association (*WMA*) General Assembly. (1964). *Declaration of Helsinki—Ethical principles for medical research involving human subjects.* http://www.wma.net/en/30publications/10policies/b3/ (Accessed on July 23, 2016).

66. Yin, G., Li, Y., Ji, Y. (2006). Bayesian dose-finding in phase I/II clinical trials using toxicity and efficacy odds ratios. *Biometrics* 62, 777–787.

67. Yin, G., Yuan, Y. (2009). Bayesian model averaging continual reassessment method in phase I clinical trials. *Journal of the American Statistical Association* 104(487), 954–968.

68. Yin, G., Zheng, S., Xu, J. (2013). Two-stage dose finding for cytostatic agents in phase I oncology trials. *Statistics in Medicine* 32, 644–660.

69. Yuan, Y., Nguyen, H. Q., Thall, P. F. (2016). *Bayesian Designs for Phase I/II Clinical Trials*. CRC Press, Boca Raton, FL.

70. Yuan, Y., Yin, G. (2009). Bayesian dose finding by jointly modeling toxicity and efficacy as time-to-event outcomes. *Applied Statistics* 58(5), 719–736.

71. Zang, Y., Lee, J. J., Yuan, Y. (2014). Adaptive designs for identifying optimal biologic dose for molecularly targeted agents. *Clinical Trials* 11(3), 319–327.

72. Zhang, W., Sargent, D. J., Mandrekar, S. (2006) An adaptive dose-finding design incorporating both toxicity and efficacy. *Statistics in Medicine* 25, 2365–2383.

73. Zhong, W., Carlin, B. P., Koopmeiners, J. S. (2013). Flexible link continual reassessment methods for trivariate binary outcome phase I/II trials. *Journal of Statistical Theory and Practice* 7, 442–455.

74. Zhong, W., Koopmeiners, J. S., Carlin, B. P. (2012). A trivariate continual reassessment method for phase I/II trials of toxicity, efficacy, and surrogate efficacy. *Statistics in Medicine* 30, 3885–3895.

75. Zhou, Y., Whitehead, J., Bonvini, E., Stevens, J. W. (2006). Bayesian decision procedures for binary and continuous bivariate dose-escalation studies. *Pharmaceutical Statistics* 5, 125–133.

76. Zohar, S., Chevret, S. (2007). Recent developments in adaptive designs for phase I/II dose-finding studies. *Journal of Biopharmaceutical Statistics* 17, 1071–1083.

77. Zohar, S., O'Quigley, J. (2006). Identifying the most successful dose (MSD) in dose-finding studies in cancer. *Pharmaceutical Statistics* 5, 187–199.

78. Zohar, S., O'Quigley, J. (2006). Optimal designs for estimating the most successful dose. *Statistics in Medicine* 25, 4311–4320.

6

Designing Early-Phase Drug Combination Trials

Ying Yuan

The University of Texas MD Anderson Cancer Center

Liangcai Zhang

Rice University

CONTENTS

Drug combination therapy has become the mainstream approach to cancer treatment. It provides the means by which treatment efficacy is improved and the resistance to treatment that impedes cancer monotherapy is overcome. The objectives of using drug combination are to induce a synergistic treatment effect, increase the joint dose intensity with nonoverlapping toxicities, and target various tumor cell susceptibilities and disease pathways. A search on PubMed with the keyword "drug combination" identified more than 88,000 publications from 2010 to 2015. However, despite the enormous importance and apparent popularity of combination therapies, in terms of the designs used in actual trials of drug combinations, the current status is far from desirable. Riviere et al. [1] reviewed 162 trials published between 2011 and 2013 and found that 88% of the trials used the conventional $3 + 3$ design, which has been widely criticized for its poor operating characteristics, even when used for single-agent trials. They found only one trial that used a new design for combination trials, despite the availability of more than a dozen novel combination trial designs in the (mainly statistical) literature. As we describe herein, the design of drug combination trials is more complicated and challenging than that of single-agent trials. The goal of this chapter is to clarify some challenges (Section 6.1) and misconceptions on designing combination trials (Section 6.2) and provide practical guidance and designs to practitioners for conducting drug combination trials (Section 6.3).

6.1   Challenges of Designing Combination Trials

6.1.1   Partial order in toxicity

A major challenge in designing combination trials is that combinations are only partially ordered according to their toxicity probabilities. Consider a trial combining J doses of agent A, denoted as $A_1 < A_2 < \cdots < A_J$, and K doses of agent B, denoted as $B_1 < B_2 < \cdots < B_K$. Let $A_j B_k$ denote the combination of A_j and B_k, and p_{jk} denote the probability of dose-limiting toxicity (DLT) for $A_j B_k$. It is typically reasonable to assume that when the dose of one agent (say agent A) is fixed, the toxicity of the combination increases as the dose of the other agent increases (i.e., agent B). In other words, as shown in Figure 6.1, in the dose matrix, the rows and columns are ordered, with the probability of DLT increasing along with the dose. However, in other directions of the dose matrix, e.g., along the diagonals from the upper left corner to the lower right corner, the toxicity order is unknown due to unknown drug–drug interactions. For example, between $A_2 B_2$ and $A_1 B_3$, we do not know which drug is more toxic because the first combination has a higher dose of agent A, whereas the second combination has a higher dose of agent B. Thus, we cannot fully rank $J \times K$ combinations from low to high in terms of their DLT rates. This is distinctly different from single-agent trials, for which the dose can be unambiguously ranked, assuming that higher dosage yields higher probability of DLT. The implication of such a partial ranking is that conventional single-agent dose-finding designs cannot be directly used for finding the maximum tolerated dose (MTD) in drug combination trials.

6.1.2   MTD contour

Another important feature for combination trials is the existence of the MTD contour in the two-dimensional dose space, as shown in Figure 6.2. As a result, multiple MTDs may exist in the $J \times K$ dose matrix. The implication of the MTD contour is that when designing a drug combination trial, the first and most important question requiring careful consideration is "Are we interested in finding one MTD or multiple MTDs?"

As we describe below, the answer to this question determines the choice of different design strategies for drug combination trials. This important issue, unfortunately, is largely overlooked by existing trial designs.

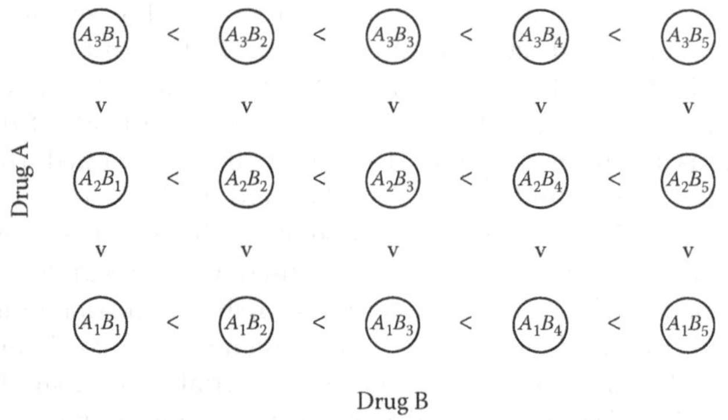

FIGURE 6.1
Partial order in toxicity for drug combinations.

6.2 Designing Drug Combination Trials to Find One MTD

6.2.1 Model-based designs

Numerous designs have been proposed to find a single MTD for drug combinations. For example, Conaway et al. [2] proposed a drug combination dose-finding method based on the order of the restricted inference. Yin and Yuan [3, 4] proposed Bayesian dose-finding designs based on latent contingency tables [3] and a copula-type model [4] for drug combination trials. Braun and Wang [5] developed a dose-finding method based on a Bayesian hierarchical model. Wages et al. [6] extended the continual reassessment method (CRM) [7] based on partial ordering of the dose combinations. Braun and Jia [8] generalized the CRM to handle drug combination trials. Riviere et al. [9] proposed a Bayesian dose-finding design based on the logistic model. Cai et al. [10] and Riviere et al. [11] proposed Bayesian adaptive designs for drug combination trials involving molecularly targeted agents. Albeit very different, most of these designs adopt a common dose-finding strategy similar to the CRM: devise a model to describe the dose–toxicity surface, and then, based on the accumulating data, continuously update the model estimate and make the decision of dose assignment for the new patient, typically by assigning the new patient to the dose for which the estimated toxicity is closest to the MTD.

Although these designs perform reasonably well, they are rarely used in practice for several reasons. First, these designs are statistically and computationally complicated, leading many practitioners to perceive that decisions of dose allocation arise from a "black box." Lack of easy-to-use software further hinders the adoption of these designs in practice. Riviere et al. [11] found only one trial that used a new model-based design in their review of 162 drug combination trials. Robustness is another potential issue for model-based drug combination trial designs. Since these designs use a model-based strategy similar to that of the CRM, we may expect them to share the robustness of the CRM, e.g., consistent under misspecified models [12]. Unfortunately, that is not the case in general. The consistency of the CRM under misspecified models requires several assumptions [12]. A critical one is monotonicity (toxicity monotonically increases with the dose), which does not hold for drug combinations. Based on our experience, model-based drug combination trial designs are substantially more delicate, and it is not difficult to find some scenarios where these designs do not perform well. One reason is that in the two-dimensional dose space, the dose-finding scheme is much more likely to become stuck at local "suboptimal" doses. Some strategies (e.g., giving high priority to exploring new doses [10] and randomization [11]) have been proposed to alleviate this issue, but given the small sample size of early-phase trials, this remains an issue that affects the robustness of drug combination trial designs. The robustness of the model-based drug combination trial designs warrants further research. Because of the aforementioned issues, we will not further discuss these model-based approaches. Instead, in what follows, we focus on two simple and robust approaches that can be easily implemented using an existing R package, making them more likely to be used in practice.

6.2.2 Linearization approach

When the goal is to find a single MTD, a much simpler, robust approach to drug combination trials is available. The key observation is that there is no need to search the whole (partially ordered) dose matrix. As demonstrated in Figure 6.2, we can select a certain ordered path (i.e., a sequence of combinations), which starts from a low-dose combination (e.g., lower left corner) and ends at a high-dose combination (e.g., upper right corner), to find the MTD. This approach, we call it *"linearization,"* has been widely used in practice to design

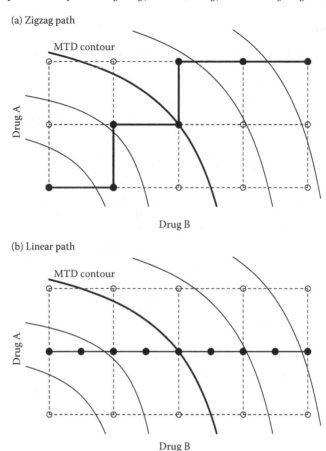

FIGURE 6.2

Illustration of the linearization approach to find a single MTD for drug combination trials using a (a) zigzag or (b) linear path. The lattices of dotted lines denote the dose combination matrix. The solid curved lines indicate the toxicity contours, and the solid line with solid circles indicates the linear path for dose finding.

drug combination trials. One may argue that compared to searching the dose matrix, the linearization approach is more likely to miss the MTD because the MTD is less likely to be in the selected linear path than in the whole dose matrix. That occurs simply because the dose matrix contains more doses to be investigated. For example, a 4 × 4 drug combination matrix contains 16 investigational doses. In the linearization approach, if we specify the same number of, say 16, doses (on a finer grid), there is little reason for the linear path to be less likely than the dose matrix to contain the MTD. This is because in principle, as the number of doses increases, the linear path will eventually hit the MTD contour (see Figure 6.2). Actually, given a prespecified $J \times K$ dose matrix, there is also no guarantee that it contains the MTD. The same argument applies to traditional single-agent dose finding as well. (In this chapter, we use the terms one-dimensional dose finding and single-agent dose finding to indicate the same thing.) Recently, Chu et al. [13] proposed a method to adaptively add new doses when the trial data indicate that none of the prespecified doses are close to the target toxicity rate. That method can be used with the linearization approach to address the concern that none of the doses are close to the MTD.

The beauty of linearization is that it converts a complex, partially ordered dose combination matrix into a sequence of ordered combinations. Therefore, the existing single-agent dose-finding methods, for example the CRM or the Bayesian optimal interval design (BOIN), can be directly used to find the MTD. Depending on the clinical setting, different linearization paths can be used. For example, if drug A is the standard treatment and serves as the backbone of the combination treatment, we may prefer to fix A at its standard dose and vary the dose of drug B (see Figure 6.2b). In other settings, such as when two drugs are similarly important, we may prefer to alternatively increase the doses of A and B, which results in a zigzag line in the dose surface (see Figure 6.2a).

After linearization, we obtain a sequence of ordered doses. Although any reasonable single-agent dose-finding trial design now can be used to find the MTD, here we focus on the BOIN design [14, 15] because of its simplicity for implementation in practice and its superior performance. The BOIN design can be implemented in a simple way that is similar to that of the traditional "3 + 3" design, but it yields good operating characteristics that are comparable to those of the well-known CRM [14]. The BOIN is also ethically attractive because it optimizes patient ethics by minimizing the chance of incorrect dose escalation and de-escalation (i.e., inappropriate dosing) during the trial conduct.

Given a sequence of L ordered doses, the BOIN design can be described as follows:

1. Patients in the first cohort are treated at the lowest dose level or at a prespecified intermediate dose.

2. At the current dose level ℓ, we assume that a total (or the cumulative number) of n_ℓ patients have been treated, and m_ℓ of them have experienced DLT. Let $\hat{p}_\ell = m_\ell/n_\ell$ denote the observed DLT rate at dose level ℓ. To assign a dose to the next cohort of patients, we use the following three decision rules. Given that λ_1 and λ_2 are prespecified dose escalation and de-escalation boundaries respectively,

   - If $\hat{p}_\ell \leq \lambda_1$, we escalate the dose level to $\ell + 1$.
   - If $\hat{p}_\ell \geq \lambda_2$, we de-escalate the dose level to $\ell - 1$.
   - Otherwise, i.e., $\lambda_1 < \hat{p}_\ell < \lambda_2$, we retain the same dose level ℓ.

3. This process continues until the maximum sample size is reached or the trial is terminated due to excessive toxicity, as described below.

We can see that the BOIN design shares the simplicity of the 3 + 3 design. The 3 + 3 design makes the decision of dose escalation/de-escalation by comparing the observed DLT rate $\hat{p}_\ell$ with 0/3, 1/3, 2/3, 0/6, 1/6, and 2/6, while the BOIN design makes the decision by comparing $\hat{p}_\ell$ with two fixed boundaries λ_1 and λ_2, which is arguably even simpler. Table 6.1 provides the values of λ_1 and λ_2 for common target DLT rates. For example, given the target DLT rate $\theta = 30\%$, the corresponding escalation threshold $\lambda_1 = 0.236$ and the de-escalation threshold $\lambda_2 = 0.358$. The theory and derivation of λ_1 and λ_2 can be found in Liu and Yuan [14].

To protect patients from overly toxic doses, the BOIN design imposes the following dose elimination rule during trial conduct:

If $\Pr(p_\ell > \theta | m_\ell, n_\ell) > 0.95$ and $n_\ell \geq 3$, dose levels ℓ and higher are eliminated from the trial, and the trial is terminated if the first dose level is eliminated

where θ is the target DLT rate, and $\Pr(p_\ell > \theta | m_\ell, n_\ell) > 0.95$ can be evaluated on the basis of a beta-binomial model, assuming that m_ℓ follows a binomial distribution (with size and probability parameters n_ℓ and p_ℓ, respectively) and p_ℓ follows a vague beta prior, e.g., $p_\ell \sim beta(1,1)$. The eliminated doses cannot be used to treat patients and

TABLE 6.1

Escalation and de-escalation boundaries λ_1 and λ_2 for the BOIN design under different target DLT rates.

Boundaries	Target DLT Rate θ					
	0.15	0.2	0.25	0.3	0.35	0.4
λ_1	0.118	0.157	0.197	0.236	0.276	0.316
λ_2	0.179	0.238	0.298	0.358	0.419	0.479

are not selected as the MTDs. Based on our experience, rather than repeatedly evaluating the above dose elimination rule in real time during trial conduct, medical researchers often prefer to enumerate the dose elimination boundaries for each possible value of n_ℓ before the initiation of the trial and include these boundaries in the trial protocol. Therefore, when conducting the trial, they can determine dose elimination by simply examining whether the number of patients who experience DLT at the current dose, i.e., m_ℓ, reaches the elimination boundaries. For example, given the cohort size of 3 and target DLT rate $\theta = 30\%$, a dose should be eliminated if (# of DLT)/(# of patients treated) $\geq 3/3$, $4/6$, $5/9$, $7/12$, $8/15$, $9/18$.

After the trial has been completed, the MTD is selected based on $\{\tilde{p}_\ell\}$, the isotonically transformed values of the observed DLT rates $\{\hat{p}_\ell\}$. Specifically, we select as the MTD dose ℓ^*, for which the isotonic estimate of DLT rate $\tilde{p}_{\ell^*}$ is closest to the target DLT rate θ. If there are ties for $\tilde{p}_{\ell^*}$, we select from the ties the highest dose level when $\tilde{p}_{\ell^*} < \theta$ or the lowest dose level when $\tilde{p}_{\ell^*} > \theta$. The isotonic estimates $\{\tilde{p}_\ell\}$ can be obtained by applying the pooled adjacent violators algorithm [16] to $\{\hat{p}_\ell\}$. Operatively, the pooled adjacent violators algorithm replaces any adjacent $\hat{p}_j$'s that violate the nondecreasing order by their (weighted) average so that the resulting estimates $\tilde{p}_\ell$ become monotonic. In the case in which the observed DLT rates are monotonic, $\tilde{p}_\ell$ and $\hat{p}_\ell$ are equivalent.

6.2.3 BOIN drug combination design

Unlike the linearization approach that requires users to select a specific ordered path in the dose combination matrix, the BOIN drug combination design [17] provides a simple, well-performing method to find a single MTD directly in the two-dimensional dose matrix. The BOIN drug combination design makes the decision of dose escalation/de-escalation based on the same rule as the single-agent BOIN design described previously. The only difference is that, in combination trials, when we decide to escalate or de-escalate the dose, there is more than one neighbor dose to which we can move. For example, when we escalate/de-escalate the dose, we can escalate/de-escalate either the dose of drug A or the dose of drug B. The BOIN drug combination design makes this choice based on $\Pr(p_{jk} \in (\lambda_1, \lambda_2)|\text{data})$, which measures how likely a dose combination is located within (λ_1, λ_2) given the observed data. The beta-binomial model described above can be easily used to evaluate $\Pr(p_{jk} \in (\lambda_1, \lambda_2)|\text{data})$.

Let $\hat{p}_{jk} = m_{jk}/n_{jk}$ denote the observed DLT rate at dose combination $A_j B_k$, where m_{jk} and n_{jk} denote the number of toxicities and patients treated at $A_j B_k$, respectively. Define an admissible dose escalation set as $\mathcal{A}_E = \{A_{j+1}B_k, A_j B_{k+1}\}$ and an admissible dose de-escalation set as $\mathcal{A}_D = \{A_{j-1}B_k, A_j B_{k-1}\}$. The BOIN drug combination design can be described as follows:

1. Patients in the first cohort are treated at the lowest dose combination A_1B_1 or a prespecified dose combination.

2. Suppose that the current cohort is treated at dose combination A_jB_k, to assign a dose to the next cohort of patients:

   - If $\hat{p}_{jk} \leq \lambda_1$, we escalate the dose to the combination that belongs to $\mathcal{A}_E$ and has the largest value of $\Pr\{p_{j'k'} \in (\lambda_1, \lambda_2)|\text{data}\}$.
   - If $\hat{p}_{jk} \geq \lambda_2$, we de-escalate the dose to the combination that belongs to $\mathcal{A}_D$ and has the largest value of $\Pr\{p_{j'k'} \in (\lambda_1, \lambda_2)|\text{data}\}$.
   - Otherwise, if $\lambda_1 < \hat{p}_{jk} < \lambda_2$, then the dose stays at the same combination A_jB_k.

3. This process is continued until the maximum sample size is reached or the trial is terminated because of excessive toxicity.

Here, λ_1 and λ_2 are the escalation and de-escalation boundaries same as these for single-agent BOIN design. During dose escalation and de-escalation, if the two combinations in $\mathcal{A}_E$ or $\mathcal{A}_D$ have the same value of $\Pr\{p_{j'k'} \in (\lambda_1, \lambda_2)|\text{data}\}$, we randomly choose one with equal probability. If no dose combinations exist in the sets of $\mathcal{A}_E$ and $\mathcal{A}_D$ (i.e., we are at the boundaries of the dose matrix), we retain the current dose combination. After the trial is completed, the MTD is selected as the dose combination with the estimated toxicity rate closest to θ. The estimates of toxicity rates are obtained using isotonic regression as described previously, but in a matrix form. More details on the BOIN drug-combination design can be found in Lin and Yin [17].

6.3 Designing Drug Combination Trials to Find Multiple MTDs

The primary motivation for combining drugs is to achieve synergistic treatment effects. Because of the existence of the MTD contour and the fact that doses on the MTD contour may have different efficacy due to drug–drug interactions, for many drug combination trials, it is of intrinsic interest to find multiple MTDs. The efficacy of the MTDs can be evaluated in subsequent phase II trials or simultaneously in phase I–II trials. Given a prespecified $J \times K$ dose matrix, finding the MTD contour is equivalent to finding an MTD, if it exists, in each row of the dose matrix. Without loss of generality, we assume that $J \leq K$. That is, drug B has more dose levels than drug A.

Finding the MTD contour is substantially more challenging than finding a single MTD. This is because, in order to find all MTDs in the dose matrix, we must explore the whole dose matrix using the limited sample size that is characteristic of phase I trials; otherwise, we risk missing some MTDs. A general strategy for finding multiple targets is to divide and conquer:

> Divide the two-dimensional dose-finding problem into a series of simpler one-dimensional dose-finding problems that can be easily conquered by existing single-agent dose-finding methods.

Taking that strategy, Yuan and Yin [18] proposed a sequential dose-finding design that partitions the dose matrix into a series of blocks (i.e., groups of doses), within which the doses are fully ordered. Specifically, Yuan and Yin [18] suggested using each row of the dose matrix as a block. Within each block, as the doses are fully ordered, any existing single-agent dose-finding method can be used to find the MTD. These MTDs form the MTD contour. For convenience, we call dose finding within a block a "subtrial." A key feature of the sequential design of Yuan and Yin [18] is that the subtrials are conducted sequentially in a specific order, such that the position of the MTD identified by the current subtrial is used to remove some implausible doses (i.e., the doses that are supposed to have higher toxicity than the MTD identified in the current subtrial) from the subsequent subtrials. By shrinking the dose space, the design saves sample size and achieves more efficient dose finding. When we have used that design in practice, the clinicians have raised several practical issues. First, the sequential design starts the trial at the second lowest dose A_2B_1, rather than the lowest dose. In practice, clinicians strongly favor starting the trial at the lowest dose A_1B_1. Second, removing some doses on the basis of the MTD identified in the previous subtrial is too stringent. Due to the small sample size, the MTD identified in a subtrial may be incorrect. As a result, the true MTD may be incorrectly removed from the subsequent subtrials.

To address these concerns, we introduce a new dose-finding design called the *waterfall design* [19]. The name "waterfall" is used to characterize the design as finding the MTD contour sequentially from the top of the dose matrix to the bottom, as described later. The waterfall design is based on the divide-and-conquer strategy. A new partition scheme is used to partition the dose matrix into blocks such that the trial always starts with the lowest dose. In addition, the results from the prior subtrial are used only to set the starting dose rather than to directly shrink the dose space for the subsequent trial, which gives the design more flexibility to move around and identify the MTD more precisely.

In contrast to numerous drug combination designs for finding a single MTD, a very limited number of designs have been proposed to find the MTD contour. Thall et al. [20] proposed a drug combination design to find three MTDs, but that design assumes that the doses are continuous and can be freely changed during the trial, which is not common in practice. Wang and Ivanova [21] proposed a design to find the MTD contour based on a parametric model, assuming that the logarithm of the toxicity probability of a drug combination is a linear function of the doses of the two drugs. Recently, Mander and Sweeting [22] proposed a product of independent beta probabilities escalation (PIPE) design to find the MTD contour based on Bayesian model averaging, without assuming a parametric form on the dose–toxicity curve.

6.3.1   Waterfall design

6.3.1.1   Partition scheme

As illustrated in Figure 6.3, the waterfall design partitions the $J \times K$ dose matrix into J subtrials (or blocks), within which the doses are fully ordered. These subtrials are conducted sequentially from the top of the matrix to the bottom, which is why we refer to the design as the waterfall design. The goal of the design is to find the MTD contour, which is equivalent to finding the MTD, if it exists, in each row of the dose matrix. The waterfall design can be described as follows:

1. Divide the $J \times K$ dose matrix into J subtrials $S_J, \dots, S_1$, according to the dose level of drug A:

$$S_J = \{A_1B_1, \dots, A_JB_1, A_JB_2, \dots, A_JB_K\},$$
$$S_{J-1} = \{A_{J-1}B_2, \dots, A_{J-1}B_K\},$$
$$S_{J-2} = \{A_{J-2}B_2, \dots, A_{J-2}B_K\},$$
$$\dots$$
$$S_1 = \{A_1B_2, \dots, A_1B_K\}.$$

Note that subtrial S_J also includes lead-in doses $A_1B_1, A_2B_1, \dots, A_JB_1$ (the first column of the dose matrix) to impose the practical consideration that the trial

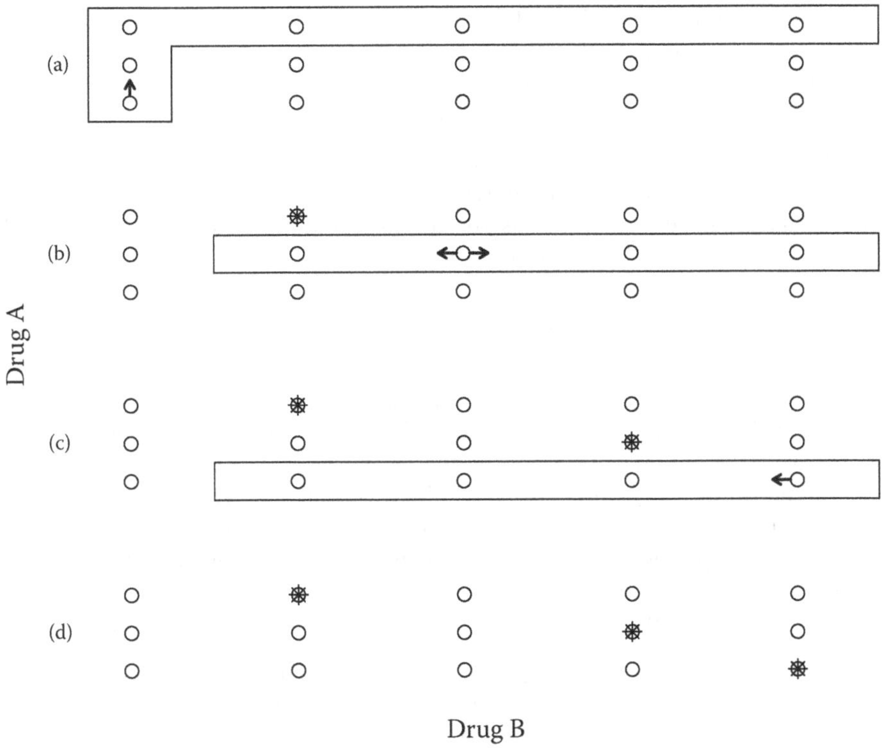

FIGURE 6.3

Illustration of the waterfall design for a 3×5 combination trial. The doses in the rectangle form a subtrial, and the asterisks denote the candidate MTDs. As shown in panel (a), the trial starts by conducting the first subtrial with the starting dose A_1B_1. After the first subtrial identified A_3B_2 as the candidate MTD, we then conduct the second subtrial with the starting dose A_2B_3 (see panel b). After the second subtrial identified A_2B_4 as the candidate MTD, we conduct the third subtrial with the starting dose A_1B_5 (see panel c). After all subtrials are completed, we select the MTD contour based on the data from all subtrials, as shown in panel (d).

starts at the lowest dose. Within each subtrial, the doses are fully ordered with monotonically increasing toxicity.

2. Conduct the subtrials sequentially using the BOIN design (or other single-agent dose-finding method) as follows:

   (a) Conduct subtrial S_J, starting from the lowest dose combination A_1B_1, to find the MTD. We call the dose selected by the subtrial the "candidate MTD" to highlight that the dose selected by the individual subtrial may not be the "final" MTD that we will select at the end of the trial. The final MTD selection will be based on the data collected from all of the subtrials. The objective of finding the candidate MTD is to determine which subtrial will be conducted next and the corresponding starting dose.

   (b) Assuming that subtrial S_J selects dose $A_{j^*}B_{k^*}$ as the candidate MTD, next, conduct subtrial S_{j^*-1} with the starting dose $A_{j^*-1}B_{k^*+1}$. That is, the next subtrial to be conducted is the one with the dose of drug A that is one level lower than the candidate MTD found in the previous subtrial. After identifying the candidate MTD of subtrial S_{j^*-1}, the same rule is used to determine the next subtrial and its starting dose. See Figure 6.3 for an example.

(c) Repeat step (b) until subtrial S_1 is completed.

3. Estimate the toxicity probability $R(A_j B_k)$ based on the toxicity data collected from all of the subtrials using matrix isotonic regression [23]. For each row of the dose matrix, select the MTD as the dose combination that has the estimate of toxicity probability that is closest to the target toxicity rate θ unless all combinations in that row are overly toxic.

In step 2, the reason that subtrial S_{j^*-1} starts with dose $A_{j^*-1}B_{k^*+1}$ rather than the lowest dose in that subtrial (i.e., $A_{j^*-1}B_2$) is that $A_{j^*-1}B_{k^*+1}$ is the lowest dose that is potentially located at the MTD contour. Starting from $A_{j^*-1}B_{k^*+1}$ allows us to quickly reach the MTD. Using Figure 6.3 as an example, the first subtrial S_3 identified the dose $A_3 B_2$ as the MTD, and thus, the second subtrial S_2 starts from the dose $A_2 B_3$. It is not desirable to start from the lowest dose $A_2 B_2$ because the partial ordering informs us that $A_2 B_2$ is below the MTD. Starting at the lowest dose in this example will waste patient resources and expose patients to low doses that may be subtherapeutic.

6.3.1.2   Conducting subtrials

As the doses in each subtrial are strictly ordered, applying the BOIN design to the subtrial is straightforward. The key issue is to determine when we should end the current subtrial and initiate the next one. One straightforward way is to prespecifiy a maximum sample size for each subtrial. When the maximum sample size is reached, we stop the subtrial, determine the candidate MTD, and initiate the next subtrial. This approach works well for standard phase I one-dimensional dose finding, but it is not efficient for conducting multiple subtrials. This is because, depending on the distance between the starting dose and the MTD, as well as the shape of the dose–toxicity curve, the subtrials often require different sample sizes to identify the MTD. Based on this consideration, we propose and recommend the following stopping rule for subtrials:

At any time of the subtrial, if the total number of patients treated at the current dose reaches a certain prespecified number of, say n.earlystop, patients, we stop the subtrial and select the candidate MTD and initiate the next subtrial.

The rationale for the stopping rule is that when the patient allocation concentrates at a dose, it indicates that the dose finding might have converged to the MTD, and thus, we can stop the trial and claim the MTD. This stopping rule allows the sample size of subtrials to be automatically adjusted according to the difficulty of the dose finding (e.g., the distance between the starting dose and the MTD, and the shape of the dose–toxicity curve). Another attractive feature of the above approach is that it automatically ensures that a certain number of patients are treated at the MTD. Conventionally, we achieve this by adding cohort expansion after identifying the MTD. In practice, we recommend n.earlystop > 9 to ensure reasonable operating characteristics. Although the above stopping rule provides an automatic, reasonable way to determine the sample size for a subtrial, in some cases, it is desirable to put a cap on the maximum sample size of subtrials. This can be done by adding an extra stopping rule:

Stop the subtrial j if its sample size reaches $N_j^{\max}$, where $N_j^{\max}$ is the prespecified maximum sample size for subtrial j.

As a rule of thumb, we recommend $N_j^{\max} = 4 \times$ (the number of doses in the jth subtrial), for $j = 1, \ldots, J$. This means that given a $J \times K$ dose combinations, the maximum total sample size for the trial is $4 \times J \times K$. For example, for a 3×5 combination, as shown in Figure 6.3, the first subtrial contains seven doses, and the second and third subtrials contain four doses each. The recommended sample sizes are 28, 16, and 16 for three subtrials, respectively, resulting in a total sample size of 60 patients. This may seems large; however, given that there are a total of 15 doses, 60 patients actually is not a very large sample size. To see this, considering a single-agent trial with 15 doses, the maximum sample size under the 3 + 3 design is 90 patients. In practice, the recommended sample sizes n.earlystop and $N_j^{\max}$ should be further calibrated using simulation until attaining desirable operating characteristics, which can be readily done using R package "BOIN" described later.

An alternative stopping rule is based on the confidence interval (CI) of the estimate of toxicity probabilities. For example, stop the subtrial when the CI of a dose contains the target toxicity probability θ and its width is narrower than a certain value. Our numerical study shows that after appropriate calibration, these two approaches have virtually the same performance. This is somewhat expected because the width of the CI is essentially determined by the sample size (i.e., n.earlystop). Thus, we recommend the stopping rule that is based on the number of patients treated because it is more transparent, in particular to clinicians, and is easy to implement.

6.4 Software

The BOIN (with linearization), BOIN drug combination, and waterfall designs can be easily implemented using the R package "BOIN," which is freely available from CRAN. The manual for the package can be found in https://cran.r-project.org/web/packages/BOIN/index.html, and a statistical tutorial for using the package to design drug combination trials can be found in http://odin.mdacc.tmc.edu/~yyuan/index_code.html. Here, we provide a brief overview of the related functions.

- BOIN design to find a single MTD using linearization

    - get.boundary(···): This function is used to generate escalation and de-escalation boundaries for conducting trials.
    - select.mtd(···): This function is used to select the MTD at the end of the trial based on isotonically transformed estimates.
    - get.oc(···): This function is used to generate the operating characteristics of the BOIN design.

- BOIN drug combination design to find a single MTD

    - get.boundary(···): This function is used to generate escalation and de-escalation boundaries for conducting trials.
    - next.comb(···): This function is used to determine the dose combination for the next cohort of new patients given the currently observed data.
    - select.mtd.comb(···): This function (with argument MTD.contour=FALSE) is used to select the MTD at the end of the trial based on isotonically transformed estimates.
    - get.oc.comb(···): This function (with argument MTD.contour=FALSE) is used to generate the operating characteristics of the BOIN drug-combination design.

- Waterfall design to find the MTD contour

    - get.boundary(···): This function is used to generate escalation and de-escalation boundaries for conducting subtrials.

– `next.subtrial(···)`: This function is used to obtain the dose range and the starting dose for the next subtrial when the current subtrial is completed.

– `select.mtd.comb(···)`: This function (with argument `MTD.contour=TRUE`) is used to select the MTD contour at the end of the trial based on isotonically transformed estimates.

– `get.oc.comb(···)`: This function (with argument `MTD.contour=TRUE`) is used to generate the operating characteristics of the waterfall design for drug combination trials.

6.5   Trial Examples

Example 6.1: Drug Combination Trial to Find a Single MTD Using Linearization

Consider a phase I dose-finding trial of checkpoint kinase inhibitor MK-8776 in combination with gemcitabine in patients with advanced solid tumor malignancies [24]. Taking the linearization approach, the trial investigated five dose levels of MK-8776 (i.e., 10, 20, 40, 80, or 112 mg/m^2) combined with gemcitabine at 800 mg/m^2. The objective is to find the MTD with a target DLT rate of 0.3. The maximum sample size is 30 patients, treated in cohort sizes of 3. To design and conduct this trial, we first ran function

```
R> get.boundary(target=0.3, ncohort=10, cohortsize=3),
```

yielding the dose–escalation and de-escalation boundaries as shown in Table 6.2.

The trial started by treating the first cohort of three patients at dose level 1, and none of the patients had DLT. According to the dose-escalation and de-escalation rule provided in Table 6.2, we escalated the dose to level 2 to treat the second cohort of three patients, none of whom experienced DLT. Thus, we escalated the dose to level 3 and treated the third cohort of patients, two of whom experienced DLT. Based on Table 6.2, we de-escalated the dose back to level 2 and treated the fourth cohort of patients, one of whom experienced DLT. We then escalated the dose to level 3 and treated the fifth cohort of patients, none of whom experienced DLT. Therefore, the sixth cohort was also treated at dose level 3. Figure 6.4 shows the dose assignment for all 30 patients. At the end of the trial, the number of patients and the number of DLTs at the five doses were `n=c(3, 6, 18, 3, 0)` and `y=c(0, 1, 5, 3, 0)`, respectively. We called function

```
R> select.mtd(target=0.3, ntox=y, npts=n),
```

which recommended dose level 3 as the MTD, with the estimated DLT rate = 28.0% and the 95% CI = (0.10, 0.50).

TABLE 6.2
Dose escalation and de-escalation rule for the BOIN design.

	Number of Patients Treated									
	3	6	9	12	15	18	21	24	27	30
Escalate if # of DLT $\leq$	0	1	2	2	3	4	4	5	6	7
De-escalate if # of DLT $\geq$	2	3	4	5	6	7	8	9	10	11
Eliminate if # of DLT $\geq$	3	4	5	7	8	9	10	11	12	14

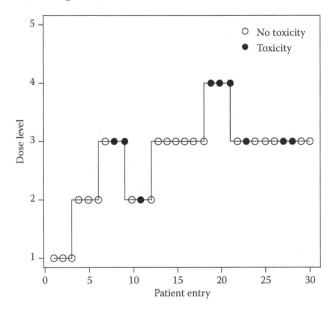

FIGURE 6.4
Illustration of a drug combination trial using the BOIN linearization design with a cohort of 3.

Example 6.2: Drug Combination Trial to Find a Single MTD Using BOIN Drug Combination Design

Consider the drug combination trial that combines three doses of gemcitabine (i.e., 600, 800, or 1,000 mg/m^2) and five doses of MK-8776 (i.e., 10, 20, 40, 80, or 112 mg/m^2). The objective is to find a MTD with a target DLT rate of 0.3, among a total of 15 dose combinations. The maximum sample size is 30 patients, treated in a cohort size of three.

Using the BOIN drug combination design, the trial started by treating the first cohort of three patients at the lowest dose combination (1,1), at which no DLT was observed. The observed data were

$$n = \begin{pmatrix} 3 & 0 & 0 & 0 & 0 \\ 0 & 0 & 0 & 0 & 0 \\ 0 & 0 & 0 & 0 & 0 \end{pmatrix}, \quad y = \begin{pmatrix} 0 & 0 & 0 & 0 & 0 \\ 0 & 0 & 0 & 0 & 0 \\ 0 & 0 & 0 & 0 & 0 \end{pmatrix},$$

where n records the number of patients treated at each dose combination, and y records the number of patients who experienced DLT at each dose combination. In matrixes y and n, entry (j, k) records the data associated with combination (j, k). To determine the dose for the second cohort of patients, we called function

```
R> next.comb(target=0.3, npts=n, ntox=y, dose.curr=c(1, 1)),
```

which recommended to escalate the dose to combination (1, 2). Therefore, we treated the second cohort of patients at dose combination (1, 2). In the second cohort, one patient experienced DLT, so the updated data matrices became

$$n = \begin{pmatrix} 3 & 3 & 0 & 0 & 0 \\ 0 & 0 & 0 & 0 & 0 \\ 0 & 0 & 0 & 0 & 0 \end{pmatrix}, \quad y = \begin{pmatrix} 0 & 0 & 0 & 0 & 0 \\ 0 & 0 & 0 & 0 & 0 \\ 0 & 0 & 0 & 0 & 0 \end{pmatrix}.$$

To determine the dose for the third cohort of patients, we again called

```
next.comb(target=0.3, npts=n, ntox=y, dose.curr=c(1, 2))
```

with updated y, n, and `dose.curr`. The function recommended escalating the dose to $(1, 3)$ for treating the third cohort of patients. We repeated this procedure until the maximum sample size was reached. Figure 6.5 shows the dose assignments for all 30 patients. For example, at dose combination $(3, 4)$ when completing the eighth cohort, there were two DLTs, based on the accumulating toxic information on this dose combination level, the function recommended de-escalating the dose to combination $(3, 3)$. When the trial was completed, the number of patients treated at each dose combination and the corresponding number of patients who experienced toxicity at each dose combination were

$$
n = \begin{pmatrix} 3 & 3 & 3 & 0 & 0 \\ 0 & 0 & 3 & 0 & 0 \\ 0 & 0 & 12 & 6 & 0 \end{pmatrix}, \qquad y = \begin{pmatrix} 0 & 0 & 0 & 0 & 0 \\ 0 & 0 & 0 & 0 & 0 \\ 0 & 0 & 4 & 4 & 0 \end{pmatrix}.
$$

We called function

```
R> select.mtd.comb(target=0.3, npts=n, ntox=y, MTD.contour=FALSE),
```

which recommended dose combination $(3, 3)$ as the MTD.

Example 6.3: Drug-combination trial to find the MTD contour using waterfall design

Consider a drug combination trial similar to Example 6.2, which combines three doses of gemicitabine (i.e., drug A) and five doses of MK-8776 (i.e., drug B). The objective now is to find the MTD contour (multiple MTDs) with a target DLT rate of 0.25. As shown

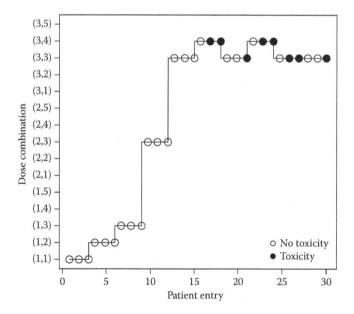

FIGURE 6.5
Illustration of a 3×5 combination trial using the BOIN drug combination design with a cohort of three.

in Figure 6.3, using the waterfall design, the trial started with the first subtrial, which consisted of seven ordered combinations $\{A_1B_1 \rightarrow A_2B_1 \rightarrow A_3B_1 \rightarrow A_3B_2 \rightarrow A_3B_3 \rightarrow A_3B_4 \rightarrow A_3B_5\}$. This subtrial was conducted using the BOIN design in a way similar to those as described in Example 6.1. The starting dose for this subtrial was A_1B_1, and n.earlystop was set as 12 such that the subtrial stopped when the number of patients treated at any of the doses reached 12. The first subtrial resulted in the following data:

$$n = \begin{pmatrix} 6 & 0 & 0 & 0 & 0 \\ 6 & 0 & 0 & 0 & 0 \\ 9 & 12 & 0 & 0 & 0 \end{pmatrix}, \qquad y = \begin{pmatrix} 0 & 0 & 0 & 0 & 0 \\ 1 & 0 & 0 & 0 & 0 \\ 1 & 3 & 0 & 0 & 0 \end{pmatrix}.$$

Based on the data, we called function next.subtrial($\cdot$) to obtain the doses for the next subtrial.

```
R> n <- matrix(c(6, 0, 0, 0, 0, 6, 0, 0, 0, 0, 9, 12, 0, 0, 0), ncol=5, byrow=TRUE)
R> y <- matrix(c(0, 0, 0, 0, 0, 1, 0, 0, 0, 0, 1, 3, 0, 0, 0), ncol=5, byrow=TRUE)
R> next.subtrial(target=.25, npts=n, ntox=y)

Next subtrial includes doses: (2, 2), (2, 3), (2, 4), (2, 5)
The starting dose for this subtrial is: (2, 3)
```

Therefore, we conducted the second subtrial with doses $\{A_2B_2 \rightarrow A_2B_3 \rightarrow A_2B_4 \rightarrow A_2B_5\}$ using the BOIN design with the starting dose A_2B_3. After the second subtrial was completed, the observed data were

$$n = \begin{pmatrix} 6 & 0 & 0 & 0 & 0 \\ 6 & 0 & 3 & 12 & 0 \\ 9 & 12 & 0 & 0 & 0 \end{pmatrix}, \qquad y = \begin{pmatrix} 0 & 0 & 0 & 0 & 0 \\ 1 & 0 & 0 & 3 & 0 \\ 1 & 3 & 0 & 0 & 0 \end{pmatrix}.$$

We called next.subtrial($\cdot$) again using the above updated data to obtain the doses for the third subtrial.

```
R> n <- matrix(c(6, 0, 0, 0, 0, 6, 0, 3, 12, 0, 9, 12, 0, 0, 0), ncol=5, byrow=TRUE)
R> y <- matrix(c(0, 0, 0, 0, 0, 1, 0, 0, 3, 0, 1, 3, 0, 0, 0), ncol=5, byrow=TRUE)
R> next.subtrial(target=.25, npts=n, ntox=y)

Next subtrial includes doses: (1, 2), (1, 3), (1, 4), (1, 5)
The starting dose for this subtrial is: (1, 5)
```

The third subtrial included doses $\{A_1B_2 \rightarrow A_1B_3 \rightarrow A_1B_4 \rightarrow A_1B_5\}$, with starting dose A_1B_5. After completing the third subtrial using the BOIN, the trial was completed and resulted in the following final data:

$$n = \begin{pmatrix} 6 & 0 & 0 & 6 & 12 \\ 6 & 0 & 3 & 12 & 0 \\ 9 & 12 & 0 & 0 & 0 \end{pmatrix}, \qquad y = \begin{pmatrix} 0 & 0 & 0 & 1 & 3 \\ 1 & 0 & 0 & 3 & 0 \\ 1 & 3 & 0 & 0 & 0 \end{pmatrix}.$$

Based on the final data, we ran select.mtd.comb($\cdot$) to select the MTD contour:

```
R> select.mtd.comb(target=0.25, npts=n, ntox=y, MTD.contour=TRUE)

The MTD contour includes dose combinations (1, 5) (2, 4) (3, 2)
Isotonic estimates of toxicity probablities for combinations are:
            0.01 NA NA 0.17 0.25
            0.12 NA 0.12 0.25 NA
            0.12 0.25 NA NA NA
```

```
NOTE: no estimate is provided for the doses at which no patient
was treated.
```

Thus, we selected dose combinations A_1B_5, A_2B_4, and A_3B_2 as the MTD contour, which had the estimated toxicity rate of 0.25.

6.6   Discussion

We have provided practical guidance and strategies to design phase I drug combination trials. We showed that the choice of design for drug combination trials critically depends on whether the goal of the trial is to find one MTD or multiple MTDs (i.e., the MTD contour). When the goal of the drug combination trial is to find a single MTD, the BOIN linearization approach and BOIN drug combination design provide simple, practical, and robust ways to find the MTD. When the goal of the combination trial is to find the MTD contour, the waterfall design is a good choice. The waterfall design is based on rules (or algorithms) and does not need complicated calculations and model fitting, which makes the design more likely to be used in practice by clinical investigators. The BOIN linearization, BOIN drug combination and waterfall designs can be easily implemented using freely available R package "BOIN."

A natural extension of the waterfall design is to seamlessly combine it with a phase II trial, resulting in a seamless phase I–II waterfall design. Specifically, after identifying the MTD contour using the waterfall design, we can seamlessly move the identified MTDs to phase II, where we randomize patients to these MTDs and identify the most efficacious MTD for further confirmative phase III trials. Details on this phase I–II approach and related software are provided by Zhang and Yuan [19] and Yuan and Yin [25].

References

1. M. K. Riviere, F. Dubois, and S. Zohar. Competing designs for drug combination in phase I dose-finding clinical trials. *Statistics in Medicine*, 34(1):1–12, 2015.

2. M. R. Conaway, S. Dunbar, and S. D. Peddada. Designs for single- or multiple-agent phase I trials. *Biometrics*, 60(3):661–669, 2004.

3. G. Yin and Y. Yuan. A latent contingency table approach to dose finding for combinations of two agents. *Biometrics*, 65(3):866–875, 2009.

4. G. Yin and Y. Yuan. Bayesian dose finding in oncology for drug combinations by copula regression. *Journal of the Royal Statistical Society: Series C (Applied Statistics)*, 58(2):211–224, 2009.

5. T. M. Braun and S. F. Wang. A hierarchical Bayesian design for phase I trials of novel combinations of cancer therapeutic agents. *Biometrics*, 66(3):805–812, 2010.

6. N. A. Wages, M. R. Conaway, and J. O'Quigley. Continual reassessment method for partial ordering. *Biometrics*, 67(4):1555–1563, 2011.

7. J. O'Quigley, M. Pepe, and L. Fisher. Continual reassessment method: A practical design for phase I clinical trials in cancer. *Biometrics*, 46:33–48, 1990.

8. T. M. Braun and N. Jia. A generalized continual reassessment method for two-agent phase I trials. *Statistics in Biopharmaceutical Research*, 5:105–115, 2013.

9. M. K. Riviere, Y. Yuan, F. Dubois, and S. Zohar. A Bayesian dose-finding design for drug combination clinical trials based on the logistic model. *Pharmaceutical Statistics*, 13(4):247–257, 2014.

10. C. Y. Cai, Y. Yuan, and Y. Ji. A Bayesian phase I/II design for oncology clinical trials of combining biological agents. *Journal of the Royal Statistical Society: Series C*, 63:159–173, 2014.

11. M. K. Riviere, Y. Yuan, F. Dubois, and S. Zohar. A Bayesian dose-finding design for clinical trials combining a cytotoxic agent with a molecularly yargeted agent. *Journal of the Royal Statistical Society: Series C*, 64:215–229, 2015.

12. J. O'Quigley and L. Z. Shen. Continual reassessment method: A likelihood approach. *Biometrics*, 52(2):673–684, 1996.

13. Y. Chu, H. Pan, and Y. Yuan. Adaptive dose modification for phase I clinical trials. *Statistics in Medicine*, 35(20):3497–3508, 2016.

14. S. Y. Liu and Y. Yuan. Bayesian optimal interval designs for phase I clinical trials. *Journal of the Royal Statistical Society: Series C (Applied Statistics)*, 64(3):507–523, 2015.

15. Y. Yuan, K. R. Hess, S. G. Hilsenbeck, and M. R. Gilbert. Bayesian optimal interval design: A simple and well-performing design for phase I oncology trials. *Clinical Cancer Research*, 22:4291–4301, 2016.

16. R. E. Barlow, D. J. Bartholomew, J. M. Bremner, and H. D. Brunk. *Statistical inference under order restrictions: The theory and application of isotonic regression*. John Wiley & Sons, New York, 1972.

17. R. Lin and G. Yin. Bayesian optimal interval design for dose finding in drug-combination trials. *Statistical Methods in Medical Research*, 2015. doi:10.1177/0962280215594494.

18. Y. Yuan and G. Yin. Sequential continual reassessment method for two-dimensional dose finding. *Statistics in Medicine*, 27(27):5664–5678, 2008.

19. L. Zhang and Y. Yuan. A simple Bayesian design to identify the maximum tolerated dose contour for drug-combination trials. *Statistics in Medicine*, 2016. doi:10.1002/sim.7095.

20. P. F. Thall, R. E. Millikan, P. Mueller, and S. J. Lee. Dose-finding with two agents in phase I oncology trials. *Biometrics*, 59(3):487–496, 2003.

21. K. Wang and A. Ivanova. Two-dimensional dose finding in discrete dose space. *Biometrics*, 61(1):217–222, 2005.

22. A. P. Mander and M. J. Sweeting. A product of independent β probabilities dose escalation design for dual-agent phase I trials. *Statistics in Medicine*, 34(8):1261–1276, 2015.

23. B. Gordon, D. Richard, P. Carolyn, and R. Tim. Isotonic regression in two independent variables. *Journal of the Royal Statistical Society: Series C (Applied Statistics)*, 33(3):352–357, 1984.

24. A. I. Daud, M. T. Ashworth, J. Strosberg, J. W. Goldman, et al. Phase I dose-escalation trial of checkpoint kinase 1 inhibitor MK-8776 as monotherapy and in combination with gemcitabine in patients with advanced solid tumors. *Journal of Clinical Oncology*, 33(9):10601066, 2015.

25. Y. Yuan and G. Yin. Bayesian phase I/II adaptively randomized oncology trials with combined drugs. *Annal of Applied Statistics*, 5(2A):924–942, 2011.

7

Dose–Schedule Finding in Early-Phase Clinical Trials

Nolan A. Wages

University of Virginia

CONTENTS

7.1 Background

It is sometimes the case in phase I dose-finding studies in cancer that there exist more than one treatment schedule. The doses of a single agent can be expressed in multiple ways based on how the treatment will be given and the frequency in which it is administered. For instance, whether a dose is given once a day for 3 days in a particular week or given once that week is likely to have an impact on the probability of observing dose-limiting toxicity (DLT) for that dose. Each of these "courses of therapy" can be considered a distinct combination of schedule and dose. For these trials, finding an acceptable dose and schedule becomes a two-dimensional dose-finding problem, where one dimension is the dose level of the agent and the other is the course of therapy. The goal becomes to find a dose–schedule combination with tolerable toxicity.

In the limited statistical literature on dose–schedule finding, there have been two different definitions of schedule. The first is based on the optimization of the number of cycles given to a patient, combined with the dose administered under each cycle. In this sense, "schedule" is defined in terms of the number of treatment cycles. For methods handling this type of problem, we refer the reader to several papers published over the past decade [1–5]. The approach of Braun et al. [2] was used to design a dose and schedule finding study of de Lima et al. [6]. In this work, we focus on a second definition of schedule, which is based on the dose per administration along with the frequency of administration within a cycle based on a given total dose per cycle. Using this "schedule" definition, Wages et al. [7] proposed a method for finding a maximum tolerated dose–schedule (MTDS) combination, based on a binary toxicity endpoint. The designs of Li et al. [8] and Guo et al. [9] develop methods that aim to find the optimal dose–schedule combination based on two binary (toxicity/efficacy) endpoints. We review each of these methods in the following sections.

7.2   Dose–Schedule Finding Based on Single Toxicity Endpoint

7.2.1   Example

As an example of a dose–schedule finding problem, consider the study of Graux et al. [10]. In this trial, eight doses of MSC1992371A, an oral inhibitor of aurora and other kinases, were administered under one of two different schedules. In Schedule 1, patients received escalating doses of MSC1992371A on days 1–3 and 8–10 of a 21-day cycle. In Schedule 2, patients received escalating doses of the agent on days 1–6 of a 21-day cycle. The per administration dose, as well as the total amount of the drug given during the DLT assessment window, is the same for each schedule, although the authors refer to Schedule 2 as the "more intense" schedule. By "more intense," it is anticipated that doses administered under Schedule 2 will have greater probability of DLT than the same dose given under Schedule 1, so we have ordered schedules. The trial consists of $2 \times 8 = 16$ (schedule, dose) combinations $\{(1,3),(1,6),(1,10),\dots,(2,3),(2,6),\dots,(2,47)\}$. For simplicity, we are going to label each of the 16 combinations, $\{d_{11},\dots,d_{28}\}$, and we have a matrix of combinations of dose and schedule as displayed in Table 7.1. The primary objective of the trial is to identify a MTDS combination based on an acceptable toxicity profile.

A reasonable assumption to be made in these type of studies is that toxicity increases monotonically with dose within each schedule. In this case, we say that the DLT probabilities follow a *simple* order in that the order relationship between all DLT probabilities for a certain schedule is completely known. Suppose that a study is investigating I schedules and J dose levels under each schedule. Denote the combination of dose j; $j = 1,\dots,J$, administered under schedule i; $i = 1,\dots,I$, as d_{ij}, and the true probability of DLT at d_{ij} by $R(d_{ij})$. In Schedule 2, $R(d_{21}) < R(d_{22}) < \dots < R(d_{28})$. An assumption being made here is that the probability of toxicity for schedule increases monotonically when the dose is being held fixed. In this case, we say that the DLT probabilities follow a simple order for a certain

TABLE 7.1

Treatment labels for dose–schedule combinations.

Schedule	Doses (mg/m^2/day)							
	3	**6**	**10**	**15**	**21**	**28**	**37**	**47**
2	d_{21}	d_{22}	d_{23}	d_{24}	d_{25}	d_{26}	d_{27}	d_{28}
1	d_{11}	d_{12}	d_{13}	d_{14}	d_{15}	d_{16}	d_{17}	d_{18}

dose and increase as the schedule moves from 1 to 2. This assumption is reasonable in the Graux et al. [10] example in which Schedule 2 is considered more intense. Therefore, for dose 6 mg/m^2/day, we assume $R(d_{12}) < R(d_{22})$. This ordering information corresponds to completely knowing the order relationship between DLT probabilities across all rows and up all columns of the dose–schedule combination matrix. The ordering of combinations along the diagonals of the matrix in Table 7.1 is unknown. It may be clear that d_{16} is more toxic than d_{15}, but we may not know the ordering between d_{16} and d_{25}. Moving from d_{16} to d_{25} corresponds to decreasing the dosage of the agent from 28 to 21 mg/m^2/day but increasing the intensity of the schedule. With regard to probability, it could be that $R(d_{16}) < R(d_{25})$ or $R(d_{16}) > R(d_{25})$, creating a *partial* order [11].

One approach to this two-dimensional problem is to preselect combinations with a known toxicity order and apply a single-agent design by escalating and de-escalating along a chosen path. This could be done by, a priori, prespecifying a subset of combinations for which we know the toxicity ordering. For instance, in the 2 × 8 grid in Table 7.1, a selected subset of combinations that satisfy the monotonicity assumption is given by

$$d_{11} \longrightarrow d_{12} \longrightarrow d_{13} \longrightarrow d_{14} \longrightarrow d_{24} \longrightarrow d_{25} \longrightarrow d_{26} \longrightarrow d_{27} \longrightarrow d_{28}.$$

This approach transforms the two-dimensional dose-finding space into a one-dimensional space. The disadvantage of this approach is that it limits the number of combinations that can be considered and it can potentially miss promising dose–schedule combinations located outside of the path. Rather than work with a single ordering, another approach to dealing with added complexity is to specify multiple possible orderings and appeal to established model selection techniques, an approach employed by the partial-order continual reassessment method (POCRM).

7.2.2 Partial-order continual reassessment method

7.2.2.1 Choosing a small subset of possible orderings

Taking into account the subset of combinations for which we know the toxicity order, the POCRM aims to formulate possible simple orders of the toxicity profile. Considering all possible simple orders may be unreasonable in some studies due to the large number of possibilities. A reasonable approach to take is to select a plausible subset of possible orderings, according to the known information among combinations. This approach was taken by Wages and Conaway [12] for drug combination trials by formulating possible orderings according to the rows, columns, and diagonals of the matrix of combinations. Suppose that, in general, we are going to consider a subset of M possible orderings indexed by m, $m = 1, \dots, M$. Let us begin by ordering the treatments across rows and up columns of the matrix. Therefore, two reasonable possibilities for the toxicity orderings are

1. Across rows [$m = 1$]
   $R(d_{11}) < R(d_{12}) < R(d_{13}) < R(d_{14}) < R(d_{15}) < R(d_{16}) < \cdots$

2. Up columns [$m = 2$]
   $R(d_{11}) < R(d_{21}) < R(d_{12}) < R(d_{22}) < R(d_{13}) < R(d_{23}) < \cdots$

There are many ways to arrange the treatments according to the diagonals of the matrix. For the sake of simplicity and in order to reduce the dimension of the problem as much as possible, we are going to restrict possible movements along diagonals to "up" movements and "down" movements. These two movements would result in the following possible orderings of the DLT probabilities.

3. Up diagonals $[m = 3]$
   $$R(d_{11}) < R(d_{21}) < R(d_{12}) < R(d_{22}) < R(d_{13}) < R(d_{23}) < \cdots$$

4. Alternating down–up diagonals $[m = 4]$
   $$R(d_{11}) < R(d_{12}) < R(d_{21}) < R(d_{22}) < R(d_{13}) < R(d_{14}) < \cdots$$

5. Alternating up–down diagonals $[m = 5]$
   $$R(d_{11}) < R(d_{21}) < R(d_{12}) < R(d_{13}) < R(d_{22}) < R(d_{23}) < \cdots$$

The dimension of the problem makes it difficult to practically consider much more information than what we have captured in these orderings. We have a way of choosing a reasonable subset that is consistent with the partially known ordering information among dose–schedule combinations, and that is independent of the dimension of the matrix. The design outlined in the following sections can certainly accommodate a larger number of orderings, should we have more or less ordering information at our disposal. If, however, the only information we have is the assumption of a monotonicity across rows and up columns of the matrix, then we can use the subsequent method based on this "default" subset of orderings and have confidence in its performance.

7.2.2.2 Modeling toxicity

The CRM for partial orders is based on utilizing a class of working models that correspond to possible orderings of the toxicity probabilities for the combinations. Specifically, suppose that there are M possible orderings being considered. For a particular ordering m, we model the true probability of toxicity at dose–schedule combination d_{ij} via

$$R(d_{ij}) \approx \psi_m(d_{ij}, a) = [\alpha_{ij}(m)]^{\exp(a)},$$

where the $\alpha_{ij}(k)$ represents the skeleton of the model under working model m and $a \in (-\infty, \infty)$. There is little difference in the operating characteristics among the various model choices common to the CRM class, such as a hyperbolic tangent function or a one-parameter logistic model.

   We let the plausibility of each working model under consideration be described by a set of prior weights $\pi = \{\pi(1), \ldots, \pi(M)\}$, where $\pi(m) \geq 0$ and $\sum \pi(m) = 1$; $m = 1, \ldots, M$. Suppose that at a certain point in the trial, y_{ij} DLTs have been observed among the n_{ij} subjects treated on dose–schedule combination d_{ij}. Using the data for k included patients $\Omega_k = \{(y_{ij}, n_{ij}); i = 1, \ldots, I, j = 1, \ldots, J\}$, the likelihood under working model m is given by

$$\mathcal{L}_m(a | \Omega_k) = \prod_{i=1}^{I} \prod_{j=1}^{J} \left\{ [\alpha_{ij}(k)]^{\exp(a)} \right\}^{y_{ij}} \left\{ 1 - [\alpha_{ij}(k)]^{\exp(a)} \right\}^{n_{ij} - y_{ij}},$$

which, for each ordering, can be used to generate the maximum likelihood estimate (MLE), $\widehat{a}_m$, for the parameter a. Wages et al. [7] propose an escalation method that first chooses the ordering that maximizes the updated model weight

$$\omega(m) = \frac{\mathcal{L}_m(\widehat{a}_m \mid \Omega_i) \, \pi(m)}{\displaystyle\sum_{m=1}^{M} \mathcal{L}_m(\widehat{a}_m \mid \Omega_i) \, \pi(m)}$$

before each patient inclusion, where $\mathcal{L}_m(\widehat{a}_m \mid \Omega_i)$ is the value of the likelihood evaluated at $\widehat{a}_m$. The prior weights, π, for the working models are updated by the toxicity data Ω. It is expected that the more the data support working model m, the larger its posterior model probability will be. When a new patient is to be enrolled, we choose a single working model, $h \in \{1, \dots, M\}$, that maximizes the updated model weights such that

$$h = \arg \max_m \omega(m).$$

Given the ordering h and the working model $\psi_h(d_{ij}, \widehat{a}_h)$, we can generate DLT probability estimates at each dose–schedule combination. The posterior probability of a DLT is generated via

$$\widehat{R}(d_{ij}) = \psi_h(d_{ij}, \widehat{a}_h), \ i = 1, \dots, I; j = 1, \dots, J,$$

from which we can make allocation decisions for the next cohort of patients accrued to the study, according to the following dose-schedule-finding algorithm.

7.2.2.3   Dose-schedule-finding algorithm in Wages et al. [7]

Stage 1: Wages et al. [13] made the case for using an initial escalation stage in drug combination trials and discussed the need for a variant of the traditional escalation schemes due to the fact that, in partially ordered trials, the most appropriate dose to which the trial should escalate could consist of more than one treatment combination. In the first stage, we make use of "zoning" the matrix of dose–schedule combinations according to the diagonals of the matrix in Table 7.1. The trial could begin in the zone $Z_1 = \{d_{11}\}$ and the first cohort of patients be enrolled on this "lowest" combination. At the first observation of a toxicity in one of the patients, the first stage is closed and the second stage, which is model based, is opened. As long as no toxicities occur, cohorts of patients are examined at each dose within the currently occupied zone before escalating to the next highest zone. If d_{11} was tried and deemed "safe," the trial would escalate to zone $Z_2 = \{d_{12}, d_{21}\}$. If more than one dose is contained within a particular zone, we sample without replacement from the treatments available within the zone. Therefore, the next cohort is enrolled on a dose that is chosen randomly from d_{12} and d_{21}. Without randomization early in the trial, it is possible, based on a limited amount of data, for the allocation to get "stuck" at a suboptimal combination that happened to be tried first. Information on a combination that has yet to be tried can only ever be obtained through experimentation. Therefore, randomization allows us to gain information more broadly. The trial is not allowed to advance to zone $Z_3 = \{d_{13}, d_{22}\}$ in the first stage until a cohort of patients have been observed at both combinations in Z_2. This procedure continues until a toxicity is observed or all available zones have been exhausted. These zones are simply a mechanism for getting the trial underway with a conservative initial escalation scheme.

Stage 2: Once we have at least one DLT and one non-DLT, the modeling stage begins.

1. Based on the accumulated data from k patients Ω_k, the estimated toxicity probabilities $\widehat{R}(d_{ij})$ are obtained for all dose–schedule combinations being tested, based on the procedure described above.

2. The next entered patient is then allocated to the dose–schedule combination with estimated toxicity probability closest to the target rate so that $|\widehat{R}(d_{ij}) - \theta|$ is minimized.

3. The MTDS combination is defined as d_{ij}^* such that

$$d_{ij}^* = \arg \min_{ij} |\widehat{R}(d_{ij}) - \theta|.$$

The MTDS is d_{ij}^* which is recommended for the $(n + 1)$th patient after accruing a maximum sample size of n patients to the study.

7.3 Extension to Phase I–II Setting

In oncology, several preclinical and clinical studies have established a relationship between toxicity, as well as efficacy, and schedule [14–18]. A very useful example that emphasizes this association is described in Guo et al. [9]. The authors point out that Shah et al. [19] demonstrated that dasatinib for treating chronic myelogenous leukemia was developed using a suboptimal course of therapy. A 70-mg twice-daily dosing schedule, approved by the FDA in 2006, was initially used due to its relatively short half-life, in an attempt to obtain sustained kinase inhibition and minimal toxicity [19]. A subsequent phase III trial of dasatinib in 670 patients with chronic myelogenous leukemia showed that a once-daily administration demonstrated similar efficacy to the twice-daily regimen, but the once-daily regimen significantly reduced the occurrence of treatment-related adverse events, improving the safety profile of the treatment. This example emphasizes the impact of accounting for scheduling in phase I–II trials. The methods of Li et al. [8] and Guo et al. [9] aim to find an optimal dose–schedule combination based on toxicity and efficacy in the phase I–II setting.

7.3.1 Motivating application

The following method of Li et al. [8] is motivated by a phase I–II clinical trial of a kinase inhibitor in patients with acute leukemia, myelodysplastic syndromes, or chronic myeloid leukemia in blast phase. It has been shown that these diseases associate with unregulated kinase activity, making the kinase inhibitors an important option for hematologic malignancies [20]. The study objective was to investigate $J = 5$ dose levels of a kinase inhibitor given under $I = 2$ varying schedules. Schedule 1 is a 5-day administration with a 2-day rest per week for 6 weeks. Schedule 2 is a continuous 15-day administration with a 6-day rest per 21-day cycle for two cycles.

7.3.2 Method of Li et al. [8]

7.3.2.1 Probability models

The design of Li et al. [8] extends the dose-schedule-finding problem to two binary endpoints with the aim of finding an optimal combination, defined by tolerable toxicity and high efficacy. The authors assume that $Y_k = 1$ if patient k experiences DLT; 0 otherwise, and that $V_k = 1$ if patient k experiences an efficacious response; 0 otherwise. The probability of DLT (efficacy) at dose–schedule combination d_{ij} is denoted $R(d_{ij})$ $(Q(d_{ij}))$. A global cross-ratio model [21] for the bivariate toxicity/efficacy outcomes is specified. Let $P_{yv}(d_{ij}) = \Pr(Y_k = 1, V_k = 1 \mid d_{ij})$; $y, v = 0$, where 1 is the joint probability of toxicity and efficacy, and define the association between the two outcomes by

$$P(d_{ij}) = \frac{P_{00}(d_{ij})\, P_{11}(d_{ij})}{P_{01}(d_{ij})\, P_{10}(d_{ij})}.$$

We can use $R(d_{ij}), Q(d_{ij})$, and $P(d_{ij})$ to generate the cell probabilities $P_{yv}(d_{ij})$ via

$$
\begin{aligned}
P_{11}(d_{ij}) &= \begin{cases} (a_{ij} - \sqrt{a_{ij}^2 + b_{ij}})/\{2(P(d_{ij}) - 1\}, & P(d_{ij}) \neq 1 \\ R(d_{ij}) \times Q(d_{ij}), & P(d_{ij}) = 1, \end{cases} \\
P_{10}(d_{ij}) &= R(d_{ij}) - P_{11}(d_{ij}), \\
P_{01}(d_{ij}) &= Q(d_{ij}) - P_{11}(d_{ij}), \\
P_{00}(d_{ij}) &= 1 - R(d_{ij}) - Q(d_{ij}) + P_{11}(d_{ij}),
\end{aligned}
\tag{7.1}
$$

where $a_{ij} = 1 + (R(d_{ij}) + Q(d_{ij}))(P(d_{ij}) - 1)$ and $b_{ij} = -4P(d_{ij})(P(d_{ij}) - 1)R(d_{ij})Q(d_{ij})$. Furthermore, the authors define μ_{ij} and γ_{ij} such that

$$\mu(d_{ij}) = \text{logit}(R(d_{ij})) \quad \text{and} \quad \gamma(d_{ij}) = \text{logit}(Q(d_{ij})).$$

If we let $\boldsymbol{\mu} = (\mu(d_{11}), \dots, \mu(d_{I1}), \mu(d_{12}), \dots, \mu(d_{I2}))'$, $\boldsymbol{\gamma} = (\gamma(d_{11}), \dots, \gamma(d_{I1}), \gamma(d_{12}), \dots, \gamma(d_{I2}))'$, and $\boldsymbol{P} = (P(d_{11}), \dots, P(d_{I1}), P(d_{12}), \dots, P(d_{I2}))'$, then the contribution to the likelihood of patient k treated at d_{ij} is given by

$$L_k(\boldsymbol{\mu}, \boldsymbol{\gamma}, \boldsymbol{P}) = \{P_{00}(d_{ij})\}^{(1-y_k)(1-v_k)} \{P_{10}(d_{ij})\}^{y_k(1-v_k)}$$
$$= \{P_{01}(d_{ij})\}^{(1-y_k)v_k} \{P_{11}(d_{ij})\}^{y_k v_k} \tag{7.2}$$

where y_k and v_k are the observed toxicity/efficacy responses for the kth patient treated at d_{ij}. The full likelihood is given by $L(\boldsymbol{\mu}, \boldsymbol{\gamma}, \boldsymbol{P}) = \prod L_k(\boldsymbol{\mu}, \boldsymbol{\gamma}, \boldsymbol{P})$ for the first k patients entered. For prior elicitation, Li et al. [8] assume mutual independent normal distributions so that $\mu(d_{ij}) \sim N(0, \sigma_\mu^2)$, $\gamma(d_{ij}) \sim N(0, \sigma_\gamma^2)$, and $P(d_{ij}) \sim N(0, \sigma_P^2)$, where $\sigma_\mu^2, \sigma_\gamma^2$, and σ_P^2 are prior variances taking large values such as $\sigma_\mu^2 = \sigma_\gamma^2 = 10^4$ and $\sigma_\mu^2 = 10$.

Let t_1 and t_2 be the highest tried dose in Schedules 1 and 2, repsectively, at any point in the trial. Defining $\boldsymbol{\mu}(t_1 t_2) = (\mu(d_{11}), \dots, \mu(d_{t_1 1}), \mu(d_{12}), \dots, \mu(d_{t_2 2}))'$, $\boldsymbol{\gamma}(t_1 t_2) = (\gamma(d_{11}), \dots, \gamma(d_{t_1 1}), \gamma(d_{12}), \dots, \gamma(d_{t_2 2}))'$ and $\boldsymbol{P}(t_1 t_2) = (P(d_{11}), \dots, P(d_{t_1 1}), P(d_{12}), \dots, P(d_{t_2 2}))'$, the joint distribution is given by

$$f[\boldsymbol{\mu}(t_1 t_2), \boldsymbol{\gamma}(t_1 t_2), \boldsymbol{P}(t_1 t_2) | \text{Data}] \propto L(\boldsymbol{\mu}, \boldsymbol{\gamma}, \boldsymbol{P}) \pi[\boldsymbol{\mu}(t_1 t_2)] \pi[\boldsymbol{\gamma}(t_1 t_2)] \pi[\boldsymbol{P}(t_1 t_2)],$$

where $\pi[\cdot]$ are prior densities. Based on the joint posterior, all full conditionals for the Gibbs sampling can be derived, sampling from which can be achieved using adaptive rejection Metropolis sampling (ARMS) algorithm [22].

7.3.2.2 Bayesian isotonic transformation

The probabilities $R(d_{ij})$ and $Q(d_{ij})$, as well as the $\mu(d_{ij})$'s, are assumed to adhere to the order restrictions (i.e., across rows and up columns) described in the previous section. The proposed Bayesian isotonic transformation (BIT) of Li et al. [8] is an extension of Dunson and Neelon [23] to the matrix order setting [24]. Denote the set of tried dose–schedule combinations as $C = \{d_{ij} : i = 1, 2; j = 1, \dots, t_i\}$, and define an order $\preccurlyeq$ on C such that

$$d_{i_1 j_1} \preccurlyeq d_{i_2 j_2} \quad \text{if} \quad i_1 \leq i_2 \quad \text{and} \quad j_1 \leq j_2,$$

forming a partially ordered set C [11]. The isotonic regression $\tilde{\boldsymbol{\mu}}^*$ of $\tilde{\boldsymbol{\mu}}$ is an isotonic function that minimizes the weighted sum of squares

$$\sum_{d_{ij} \in C} w_{ij} (\tilde{\boldsymbol{\mu}} - \tilde{\boldsymbol{\mu}}^*)^2$$

provided that $\tilde{\boldsymbol{\mu}}_{i_1 j_1}^* \leq \tilde{\boldsymbol{\mu}}_{i_2 j_2}^*$ whenever $d_{i_1 j_1} \preccurlyeq d_{i_2 j_2}$. The w_{ij} are weights corresponding to the posterior precisions of $\mu(d_{ij})$. In order to calculate the isotonic regression $\tilde{\boldsymbol{\mu}}^*$, the authors apply the minimum lower sets algorithm (MLSA) [11]. The following computational algorithm is required in order to carry out the Li et al. [8] approach:

1. For each d_{ij}, generate samples from posterior distributions of (μ, γ, P) using the ARMS MCMC [22].

2. For each realization $\tilde{\boldsymbol{\mu}}$ from the unconstrained joint posterior distribution of $\boldsymbol{\mu}$ obtained in step 1, use MLSA to obtain the order-restricted posterior sample $\tilde{\boldsymbol{\mu}}^*$.

3. Obtain the order-restricted posterior samples of $R(d_{ij})$ using the transformation $\text{logit}^{-1}(\tilde{\mu}_{ij}^*)$. Similarly, compute $Q(d_{ij})$ and $P(d_{ij})$.

4. Obtain posterior samples of $R_{yv}(d_{ij})$ using the samples of $R(d_{ij}), Q(d_{ij})$, and $P(d_{ij})$ for $y, v = 0, 1$ via Equation 7.1.

7.3.2.3   Dose-schedule-finding algorithm in Li et al.

The dose-schedule-finding algorithm of Li et al. [8] is based on definitions of a target dose–schedule combination using specifications of an upper toxicity limit θ_T and a lower efficacy limit θ_E. Based on these specifications, the objective of the trial is to identify a dose–schedule combination that maximizes the posterior probability $\Pr[R(d_{ij}) \leq \theta_T, Q(d_{ij}) \geq \theta_E | \text{Data}]$. The allocation algorithm is also based on the following categories of dose–schedule combinations:

- d_{ij} has *negligible toxicity* if $\Pr[R(d_{ij}) \leq \theta_T | \text{Data}] > r_n$, where r_n is a chosen probability cutoff with a relatively large values (i.e., $r_n = 0.5$).

- d_{ij} has *acceptable toxicity* if $\Pr[R(d_{ij}) \leq \theta_T | \text{Data}] > r_a$, where r_a is a probability cutoff smaller than r_n (i.e., $r_a = 0.05$).

- d_{ij} has *unacceptable toxicity* if $\Pr[R(d_{ij}) \leq \theta_T | \text{Data}] \leq r_a$, where r_a is a chosen probability cutoff with relatively large values (i.e., $r_a = 0.5$).

- d_{ij} has *acceptable efficacy* $\Pr[Q(d_{ij}) \geq \theta_E | \text{Data}] > q_a$ for some small probability cutoff $q_a \in (0, 1)$.

- d_{ij} is **acceptable** if it has both acceptable toxicity *and* efficacy.

For example, in the motivating application [20] for the Li et al. [8] method, the upper toxicity limit and the lower efficacy limit were set to $\theta_T = \theta_E = 0.3$, with chosen probability cutoffs of $r_n = 0.5, r_a = 0.05$, and $q_a = 0.02$. Let $\mathcal{A}$ be the set of all acceptable dose–schedule combinations that have been tried such that

$$\mathcal{A} = \{d_{ij} : d_{ij} \text{ is acceptable}, 1 \leq j \leq t_i; i = 1, 2\}.$$

Let $\widehat{P}_{01}(d_{ij}) = \widehat{Q}(d_{ij}) - \widehat{P}_{11}(d_{ij})$ denote the estimate $P_{01}(d_{ij})$, where $\widehat{Q}(d_{ij})$ is the posterior mean of $Q(d_{ij})$ and $\widehat{P}_{11}(d_{ij})$ is a plug-in estimate of $P_{11}(d_{ij})$. The dose–schedule finding algorithm is as follows;

1. If d_{11} has unacceptable toxicity or the maximum sample size is exhausted, the trial is stopped. For a given schedule, a dose is never skipped. For a given dose, a schedule is never skipped. If $\mathcal{A}$ is empty, the trial is stopped.

2. The trial begins at d_{11}. If d_{11} has negligible toxicity, treat the next patient cohort at d_{12}.

3. In the case that $t_1 < J$ and $t_2 < J$,

   - If $d_{t_1 1}$ and $d_{t_2 2}$ both have negligible toxicity, the next patient cohort is treated at $d_{t_1+1,1}$ or $d_{t_2+1,2}$ with the larger posterior probability $\Pr[R(d_{t_i j}) \leq \theta_T | \text{Data}]$, $i = 1, 2$.

   - If only $d_{t_1 1}$ has negligible toxicity, the next cohort is assigned $d_{t_1+1,1}$. Rather, if only $d_{t_2 2}$ has negligible toxicity, the next cohort is assigned $d_{t_2+1,2}$.

   - If neither $d_{t_1 1}$ nor $d_{t_2 2}$ has negligible toxicity, the next patient cohort is treated at $d_{ij} \in \mathcal{A}$ with the largest value of $\widehat{P}_{01}(d_{ij})$.

4. In the case that $t_1 = J$ and $t_2 < J$, if $d_{t_2 2}$ has negligible toxicity, the next cohort is treated at $d_{t_2+1,2}$. Otherwise, the next patient cohort is treated at $d_{ij} \in \mathcal{A}$ with the largest value of $\widehat{P}_{01}(d_{ij})$.

5. In the case that $t_1 = t_2 = J$, the next cohort is treated at $d_{ij} \in \mathcal{A}$ with the largest value of $\widehat{P}_{01}(d_{ij})$.

6. At study conclusion, the $d_{ij} \in \mathcal{A}$ with the largest value of $\Pr\left[R(d_{ij}) \leq \theta_T, Q(d_{ij}) \geq \theta_E \mid \text{Data}\right]$ is recommended as the optimal dose–schedule combination.

7.3.3 Method of Guo et al. [9]

Li et al. [8] developed a method based on a strong assumption that a prolonged administration of the study drug would not increase the DLT probability in patients, an assumption that may not always hold [17]. The method of Guo et al. [9] is a phase I–II method that does not rely on such a strong ordering assumption. In general, dose-finding designs have been based on the assumption that both toxicity and efficacy increase as the dose increases, and the impact that varying schedules will have on the relationships is complex. It may be the case that, for the same total dose, a more frequent, or prolonged, administration could be associated with lower toxicity. Blomqvist et al. [15] demonstrated that, in the combination of fluorouracil, epirubicin, and cyclophosphamide, toxicity was decreased when the standard dosing regimen of every 4 weeks was divided into four weekly doses. Similar findings were made in Gyergyay et al. [18], yet Shah et al. [17] showed that a prolonged administration of dasatinib may lead to higher toxicity in patients with chronic-phase myelogeneous leukemia. Similar contradictions were found with regard to the complexity of efficacy–schedule relationships in Clark et al. [25] and Blomqvist et al. [15]. The authors [9] specify probability models that are based on a trinary outcome Y, rather than bivariate binary toxicity and efficacy. Let $Y = 0$ if no toxicity and no efficacy; $Y = 1$ if efficacy and no toxicity; and $Y = 2$ if toxicity. This specification renders an efficacious response irrelevant in the presence of an observed DLT.

7.3.3.1 Probability models

We let $R(d_{ij})$ denote the probability that $Y = 2$ (toxicity), and $P(d_{ij})$ the probability that $Y = 1$ (efficacy and no toxicity). Guo et al. [9] model a transformation of $R(d_{ij})$ and $P(d_{ij})$ such that

$$\phi_{ij} = \eta[R(d_{ij})], \quad \lambda_{ij} = \eta[P(d_{ij}) + R(d_{ij})],$$

in which $\eta(\cdot)$ is a transformation mapping $(0,1)$ to $(-\infty, \infty)$, such as a logit or probit transformation. Based on the complexity associated with the ordering of dose–schedule–toxicity and dose–schedule–efficacy relationships described above, Guo et al. [9] propose a flexible Bayesian dynamic model such that

$$\phi_{ij} \mid \phi_{i-1,j}, \zeta \sim N\{\phi_{i-1,j} + \zeta(d_j - d_{j-1}), \sigma^2\},$$

$$\phi_{1j} \sim N(\phi_{0j}, \sigma_0^2),$$

for $i = 2, \ldots, I$ and $j = 1, \ldots, J$, where $\zeta > 0$ denotes an "average" dose effect, σ^2 is a fixed variance, and ϕ_{0j} and σ_0^2 are hyperparameters. Rather than restricting the ordering on the dose–schedule effect, such as the monotonicity assumption of Li et al. [8], this Bayesian dynamic model is more flexible in the sense that it relaxes this assumption. In modeling λ_{ij}, the authors rely on a proportional odds model framework:

$$\lambda_{ij} = \delta + \phi_{ij},$$

where $\delta > 0$. In this framework, if a dose–schedule combination has a larger toxicity probability than another combination, then it also has a larger probability of efficacy or toxicity, a relationship that holds after transforming $\eta^{-1}(\cdot)$. The authors note that $\eta^{-1}(\phi_{ij}) = R(d_{ij}) = \Pr(Y > 1|\, d_{ij})$ and $\eta^{-1}(\lambda_{ij}) = P(d_{ij}) + R(d_{ij}) = \Pr(Y > 0|\, d_{ij})$. The method of Guo et al. [9] utilizes the probit transformation $\eta(\cdot) = \Phi^{-1}(\cdot)$ in order to lean on the sampling method of Albert and Chib [26] for the posteriors of unknown parameters.

Suppose that we have data in the form Data $= \{y_1, \ldots, y_n\}$ after n patients have been entered onto the trial. Suppose that the kth entered patient is administered $d_{i_k j_k}$ and let $\phi = \phi_{ij}$. The resulting likelihood is

$$L(\phi, \delta; \text{Data}) = \prod_{k=1}^{n} [\mathbf{1}(y_k = 0)\{1 - \Phi(\delta + \phi_{i_k j_k})\}\mathbf{1}(y_k = 1)\{\Phi(\delta + \phi_{i_k j_k})$$
$$- \Phi(\phi_{i_k j_k})\} + \mathbf{1}(y_k = 2)\Phi(\phi_{i_k j_k})]. \tag{7.3}$$

Prior distributions for δ and ζ are represented through $g(\delta)$ and $g(\zeta)$, respectively. The posterior distribution of $\Theta = (\phi, \delta, \zeta)$ is

$$f(\Theta|\, \text{Data}) \propto L(\phi, \delta; \text{Data})g(\delta)\, g(\zeta),$$

sample forms which are obtained via the Gibbs sampler.

7.3.3.2   Dose-schedule-finding algorithm in Guo et al. [9]

The overall allocation strategy in Guo et al. [9] is to assign patients to dose–schedule combinations that are safe and efficacious. The dose-schedule-finding algorithm, like that of Li et al. [8], is based on definitions of a target dose–schedule combination using specifications of an upper toxicity limit θ_T and a lower efficacy limit θ_E. Specifically, the following definitions of *acceptable* toxicity and efficacy apply to dose–schedule combination d_{ij}:

- d_{ij} has *acceptable toxicity* if $\xi_T(d_{ij}) = \Pr[R(d_{ij}) \leq \theta_T|\, \text{Data}] > p_{2n}$, where $p_{2n} \in (0, 1)$ is a probability cutoff that depends on n.
- d_{ij} has *acceptable efficacy* $\xi_E(d_{ij}) = \Pr[P(d_{ij}) \geq \theta_E|\, \text{Data}] > p_{1n}$ for some probability cutoff $p_{1n} \in (0, 1)$ that depends on n.
- d_{ij} is *admissible* if it has both acceptable toxicity *and* efficacy.

Guo et al. [9] allow the cutoffs to be adaptive, taking on more liberal values early in the study when limited data exist, and more conservative values in the latter stages of the trial when more information has accumulated. Let n_m denote the minimum sample size at which to start implementing the above acceptability criteria, N the maximum sample size, and n the number of patients currently accrued to the study. The authors propose the following adaptive cutoffs for toxicity and efficacy:

$$p_{ln} = p_{la} + \frac{n - n_m}{N - n_m}(p_{lb} - p_{la}),$$

where $0 < p_{la} < p_{lb} < 1$, $l = 1, 2$, and the value p_{ln} linearly increases from p_{la} to p_{lb} as the sample size n increases from n_m to N.

Let $\mathcal{A}_n$ denote the set of all admissible dose–schedule combinations that have been tried in the study.

1. When escalating, a dose is never skipped under a given schedule.

2. Assign a cohort to the lowest dose under each schedule; i.e., d_{i1}; $i = 1, \ldots, I$. If the lowest dose for all schedules is too toxic, the trial is terminated for safety. The I cohorts can be randomized in several appropriate ways. For instance, single patients could be randomized to combination d_{i1} until the cohort size c patients have been accrued to each combination d_{i1}; $i = 1, \ldots, I$. Guo et al. [9] define $n_m = cI$, which is the product of the cohort size c and the number of schedules I.

3. If $\mathcal{A}_n$ is empty, the trial is terminated and declared inconclusive. If the highest tried doses under all schedules are either J or are considered too toxic, the next patient cohort is treated at $d_{ij} \in \mathcal{A}$ with the largest value of $\xi_E(d_{ij})$.

4. Otherwise, there are $s\,(1 \le s \le I)$ schedules within which the highest tried doses j_s have acceptable toxicity. In this case, the dose shall be escalated to the next highest dose $j_s + 1$ within that schedule. We then must choose among schedules, so we randomize to the dose–schedule combination d_{i,j_s+1}, with probability

$$\frac{\xi_E(d_{i,j_s+1})}{\sum \xi_E(d_{i,j_s+1})}.$$

5. The trial is stopped when N patients have been accrued to the study. The $d_{ij} \in \mathcal{A}$ with the largest value of $\xi_E(d_{ij})$ is recommended as the optimal dose–schedule combination.

7.4 Conclusion

This chapter presented methodology for identifying optimal dose–schedule combinations in early-phase oncology trials. The method of Wages et al. [7] is for use when attempting to find a MTDS combination based on safety considerations using a binary toxicity endpoint. The methods of Li et al. [8] and Guo et al. [9] are intended for trials investigating bivariate binary (toxicity/efficacy) outcomes, with the aim of estimating an optimal dose–schedule combination that is both safe and efficacious. Besides the differences in trial objectives for the phase I method and the phase I–II methods, there are also striking differences in their approach to the dose-finding problem. Wages et al. [7] take an "underparameterized" approach, making use of a class of single-parameter "CRM-like" models, and relying on Bayesian model choice to select the most appropriate model. The methods of Li et al. [8] and Guo et al. [9] employ additional parameters in an attempt to increase flexibility and model the entire dose–schedule response surface. The added mathematical complexity in using the more flexible models utilized in the phase I–II methods may hinder the implementation of these methods in practice.

References

1. T. M. Braun, Z. Yuan, and P. F. Thall. Determining a maximum-tolerated schedule of a cytotoxic agent. *Biometrics*, 61:335–343, 2013.

2. T. M. Braun, P. F. Thall, H. Q. Nguyen, and M. de Lima. Simultaneously optimizing dose and schedule of a new cytotoxic agent. *Clinical Trials*, 4:113–124, 2007.

3. C. A. Liu and T. M. Braun. Parametric non-mixture cure models for schedule finding of therapeutic agents. *Journal of the Royal Statistical Society: Series C (Applied Statistics)*, 58:225–236, 2009.

4. P. F. Thall, H. Q. Nguyen, T. M. Braun, and M. H. Qazilbash. Using joint utilities of the times to response and toxicity to adaptively optimize schedule dose regimes. *Biometrics*, 69:673–682, 2013.

5. J. Zhang and T. M. Braun. A phase I Bayesian adaptive design to simultaneously optimize dose and schedule assignments both between and within patients. *Journal of American Statistical Association*, 108:892–901, 2013.

6. M. de Lima, S. Giralt, P. F. Thall, L. de Padua Silva, U. Popat, C. Hosing, X. Wang, E. J. Shpall, R. B. Jones, M. Qazilbash, G. McCormick, B. S. Andersson, K. Komanduri, A. Alousi, A. Gulbis, T. M. Braun, H. Q. Nguyen, P. Kebriaei, R. Champlin, and G. Garcia-Manero. Maintenance therapy with low dose azacitidine after allogenic hematopoietic stem cell transplantation for recurrent acute myelogenous leukemia or myelodysplastic syndrome: A dose and schedule finding study. *Cancer*, 116:5420–5431, 2010.

7. N. A. Wages, J. O'Quigley, and M. R. Conaway. Phase I design for completely or partially ordered treatment schedules. *Statistics in Medicine*, 33:569–579, 2013.

8. Y. Li, B. N. Bekele, Y. Ji, and J. D. Cook. Dose-schedule finding in phase I/II clinical trials using a Bayesian isotonic transformation. *Statistics in Medicine*, 27:4895–4913, 2008.

9. B. Guo, Y. Li, and Y. Yuan. A dose-schedule finding design for phase I–II clinical trials. *Journal of the Royal Statistical Society: Series C (Applied Statistics)*, 65:259–272, 2016.

10. C. Graux, A. Sonet, J. Maertens, J. Duyster, J. Greiner, Y. Chalandon, G. Martinelli, D. Hess, D. Heim, F. J. Giles, K. R. Kelly, A. Gianella-Borradori, B. Longerey, E. Asatiani, N. Rejeb, and O. G. Ottman. A phase I dose-escalation study of MSC1992371A, an oral inhibitor of aurora and other kinases, in advanced hematologic malignancies. *Leukemia Research*, 37:1100–1106, 2013.

11. T. Robertson, F. T. Wright, and R. Dykstra. *Order Restricted Statistical Inference*. John Wiley and Sons, New York, 1988.

12. N. A. Wages and M. R. Conaway. Specifications of a continual reassessment method for phase I trials of combined drugs. *Pharmaceutical Statistics*, 12:217–224, 2013.

13. N. A. Wages, M. R. Conaway, and J. O'Quigley. Continual reassessment method for partial ordering. *Biometrics*, 67:1555–1563, 2011.

14. M. L. Slevin, P. I. Clark, S. P. Joel, S. Malik, R. J. Osborne, W. Gregory, D. G. Lowe, R. H. Reznek, and P. F. W. Wrigley. A randomized trial to evaluate the effect of schedule on the activity of etoposide in small-cell lung cancer. *Journal of Clinical Oncology*, 7:1333–1340, 1989.

15. C. Blomqvist, I. Elomaa, P. Rissanen, P. Hietanen, K. Nevassari, and L. Helle. Influence of treatment schedule on toxicity and efficacy of cyclophosphamide, epirubicin, and fluorouracil in metastatic breast cancer: A randomized trial comparing weekly and every-4-week administration. *Journal of Clinical Oncology*, 11:467–473, 1993.

16. R. Gervais, A. Ducolone, J. L. Breton, D. Braun, B. Lebeau, F. Vaylet, D. Debieuvre, J. L. Pujol, J. Tredaniel, P. Clouet, and E. Quoix. Phase II randomized trial comparing docetaxel given every 3 weeks with weekly schedule as second-line therapy in patients with advanced non-small-cell lung cancer (NSCLC). *Annals of Oncology*, 16:90–96, 2005.

17. N. P. Shah, H. M. Kantarjian, D.-W. Kim, D. Rea, P. E. Dorlhiac-Llacer, J. H. Milone, C. Nicaise, J. Vela-Ojeda, R. T. Silver, H. J. Khoury, A. Charbonnier, N. Khoroshko, R. L. Paquette, M. Deininger, R. H. Collins, I. Otero, T. Hughes, E. Bleickardt, L. Strauss, S. Francis, and A. Hochhaus. Intermittent target inhibition with dasatinib 100 mg once daily preserves efficacy and improves tolerability in imatinib-resistant and -intolerant chronic-phase chronic myeloid leukemia. *Journal of Clinical Oncology*, 26:3204–3212, 2008.

18. R. Gyergyay, K. Nagyvanyi, I. Bodrogi, and Hungary National Institute of Oncology, Budapest. Decreased toxicity schedule of sunitinib in renal cell cancer: 2 weeks on/1 week off. *Journal of Clinical Oncology*, 27:suppl, abstract e16113, 2009.

19. N. P. Shah, C. Kasap, C. Weier, M. Balbas, J. M. Nicoll, E. Bleickardt, C. Nicaise, and C. L. Sawyers. Transient potent BCR-ABL inhibition is sufficient to commit chronic myeloid leukemia cells irreversibly to apoptosis. *Cancer Cell*, 14:485–493, 2008.

20. J.-P. J. Issa, G.-M. Guillermo, F. J. Giles, R. Mannari, D. Thomas, S. Faderl, E. Bayar, J. Lyons, C. S. Rosenfeld, J. Cortes, and H. M. Kantarjian. Phase I study of low-dose prolonged exposure schedules of the hypomethylating agent 5-aza-2′-deoxycytidine (decitabine) in hematopoietic malignancies. *Blood*, 103:1635–1640, 2004.

21. Dale J. R. Global cross-ratio models for bivariate, discrete, ordered responses. *Biometrics*, 42:909–917, 1986.

22. W. R. Gilks, N. G. Best, and K. K. C. Tan. Adaptive rejection Metropolis sampling within Gibbs sampling. *Journal of the Royal Statistical Society: Series C (Applied Statistics)*, 44:455–472, 1995.

23. S. Dunbar and S. Peddada. Bayesian inference on order-constrained parameters in generalized linear models. *Biometrics*, 59:286–295, 2003.

24. M. Conaway, S. Dunbar, and S. Peddada. Designs for single- or multiple-agent phase I trials. *Biometrics*, 60:661–669, 2004.

25. P. I. Clark, M. L. Slevin, S. P. Joel, R. J. Osborne, D. I. Talbot, P. W. Johnson, R. Reznek, T. Masud, W. Gregory, and P. F. W. Wrigley. A randomized trial of two etoposide schedules in small-cell lung cancer: The influence of pharmacokinetics on efficacy and toxicity. *Journal of Clinical Oncology*, 12:1427–1435, 1994.

26. J. H. Albert and S. Chib. Bayesian analysis of binary and ploytomous response data. *Journal of American Statistical Association*, 88:669–679, 1993.

8

Patient Heterogeneity in Dose-Finding Trials

Mark R. Conaway

University of Virginia

CONTENTS

8.1 Patient Heterogeneity

In some dose-finding trials, there are several groups of patients, and the goal is to estimate a maximally tolerated dose (MTD) within each group. These groups may be defined by the patients' degree of impairment at baseline [9, 16], amount of pre-treatment [17], or genetic characteristics [6]. For example, Ramanathan et al. [16] enrolled 89 patients with varying solid tumors to develop dosing guidelines for the administration of imatinib in patients with liver dysfunction. Prior to dosing, patients were stratified into none, mild, moderate, or severe liver dysfunction at baseline, according to serum total bilirubin and AST. A similar classification is used by LoRusso et al. [9]. Kim et al. [6] define three groups of patients according to the number of defective alleles, either 0, 1, or 2. In each of these cases, parallel phase I studies were conducted within each group, but they did not account for the expectation that the MTD would be lower in the more severely impaired patients at baseline, or in the subset of patients with a greater number of defective alleles. In these cases, even with an efficient design, with the sample sizes typically seen in phase I trials, ignoring the orderings among the groups can lead to reversals in the MTD estimates, meaning that the estimated MTDs in the groups can contradict what is known clinically. For example, the parallel designs might recommend a greater dose level as the MTD in the most severely impaired group compared to a less severely impaired group. Even in cases where the ordering is not known, running parallel studies can be inefficient compared to a design that uses a model to pool information from all patients across all groups in order to estimate the dose–toxicity relationship.

An example of a dose-finding study in groups is given in Ref. [21]. In the actual study, both measures of toxicity and efficacy were considered, and the dose levels under consideration differed between the groups. A simplified version of the study serves as an example. In the simplified version, there are two groups of patients, those with a poor prognosis and those with a good prognosis; toxicity is the only endpoint; and there are four doses of radiation in each group.

TABLE 8.1

An example of four doses in two ordered groups.

Group	Prognosis	Dose			
		8	10	12.5	15
2	Poor	π_{21}	π_{22}	π_{23}	π_{24}
1	Good	π_{11}	π_{12}	π_{13}	π_{14}

π denotes the probability of DLT at each group-dose combination.

O'Quigley and Paoletti [13] and O'Quigley, Shen, and Gamst [15] were the first to investigate the consequences of using parallel trials. More recently, Raphael et al. [17] discussed the use of parallel trials of heavily and lightly pretreated patients in dose-finding trials in pediatrics. Using data from a dose-finding study of irinotecan to guide the simulations, they generated parallel group trials under the assumptions ranging from no difference to a large difference in the dose–toxicity curves between the groups. They also used varied sample sizes, from 20 to 60 patients in each of the two groups. In their simulations, the single-agent continual reassessment method (CRM) [14] was conducted independently within each group. In the case of the same dose–toxicity curve between groups, the independent CRM designs found different MTDs in the two groups: 37% of the time for 60 patients per group, and increasing to 68% of the time for 20 patients per group. When there were differences between the groups, the parallel groups approach incorrectly identified the same MTD or a reversal in the MTD estimates a substantial fraction of the time. Based on these results, Raphael et al. [17] recommended that parallel trials can only be undertaken when there is a strong rationale for doing so (Table 8.1).

It is important to note that the simulation results in Ref. [17] were not based on any of the methods that will be discussed in this chapter, namely methods that explicitly account for known orderings between the groups. The simulations do, however, reflect the way that studies in heterogeneous groups of patients are being conducted at present.

To avoid the issues with running parallel groups, a number of statistical methods have been proposed for estimating MTDs when there is heterogeneity among patients. All of these methods proposed to date for dose-finding, accounting for patient heterogeneity, are generalizations of model-based methods for single-agent trials. The methods can be broadly classified as those that incorporate heterogeneity by using additional parameters in the model, or as those based on order-restricted inference, either alone or in combination with fully or underparametrized parametric models. With few exceptions, the statistical methods are developed for a binary measure of toxicity, denoted by Y, with $Y = 1$ indicating that the patient experienced a dose-limiting toxicity and $Y = 0$ otherwise. The target "acceptable" toxicity rate is denoted by θ. A set of K pre-specified doses are under consideration, $d_1, \ldots, d_K$, ordered with respect to the probability of toxicity, and patient characteristics are denoted by a m $\times$ 1 vector of covariate values z. In many cases, the patient characteristic is membership in one of G groups, and z is a set of indicator variables $(z_2, \ldots, z_G)$, with $z_g = 1$ if the patient is in group g, and $z_g = 0$ otherwise, for $g = 2, \ldots, G$. The probability of toxicity for a patient with characteristics z given dose d_i is

$$\Pr\left(Y = 1 \,|\, d_i, z, \beta\right) = \psi(d_i, \beta, z) \tag{8.1}$$

The likelihood, after l patients have been observed, is given by

$$L(\beta) = \prod_{i=1}^{l} \left[\psi(d_i, \beta, z)^{y_i} \left([1 - \psi(d_i, \beta, z)]^{(1-y_i)} \right) \right] \tag{8.2}$$

8.2 Modeling Heterogeneity via Additional Parameters

O'Quigley, Shen, and Gamst [15] proposed a generalization of the CRM [14] for two groups. The authors consider a number of models, one of which is a generalization of the CRM power model [14]:

$$\psi(d_i, a, b) = \alpha_i^{\exp(a+bz_2)}, \quad i = 1, \ldots, K \tag{8.3}$$

with prespecified values $0 < \alpha_1 < \cdots < \alpha_K < 1$, $-\infty < a < \infty$, and $-\infty < b < \infty$ and z_2 is a binary group indicator equal to 1 for a patient in group 2 and 0 for a patient in group 1. In group 1, the probability of a DLT at dose level k is $\alpha_k^{\exp(a)}$; in group 2, the probability is $\alpha_k^{\exp(a+b)}$. The parameter b governs the difference in the toxicity probabilities between groups; a value of $b = 0$ means no group effect. It is possible to induce an ordering in the groups by an appropriate constraint, such as $b > 0$, or by specifying an appropriate prior distribution for the parameter b. As data accumulated through the trial, estimates of a and b can be obtained either by maximum likelihood [19] or by using the means or medians of the posterior distributions of a and b. The estimates $\hat{a}$ and $\hat{b}$ yield estimates of the toxicity probabilities at each dose d_i in each group, $\hat{\psi}(d_i, a, b)$. If the next patient is from group g, the patient is assigned to the dose level d with an estimated toxicity probability that is closest to the prespecified target probability of toxicity, θ.

O'Quigley and Paoletti [13] consider a two-group version of the CRM in which the ordering of the group is known. The proposed designs are two-stage designs [19] with the first stage consisting of a rule-based escalation until there is heterogeneity in toxicity outcomes in each of the two groups. Several possible first-stage designs are considered, including independent escalation in each group until a toxicity is observed or pooling the groups, assuming that there is no group difference. An alternative design is a rule-based escalation that respects the known ordering in the groups. For example, supposing that patients in group 2 are known to be more susceptible to DLTs at a given dose than patients in group 1, a restriction could be imposed such that the current dose in group 2 is never more than the current dose in group 1.

Once at least one toxicity and one nontoxicity have been observed in each group, dose allocation proceeds as in Ref. [15] using model (8.3), with a noninformative prior on a. A "known ordering of unknown magnitude" can be incorporated through the prior distribution on b, using a gamma or normal model with mean μ_b and variance σ_b^2. The ordering can be rigidly imposed by choosing the prior for b to have support only on negative values, but O'Quigley and Paoletti recommend that some flexibility be allowed even in the case of strong prior beliefs. The prior for b could be chosen to have only a small amount of weight on positive values and a large part of the prior weight on negative values, reflecting a strong belief in the ordering, but the data could override the prior in the event that the assumed ordering was incorrect.

This paper also discusses estimation for "known orderings of known magnitude" in which the investigators have reason to believe that the difference in the MTDs between the groups is Δ levels. One way to incorporate this belief into the design is to choose skeleton values $\alpha_1, \ldots, \alpha_K$ such that

$$\ln \ln \alpha_{i-\Delta} - \ln \ln \alpha_i = \mu_b \tag{8.4}$$

The prior variance σ_b^2 can be used to express the strength of the prior belief that the MTDs differ by Δ levels. For either an ordering with known or unknown magnitude, once the second stage begins, model (8.3) is used to estimate the toxicity probabilities in each group, and patients are allocated sequentially to the dose nearest to the target θ.

Model (8.3) used in Refs. [15, 13] can be thought of as adding a parameter to account for patient heterogeniety to the power model for the CRM, a method for a single-agent trial with no heterogeneity among patients. This idea of accounting for heterogeneity by adding parameters to a "single agent, no heterogeneity model" is the basis of several proposed methods. Babb and Rogatko [1] extend the "escalation with overdose control" (EWOC) method [2] to allow for a continuous covariate to the original version of EWOC. The original method assumes that the true MTD is in the interval $[X_{\min}, X_{\max}]$ and is based on a two-parameter model for the probability of a DLT at dose $x \in [X_{\min}, X_{\max}]$:

$$P(DLT|dose = x) = F(\beta_0 + \beta_1 x) \tag{8.5}$$

where F is a distribution function and $\beta_1 > 0$ so that the probability of a DLT is increasing in x. A prior distribution is assumed for the pair of parameters (β_0, β_1). The first patient is assigned dose $X_{\min}$, and the dose for the jth patient is derived from the posterior distribution of (β_0, β_1), combining the prior on (β_0, β_1) and the likelihood based on the binary responses and dose allocations from the previous $j - 1$ patients. The posterior distribution on (β_0, β_1) can be written in terms of the posterior distribution on (p_0, γ), where p_0 is the probability of a DLT at dose $X_{\min}$ and γ is the MTD. Integrating over p_0 yields the marginal posterior CDF of the MTD:

$$G(\gamma|Dj - 1) = \text{Prob}(MTD \leq \gamma \mid D_{j-1}) \tag{8.6}$$

where D_{j-1} denotes all of the data up to and including patient $j - 1$. If all doses between $X_{\min}$ and $X_{\max}$ could be used, the next patient would go on the dose x such that $G(x|D_{j-1}) = \alpha$, where α is a prespecified tolerance for overdosing. That is, the patient is allocated to the dose x such that the posterior probability that the dose exceeds the MTD is equal to α. In the more practical case where a set of discrete doses $d_1, d_2, \ldots, d_K$ between $X_{\min}$ and $X_{\max}$ are available for study, the jth patient would be allocated to the discrete dose that is sufficiently close to the continuous dose choice and where the probability of an overdose is sufficiently close to α:

$$\max_{d_1, d_2, \ldots, d_K} : d_k - x \leq T_1 \quad \text{and} \quad G(d_k|D_{j-1}) - \alpha \leq T_2 \tag{8.7}$$

where T_1 and T_2 are prespecified constants. At the end of the trial, the MTD is chosen as the value that minimizes the expected loss with respect to the posterior distribution of the MTD. This loss is taken as an asymmetric loss function, penalizing overdosing more than underdosing.

In the extension to include a covariate, c, the dose–toxicity model is

$$LOGIT(\psi(d_i, \beta)) = \beta_0 + \beta_1 \ln(d_i) + \beta_2 LN(c) \tag{8.8}$$

with $\beta_1 > 0$, so that for fixed levels of the covariate c, increasing doses are associated with an increasing probability of toxicity. In their application, the covariate c was protective, with increasing levels of the covariate associated with a lower probability of a DLT, $\beta_2 < 0$. Data from a previous study of the agent allowed the investigators to set bounds on the permissible doses for a patient with covariate value c. The previous data also allowed, after transforming the model parameters to aid in interpretation, the specification of a prior distribution for the transformed parameters. As in the original EWOC, the posterior distributions of the transformed parameters are computed from the prior information from the previous study and the data that accumulate as the trial progresses. From these posterior distributions, the investigators can derive the posterior distribution of the MTD as a function of c. The next patient, with covariate value c, is assigned to the dose that minimizes the posterior expected loss with respect to a loss function that penalizes toxicity probabilities greater than the target θ, more than toxicity probabilities less than the target. In this method, patients can receive individualized doses according to their level of the covariate value c.

Tighiouart, Cook-Wiens, and Rogatko [20] took a similar approach, incorporating a binary covariate into the EWOC method. If z is a binary covariate, their model is the same as (8.8),

$$\text{logit}(\psi(d_i, \beta)) = \beta_0 + \beta_1 \ln(d_i) + \beta_2 z \tag{8.9}$$

Under model (8.9), the MTD for a population of patients with covariate value z, denoted $\gamma(z)$, is given by

$$\gamma(z) = \frac{\text{logit}(\theta) - \beta_0 - \beta_2 z}{\beta_1} \tag{8.10}$$

Model (8.9) is reparametrized in terms of $\gamma(0)$, $\gamma(1)$, and $p_{0,0}$, where $p_{0,0}$ is the toxicity probability at the lowest dose in the group defined by $z = 0$. The paper shows the transformation from the parameters $(\beta_0, \beta_1, \beta_2)$ to $(\gamma(0), \gamma(1), p_{0,0})$ and derives the likelihood in terms of $(\gamma(0), \gamma(1), p_{0,0})$. Data from previous studies are used to select priors for the transformed parameters, and posterior distributions for these parameters are found by combining the likelihood from the accumulated data with the prior. After l patients have been evaluated, the posterior cdf for the MTD in the group with covariate z is denoted by $\Pi_{z,l}$. The next, $l + 1$, patient with covariate value z is assigned to the dose closest to $\Pi_{z,l}^{-1}(f)$, where f is a prespecified feasibility bound, an upper limit on the probability that a patient will be assigned to a dose above the MTD.

The EWOC-based methods [1, 20] transform the parameters of a logit model to allow for simpler elicitation of the prior information. Legedza and Ibrahim [7] derive a dose-finding design under a general form of the dose–toxicity model and a data-based prior. With a $p \times 1$ vector z of patient covariates, the probability of a DLT at dose d_i is given by

$$\Pr\left(Y = 1 \,|\, d_i, z, \beta\right) = \Psi(\eta_z) \tag{8.11}$$

where $\Psi()$ is an inverse link function for links such as the logit or complementary log–log link, and $\eta_z = \beta_0 + \beta_1 d_i + \beta_2' z$. The use of data D_0 from previous studies is proposed as the prior, where D_0 consists of n_0 observations on toxicity, a $n_0 \times 1$ vector y_0 of binary indicators for toxicity from dose levels, and covariates d_0, X_0. The prior has the form

$$\pi(\beta_0, \beta_1, \beta_2') = \prod_{i=1}^{n_0} \left[\Psi(\eta_{zi})^{y_{0i}} \left([1 - \Psi(\eta_{zi})]^{(1-y_{0i})} \right) \right]^{a_0} \tag{8.12}$$

where a_0 is a tuning parameter, $0 \le a_0 \le 1$, which reflects how much weight the prior data should have in the current study. Combining the prior (8.12) with the likelihood (8.2) based on l observed patients, Legedza and Ibrahim compute the posterior expectations of β_0, β_1, and β_2'. The next patient, with covariate values z, is assigned to the dose closest to the solution of

$$\theta = \psi(d, z, \beta_0^*, \beta_1^*, \beta_2'^*) \tag{8.13}$$

where $(\beta_0^*, \beta_1^*, \beta_2'^*)$ are the posterior expectations of $(\beta_0, \beta_1, \beta_2')$. Bailey et al. [3] present a case study of dose-finding with covariates that has many of the features of the method in Ref. [7]. They use a logit model for the dose–toxicity curve, and the covariate z in Equation 8.11 is used to distinguish three groups of patients. The approaches of Refs. [3] and [7] differ in their specification of the prior; Bailey et al. use normal and log-normal priors for the parameters in (8.11).

All of the above methods account for heterogeneity by adding covariates to models that would be used in designs in which patient heterogeniety is not taken into account.

TABLE 8.2

Skeleton values in group 2.

Δ	d_1	d_2	d_3	d_4	d_5	d_6
			$\alpha_{i(\Delta)}$			
0	0.2	0.3	0.5	0.7	0.8	0.9
1	0.1	0.2	0.3	0.5	0.7	0.8
2	0.05	0.1	0.2	0.3	0.5	0.7
3	0.025	0.05	0.1	0.2	0.3	0.5

The "shift model," described in Refs. [10, 11] and developed more fully in Ref. [12], takes a different approach to generalizing the CRM to two ordered groups. The assumption underlying this method is that the MTD in group 2 will be Δ dose levels less than that in group 1, with $\Delta = 0, 1, 2, \ldots, K$. O'Quigley and Iasonos [12] restrict Δ to be 0, 1, 2, or 3 levels, but their method applies to any shift in the MTD. It is more convenient to write the model for the DLT probabilities in terms of the log probabilities:

$$\log \psi(d_i, a, \Delta) = \exp(a) \log \alpha_{i(\Delta)}, \alpha_{i(\Delta)} = I(z = 0)\alpha_i + I(z = 1)h_i(\Delta) \qquad (8.14)$$

where $0 < \alpha_1 < \cdots < \alpha_K < 1$ and

$$h_i(\Delta) = \alpha_{i-\Delta}I(1 + \Delta \leq i \leq K) + (\alpha_i/2)I(i = \Delta > 0)$$
$$+ (\alpha_i/4)I(i = \Delta - 1 > 0) + (\alpha_i/8)I(i = \Delta - 2 > 0), \Delta = 0, 1, 2, 3$$

As displayed in Table 8.2, with $K = 6$ dose levels, and $\alpha_1, \ldots, \alpha_6$ chosen as $(0.2, 0.3, 0.5, 0.7, 0.8, 0.9)$, there are several skeletons for the toxicity probabilities in group 2. A discrete uniform prior can be put on the values of Δ, or the prior can put unequal weight on the possible values of Δ. For example, greater prior probability can be put on $\Delta = 0$, reflecting a greater belief that the MTD is the same rather than different in the two groups. Either an informative or a noninformative prior can be used for a. After l patients have been observed, the posterior mode provides estimates of a and Δ, and estimates of the DLT probabilities in each of the groups. The next patient, from group g, is allocated to the dose level with the group-specific toxicity probability closest to the target (Table 8.2).

O'Quigley and Iasonos discuss the use of this method for studies done in groups of patients, or in "bridging" studies, in which a dose-finding trial has been completed in one population, and a subsequent dose-finding trial is conducted in a different population. Liu et al. [8] present a method for bridging studies in different ethnic populations using model (8.14), phrased in terms of multiple skeletons.

The previous methods used elements of order-restricted inference, for example, in some cases, parameter estimates were constrained to be greater than 0. Similarly, the methods of Ivanova and Wang [5] and Yuan and Chappell [22] explicitly use isotonic regression methods [18], alone or in combination with parametric models, to allow for patient heterogeneity.

Ivanova and Wang [5] use two-dimensional isotonic regression to estimate dose–toxicity probabilities in G ordered groups. The probability of a DLT at dose d_i in group $g, g = 1, \ldots, G$ is denoted by $\psi(d_i, g)$. Ivanova and Wang assume that $\psi(d_i, g) \leq \psi(d_{i'}, g)$ for $i < i'$ and $\psi(d_i, g) \leq \psi(d_i, g')$ for $g < g'$. The design is a two-stage design, with the first stage being a rule-based design that respects the ordering in the groups [13]. The second stage begins when at least one DLT and one non-DLT are observed in each group. In the second stage, the bivariate isotonic regression estimate is computed with the algorithm described in Ref. [18] to obtain toxicity probability estimates that follow the order constraints. Once these estimates are obtained, dose allocation for the next patient in group g proceeds as follows: if the current dose in group g is denoted by (d_j, g), the next patient receives dose

d_{j+1} if $\hat{\psi}(d_j, g) < \theta - \delta$, dose d_j if $\theta - \delta < \hat{\psi}(d_j, g) < \theta + \delta$, and dose d_{j-1} if $\hat{\psi}(d_j, g) \geq \theta + \delta$, where δ is a design parameter chosen prior to the study. Estimation and dose allocations continue until a prespecified number of patients have been observed.

Ivanova and Wang also consider the possibility of estimation for two unordered groups. In this case, they consider estimates $\psi^{(12)}(d_i, g)$ computed under the assumption that for a given dose, the probability of a DLT in group 1 is less than that of group 2 and $\psi^{(21)}(d_i, g)$ computed under the assumption that for a given dose, the probability of a DLT in group 2 is less than that of group 1. The choice between which of the two sets of estimates to use in the dose allocation is based on which set is "closer" to the unrestricted estimates of the toxicity probability. Specifically, if $\hat{\pi}(d_i, g)$ denotes the unrestricted estimate of the probability of toxicity for dose d_i in group g, equal to the number of observed DLTs divided by the number of patients treated with dose d_i in group g, the estimates $\psi(d_i, g)^{12}$ are used in the dose allocation if

$$\sum_{g=1}^{2} \sum_{i=1}^{K} \left[\psi^{(12)}(d_i, g) - \hat{\pi}(d_i, g) \right]^2 < \sum_{g=1}^{2} \sum_{i=1}^{K} \left[\psi^{(21)}(d_i, g) - \hat{\pi}(d_i, g) \right]^2 \tag{8.15}$$

otherwise, the estimates $\psi^{21}(d_i, g)$ are used.

Yuan and Chappell [22] propose a generalization of the CRM that is a hybrid of the single agent–single group CRM and isotonic regression methods described by Robertson, Wright, and Dykstra [18]. As in the single-agent CRM, the working model and the data within each group are used to estimate the DLT probabilities at each dose for that group. Using the bivariate isotonic regression estimator [18], the resulting DLT probability estimates within each dose level are modified so that there are no reversals, meaning no dose levels where a lower-risk group has greater DLT probability estimates than a higher-risk group. Once the isotonic estimates are computed, dose allocation proceeds as in the single-group CRM, the next patient in group g is allocated to the dose with an estimated toxicity probability in group g closest to the target θ.

Each of the previous methods focused solely on safety, using a binary measure of toxicity. Bekele et al. use an ordered categorical outcome for toxicity grade with patients stratified into G risk groups. For each of the c possible toxicity classifications, $c = 1, \ldots, C$, Bekele et al. elicit a toxicity score s_c and assume a Dirichlet prior for $\pi(c, d_i, g)$, the probability associated with toxicity category c at dose d_i in group g. Combining the observed toxicities with the prior yields the posterior distribution for $\pi(c, d_i, g)$, which has a Dirichlet distribution, and M random draws, $\pi^m(c, d_i, g), m = 1, \ldots, M$, are taken from the posterior distribution. For each of these draws, the average toxicity score is computed:

$$\text{ATS}^m(d_i, g) = \sum_{c=1}^{C} s_c \pi^m(c, d_i, g) \tag{8.16}$$

The ATS is meant to summarize the total amount of toxicity at dose d_i in group g. Bivariate isotonic regression is applied to $\text{ATS}^m(d_i, g)$ to ensure that the toxicity score is increasing in dose for a fixed group and increasing across groups for a fixed dose. Allocations are made based on the probability that the posterior distribution of the ATS exceeds a prespecified target ATS level. Methods for eliciting the target ATS score are given in Bekele and Thall [4].

8.3 Summary

With increased focus on personalized dosing, and with studies taking into account the patients' genetic characteristics, dose-finding studies in groups are becoming increasingly common. While the current standard practice is to run parallel and independent dose-finding studies among several groups, this practice can be inefficient or lead to MTD estimates that violate what is known clinically about the groups. To avoid these issues, a number of statistical methods have been proposed that allow for borrowing information across groups, either by adding parameters to a model or by using order-restricted inference.

References

1. J. Babb and A. Rogatko. Patient specific dosing in a cancer phase I clinical trial. *Statistics in Medicine*, 20:2079–2090, 2001.

2. J. Babb, A. Rogatko, and S. Zacks. Cancer phase I clinical trials: Efficient dose escalation with overdose control. *Statistics in Medicine*, 17:1103–1120, 1998.

3. S. Bailey, B. Neuenschwander, G. Laird, and M. Branson. A Bayesian case study in oncology phase I combination dose-finding using logistic regression with covariates. *Journal of Biopharmaceutical Statistics*, 19:469–484, 2009.

4. B. Bekele and P. Thall. Dose-finding based on multiple toxicities in a soft tissue sarcoma trial. *Journal of the American Statistical Association*, 99:261–35, 2004.

5. A. Ivanova and K. Wang. Bivariate isotonic design for dose-finding with ordered groups. *Statistics in Medicine*, 25:2018–2026, 2006.

6. K. Kim, H. Kim, S. Sym, K. Bae, Y. Hong, H. Chang, J. Lee, Y. Kang, J. Lee, J. Shin, and T. Kim. A UGT1A1*28 and *6 genotype-directed phase I dose-escalation trial of irinotecan with fixed-dose capecitabine in Korean patients with metastatic colorectal cancer. *Cancer Chemotherapy and Pharmacology*, 71:1609–1617, 2013.

7. A. Legedza and J. Ibrahim. Heterogeneity in phase I clinical trials: Prior elicitation and computation using the continual reassessment method. *Statistics in Medicine*, 20:867–882, 2001.

8. S. Liu, H. Pan, J. Xia, Q. Huang, and Y. Yuan. Bridging continual reassessment method for phase I clinical trials in different ethnic populations. *Statistics in Medicine*, 34:1681–1694, 2015.

9. P. LoRusso, K. Venkatakrishnan, R. Ramanathan, J. Sarantopoulos, D. Mulkerin, S. Shibata, A. Hamilton, A. Dowlati, S. Mani, M. Rudek, C. Takimoto, R. Neuwirth, D. Esseltine, and P. Ivy. Pharmacokinetics and safety of bortezomib in patients with advanced malignancies and varying degrees of liver dysfunction: Phase I NCI Organ Dysfunction Working Group Study NCI-6432. *Clinical Cancer Research*, 18(10): 1–10, 2012.

10. J. O'Quigley. Phase I and phase I/II dose finding algorithms using continual reassessment method. In *Handbook of Statistics in Clinical Oncology*, 2nd ed., J. Crowley and D. Ankherst (eds). Chapman and Hall/CRC Biostatistics Series, Boca Raton, FL, 2006.

11. J. O'Quigley and M. Conaway. Extended model-based designs for more complex dose-finding studies. *Statistics in Medicine*, 30:2062–2069, 2011.

12. J. O'Quigley and A. Iasonos. Bridging solutions in dose-finding problems. *Journal of Biopharmaceutical Statistics*, 6(2):185–197, 2014.

13. J. O'Quigley and X. Paoletti. Continual reassessment method for ordered groups. *Biometrics*, 59:430–440, 2003.

14. J. O'Quigley, M. Pepe, and L. Fisher. Continual reassessment method: A practical design for phase I clinical trials in cancer. *Biometrics*, 46(1):33–48, 1990.

15. J. O'Quigley, L. Shen, and A. Gamst. Two sample continual reassessment method. *Journal of Biopharmaceutical Statistics*, 9:17–44, 1999.

16. R. Ramanathan, M. Egorin, C. Takimoto, S. Remick, J. Doroshow, P. LoRusso, D. Mulkerin, J. Grem, A. Hamilton, A. Murgo, D. Potter, C. Belani, M. Hayes, B. Peng, and P. Ivy. Phase I and pharmacokinetic study of imatinib mesylate in patients with advanced malignancies and varying degrees of liver dysfunction: A study by the National Cancer Institute Organ Dysfunction Working Group. *Journal of Clinical Oncology*, 26:563–569, 2008.

17. M. Raphael, M.-C. Le Deley, G. Vassal, and X. Paoletti. Operating characteristics of two independent sample design in phase I trials in paediatric oncology. *European Journal of Cancer*, 46:1392–1398, 2010.

18. T. Robertson, F. T. Wright, and R. Dykstra. *Order Restricted Statistical Inference.* John Wiley & Sons, New York, 1988.

19. L. Shen and J. O'Quigley. Continual reassessment method: A likelihood approach. *Biometrics*, 52(2):673–684, 1996.

20. M. Tighiouart, G. Cook-Wiens, and A. Rogatko. Incorporating a patient dichotomous characteristic in cancer phase I clinical trials using escalation with overdose control. *Journal of Probability and Statistics*, 2012. Article ID 567819, doi:10.1155/2012/567819.

21. N. Wages, P. Read, and G. Petroni. A phase I/II adaptive design for heterogeneous groups with application to a stereotactic body radiation therapy trial. *Pharmaceutical Statistics*, 14(4):302–310, 2015.

22. Z. Yuan and R. Chappell. Isotonic designs for phase I cancer clinical trials with multiple risk groups. *Clinical Trials*, 1(6):499–508, 2004.

9

Nonparametric Optimal Design in Adaptive Dose-Finding Studies

Nolan A. Wages

University of Virginia

CONTENTS

9.1 Background

Historically, the primary objective of a dose-finding clinical trial in oncology has been to identify the maximum tolerated dose (MTD) of the agent being investigated, from a discrete set of available doses $D = \{d_1, ..., d_K\}$. Numerous phase I clinical trial designs [1–5] have been proposed for identifying the MTD for situations in which toxicity is described as a binary random variable (dose-limiting toxicity, DLT; yes/no). Since the works of Storer [1] and O'Quigley, Pepe, and Fisher [2], there has been considerable development in the statistical design and analysis of dose-finding methods, both for phase I and phase I–II trials, a recent review of which is given in Iasonos and O'Quigley [6]. Many of these approaches appeal to Bayesian techniques and involve the use of prior information. Such information is typically not informative, although sometimes attempts are made to elicit relevant information from the clinicians involved in the studies. One common criticism of the standard $3 + 3$ design in this context is that it behaves like a random walk [1] so that no real learning is taking place as more and more patients are included into a study. For model-based designs, on the other hand, there is learning taking place, and, generally, if we allow sample size to increase without bound (as a theoretical construction), then we will find the correct MTD with a probability of 1.

Large-sample properties are somewhat theoretical, and although they can help a statistician to obtain a better grasp on anticipated finite sample characteristics, their use is quite limited. Of more value are studies of finite sample behavior, and the tool of choice here is necessarily that of simulation. Some situations, corresponding to hypothesized true, yet unknown, dose–toxicity relationships, can be postulated. Any proposed method can be judged, at least to some extent, by the degree to which it performs when faced with these true, yet in principle unknown, realities. The kind of characteristics that we typically study are the PCS of the MTD, the percentage of patients treated at and close to the MTD, and, possibly, the accuracy of the recommendation itself. Yet, the problem of determining whether some given design performs less well, comparably, or better than some other design is still not an easy question to answer. Under one set of true dose–toxicity curves, we may come to a conclusion that fails to hold up under another set of curves. This is particularly so for Bayesian designs where, often, the information contained in the prior can be very difficult to assess. It happens that such information can favor performance under certain true dose–toxicity relationships and the opposite under others. The choice then of which relationships to show, which is a subjective choice, becomes difficult.

One important measure of performance of a particular design is its accuracy, which is reflected by the distribution of the dose estimated as the MTD. For instance, suppose method A recommends the true MTD 45% of the time and method B 50%. One might conclude that method B is superior to method A. However, it is also important to consider how often a method recommends doses other than the true MTD. If method A recommended either the true MTD or a neighboring dose (MTD−1, MTD+1) in a large percentage of trials, while method B tended to recommend either the MTD or doses far from the MTD, then method A could be considered the better option. A necessary component of the evaluation process is to have some concept of how well a design can possibly perform. A nonparametric optimal design was first described by O'Quigley, Paoletti, and Maccario [7] as a benchmark for identifying the MTD based on a binary toxicity endpoint. Zohar and O'Quigley [8] further developed the benchmark to account for two binary (toxicity/efficacy) endpoints.

The nonparametric optimal design is a theoretical tool for simulations and therefore not applicable in a real trial. Although it is not useful as a practical design, it can be used as a benchmark for efficiency. The authors [7, 9] showed that it is not generally possible to do better than the optimal design on the basis of the observations themselves, so it can be used as an upper bound for the performance of any dose-finding scheme. To improve on the finite sample optimal design requires extraneous knowledge. Such knowledge could come from an informative prior distribution or possibly from some parametric assumption, an assumption beyond the reasonable stipulation of monotonicity, and one that is necessarily strong and, in almost all practical cases, unverifiable. If we only allow admissible designs, then we can take the finite sample optimal design as a benchmark, noting that it is not possible, in practice, to do better than that. Designs such as "always choose dose level 2," a design that is impossible to beat even with no observations under certain situations, are not, however, admissible designs.

9.2   Nonparametric Optimal Design

During the course of a phase I trial, each patient receives a dose and is observed for the response only at that dose. Therefore, we can only observe information that is *partial*. In simulating trial data, however, we can generate each patient's latent outcome from which we can observe *complete* toxicity information at all available dose levels [7]. We will illustrate the idea of partial versus complete information through examples in a subsequent section.

9.2.1   Partial information

An assumption typically made in the standard phase I setting using a binary toxicity (DLT; yes/no) endpoint is that a patient who experiences a DLT at a particular dose level would necessarily experience a DLT at any higher level. Similarly, if a patient tolerates a given dose level, he or she would also tolerate any lower dose level. These assumptions lead to the development of complete and partial information, ideas vital to the derivation of a nonparametric optimal design. Suppose that the binary indicator Y_j takes value 1 if patient j experiences a DLT at dose d_k; 0 otherwise. The true probability of DLT at dose level d_k is denoted $R(d_k)$. The design objective is to identify the dose d_ν with DLT probability closest to a target DLT rate θ so that

$$d_\nu \equiv \arg\min_k |R(d_k) - \theta|. \tag{9.1}$$

During the course of a phase I trial, each patient receives a dose and is observed for the presence or absence of toxicity only at that dose. Therefore, we can only observe information that is incomplete. For instance, consider a trial investigating six available dose levels. Suppose that a patient is given dose level 4 and experiences a DLT. The monotonicity assumption implies that a toxicity would necessarily be observed at dose levels 5 and 6. We will not have any information regarding whether the patient would have suffered a toxic response for any dose below level 4. Conversely, should dose 3 be deemed safe for an enrolled patient, then we can infer that he or she would experience a nontoxic outcome at dose levels 1 and 2. However, any information concerning whether the patient would have had a DLT had he or she been given any dose above level 3 is unknown. Table 9.1 illustrates partial information.

9.2.2   Complete information

For each patient, if we knew the DLT outcome at each available dose level, we would have complete information. In simulating trial data, we can generate each patient's latent outcome from which we can observe DLT at all available dose levels. For example, suppose that we have a patient who experiences a DLT from dose level 3. Complete information is summarized in Table 9.2. In the simulation of DLT outcomes in a trial, the latent outcome, V_j, of each patient can be considered a uniformly distributed random variable $V_j \sim \text{Uniform}(0,1)$, which we term a patient's latent toxicity tolerance and denote v_j for the jth entered patient [7, 10]. At the dose (d_k) assigned to patient j, if the tolerance is less than or equal to its true DLT probability (i.e., $v_j \leq R(d_k)$), then patient j has a DLT; otherwise, the patient has a non-DLT outcome.

Table 9.3 presents the complete toxicity vectors of 25 simulated patients for true toxicity probabilities $R(d_1) = 0.04, R(d_2) = 0.07, R(d_3) = 0.20, R(d_4) = 0.35, R(d_5) = 0.55,$ and $R(d_6) = 0.70$. Patient 7, for instance, has a latent toxicity tolerance of $v_7 = 0.238$. Therefore, he or she will experience a non-DLT at dose levels $1, 2,$ and 3 because $v_7 > R(d_k)$ for $k = 1, 2, 3$, and will suffer a DLT at levels $4, 5,$ and 6 because $v_7 < R(d_k)$ for $k = 4, 5, 6$. The information in Table 9.3 is not obtainable from a trial due to the fact that we cannot, in reality, observe a patient's toxicity tolerance. We can, however, simulate complete vectors of toxicity information and use them to estimate the toxicity probabilities by using the sample

TABLE 9.1

Example of partial information.

Doses	d_1	d_2	d_3	d_4	d_5	d_6
Y_j	*	*	*	1	1	1
Y_j	0	0	0	*	*	*

'*' Indicates dose levels for which DLT information is not available.

TABLE 9.2

Example of complete information.

Doses	d_1	d_2	d_3	d_4	d_5	d_6
Y_j	0	0	0	1	1	1

DLT information is available at all dose levels.

TABLE 9.3

Simulated trial of complete information.

Patient	Latent Toxicity	Toxicity at Dose Level d_k					
j	v_j	d_1	d_2	d_3	d_4	d_5	d_6
1	0.004	1	1	1	1	1	1
2	0.751	0	0	0	0	0	0
3	0.563	0	0	0	0	0	1
4	0.429	0	0	0	0	1	1
5	0.198	0	0	1	1	1	1
6	0.995	0	0	0	0	0	0
7	0.238	0	0	0	1	1	1
8	0.509	0	0	0	0	1	1
9	0.381	0	0	0	0	1	1
10	0.053	0	1	1	1	1	1
11	0.005	1	1	1	1	1	1
12	0.883	0	0	0	0	0	0
13	0.944	0	0	0	0	0	0
14	0.579	0	0	0	0	0	1
15	0.241	0	0	0	1	1	1
16	0.840	0	0	0	0	0	0
17	0.060	0	1	1	1	1	1
18	0.267	0	0	0	1	1	1
19	0.688	0	0	0	0	0	1
20	0.297	0	0	0	1	1	1
21	0.196	0	0	1	1	1	1
22	0.962	0	0	0	0	0	1
23	0.578	0	0	0	0	0	1
24	0.432	0	0	0	0	1	1
25	0.657	0	0	0	0	0	1
$\widehat{R}(d_k)$		0.08	0.16	0.24	0.40	0.56	0.80

proportion of observed toxicities at each dose. That is, we can estimate $R(d_k)$; $k = 1, \ldots, K$ from the sample proportions:

$$\widehat{R}(d_k) = \frac{1}{n} \sum_{j=1}^{n} Y_j(d_k),$$

and use them to select the MTD as the dose d_ν such that

$$d_\nu = \arg \min_k |\widehat{R}(d_k) - \theta|.$$

The last row of Table 9.3 gives the sample proportions of the simulated trial. After 25 patients, the recommended dose is level 3, with an estimated toxicity probability of 0.24, which is closest to a target toxicity rate of 0.20. It can be shown that $\widehat{R}(d_k)$ is an unbiased estimator of $R(d_k)$ and that the variance of $\widehat{R}(d_k)$ achieves the Cramer–Rao lower bound. In this sense, the design can be considered optimal.

9.2.3 Design efficiency in simulation studies

The performance of the optimal design can be evaluated over many simulation runs and can be used as a benchmark for efficiency. One way to assess how well a method is performing is by simply observing in what percentage of trials a method is recommending the true MTD. This is referred to as the percentage of correct selection (PCS). A more thorough assessment will involve looking at the entire distribution of the selected doses in order to see how often a method recommends doses other than the correct one as the MTD. For instance, in order to adhere to certain ethical considerations presented by phase I trials, it is appropriate to evaluate how often a method selects doses above the MTD (i.e., overly toxic doses). It is important to have some measure of accuracy that represents the distribution of doses selected as the MTD. For instance, the accuracy index of Cheung [11] is given by

$$
\mathcal{A}_n = 1 - K \times \frac{\sum_{k=1}^{K} \rho_k \times p_k}{\sum_{k=1}^{K} \rho_k},
$$

where $p_k = \Pr\,(d_k$ is selected as the MTD) and ρ_k is a distance measure between the true probability of toxicity $R(d_k)$ at d_k and the target DLT rate θ. For example, a commonly used distance measure is absolute distance $\rho_k = |R(d_k) - \theta|$. The accuracy index, $\mathcal{A}_n$, provides a numerical measure of the distribution of MTD recommendation. Its maximum value is 1 with larger values (close to 1) indicating that the method possesses high accuracy.

How well a method is performing relative to another can be quantified by efficiency. There are many ways to measure efficiency, some of which can be found in O'Quigley, Paoletti, and Maccario [7]; Paoletti et al. [9]; and Cheung [11]. As one measure of efficiency, O'Quigley, Paoletti, and Maccario [7] summarized performance into a measure of finite sample efficiency via

$$
e(n) = \frac{\sum_k p_k(n)\,q_k(n)}{\max\left(\sum_k p_k(n)^2, \sum_k q_k(n)^2\right)},
$$

where $p_k(n)$ is the percentage recommendation for level k provided by the optimal design and $q_k(n)$ is that for any method being assessed, after exhausting a sample size of n patients. In Chapter 8 of Ref. [11], Cheung defines the efficiency of a design in terms of the ratio of average PCS for any dose-finding scheme relative to the optimal method over several true scenarios. This definition of efficiency appears to be not fully satisfactory in that it solely considers PCS, which takes into account only what happens at the MTD and ignores recommendation percentages at other levels. A more comprehensive efficiency measure may be the ratio of the accuracy index of a design to that of the optimal design, which considers recommendation percentages across the entire dose range [12].

As an illustration of how the optimal can be used to assess design performance, we present simulation results in order to get an idea of how well the two-stage, likelihood-based, continual reassessment method (CRM-L [13]) is performing when compared to the optimal design. For each simulated trial using the optimal method, complete information was generated for a fixed sample size of n patients, from which the sample proportions $\widehat{R}(d_k)$

were calculated. These values were used to select the MTD as the dose that minimizes $|\widehat{R}(d_k) - \theta|$ at the end of each trial. The distribution of MTD selection for the optimal method was calculated by tabulating the proportion of simulated trials in which d_k was selected as the MTD. The PCS is this proportion for the true MTD.

Obviously, it is not possible to look at all situations, but the true DLT probabilities chosen in Table 9.4 reflect a somewhat wide range of toxicity scenarios, in that there is a mixture of steep, flat, and intermediate dose–toxicity curves. We also varied the location of the MTD within the dose space, including curves where the MTD is at the extremes (i.e., the highest or lowest level). Another approach to take in order to ensure that things are being assessed over a broad range of dose–toxicity relations is to generate scenarios at a random class of curves [9]. For all scenarios, there are $K = 6$ dose levels, the target toxicity rate is $\theta = 0.30$, and the fixed sample size for each simulated trial is $n = 25$. In each simulated trial, escalation is restricted to no more than one level. For each scenario, 10,000 trials were simulated under the true toxicity probabilities given next to scenario number in Table 9.4, with the true MTD indicated in bold type. Overall, the simulations study the operating characteristics, in relation to the optimal method, of the following specifications for CRM-L. The power model, $\psi(d_k, a) = \alpha_k^{\exp(a)}$, is used to model toxicity probabilities, using a skeleton $\alpha_1 = 0.10, \alpha_2 = 0.20, \alpha_3 = 0.30, \alpha_4 = 0.40, \alpha_5 = 0.50$, and $\alpha_6 = 0.60$. The spacing of this skeleton was investigated in O'Quigley and Zohar [14], and it exhibited good operating characteristics across a broad range of true dose–toxicity scenarios. All simulation results for the CRM-L design were carried out using the **crmsim** function

TABLE 9.4

Compared proportions of MTD recommendation and accuracy measure for the optimal design and CRM-L after 10,000 simulated trials.

Scenario		Dose Level d_k						$\mathcal{A}_n$
		1	2	3	4	5	6	
1	$R(d_k)$	0.05	0.15	**0.30**	0.40	0.50	0.60	
	CRM-L	0.00	0.16	**0.46**	0.28	0.09	0.01	0.564
	Optimal	0.00	0.18	**0.55**	0.23	0.05	0.00	0.641
2	$R(d_k)$	0.08	0.12	0.20	**0.30**	0.42	0.53	
	CRM-L	0.00	0.05	0.24	**0.42**	0.24	0.05	0.482
	Optimal	0.00	0.03	0.25	**0.47**	0.21	0.03	0.552
3	$R(d_k)$	**0.30**	0.38	0.45	0.55	0.70	0.80	
	CRM-L	**0.63**	0.26	0.10	0.01	0.00	0.00	0.829
	Optimal	**0.65**	0.25	0.09	0.01	0.00	0.00	0.842
4	$R(d_k)$	0.02	0.05	0.10	0.15	0.23	**0.30**	
	CRM-L	0.00	0.00	0.01	0.10	0.29	**0.59**	0.758
	Optimal	0.00	0.00	0.01	0.08	0.31	**0.60**	0.771
5	$R(d_k)$	0.18	**0.28**	0.36	0.44	0.52	0.65	
	CRM-L	0.19	**0.38**	0.27	0.12	0.03	0.00	0.534
	Optimal	0.20	**0.40**	0.27	0.10	0.02	0.00	0.546
6	$R(d_k)$	0.01	0.03	0.05	0.12	**0.30**	0.46	
	CRM-L	0.00	0.00	0.00	0.14	**0.54**	0.32	0.598
	Optimal	0.00	0.00	0.00	0.12	**0.71**	0.17	0.745

Average $\mathcal{A}_n$, CRM-L = 0.628, optimal = 0.684.

The true MTD is indicated in bold type. The target toxicity rate is 30% and the fixed sample size for each trial is 25 patients.

in **R** package **dfcrm**, while an **R** shiny web app for the optimal method is available at https://uvatrapps.shinyapps.io/nonparbnch/.

The simulation results assess how well the CRM-L and the nonparametric optimal design are performing in two ways. One is by simply observing the distribution of dose selection as the MTD. The other is measured by the accuracy index described in the previous section. Table 9.4 compares the distribution of selected doses for the CRM-L and the optimal design, as well as provides the value of $\mathcal{A}_{25}$. There are scenarios (i.e., 3–5) in which the CRM-L yields a PCS approximately equal to that of the optimal method. It is interesting to note, however, that in these scenarios, the CRM-L results in a different accuracy benchmark than that of the optimal design. This indicates that it matters what doses are being recommended by a method when it fails to correctly recommend the MTD. In Scenario 4, for example, CRM-L selects the dose directly below the MTD, a dose with a DLT probability just 0.07 less than the target rate, 29% of the time, while the optimal does this 31% of the time. In other words, the optimal method missed more often on a dose that was closer to the target than did the CRM-L, which results in the different accuracy index values. Despite this fact, the accuracy indices of the CRM-L are quite close to that of the optimal, again indicating that the capacity for improvement of a design over the CRM-L is quite limited in these scenarios.

In Scenario 3, the PCS is 63% and 65% for the CRM-L and the optimal methods, respectively. The accuracy index for the CRM-L designs yielded a value of 0.829, compared to 0.842 for the optimal method. In Scenario 1, the performance of the CRM-L diminishes relative to the optimal benchmark. The difference in recommendation proportions for the CRM-L and optimal design widens. In Scenario 1, CRM-L recommends the true MTD in 46% of simulated trials, whereas the optimal method does so 55% of the time. This disparity is again reflected in measuring accuracy. Even in these cases where the CRM performs less well, it is recommending the MTD, or a neighboring dose (MTD-1 or MTD + 1), in a large percentage of trials. It is important to take into consideration how often each method is recommending doses between $(\theta \pm \delta)$ for some positive difference δ. For instance, keeping in mind that the target rate is 0.30, for $\delta = 0.10$, we would note how often each method recommends a dose as the MTD with a DLT probability between 0.20 and 0.40. In Scenario 1, CRM-L recommends, as the MTD, doses with DLT probabilities between 0.15 and 0.40 in 90% of the trials, while the optimal design does this in 96% of the trials. Table 9.5 summarizes the proportion of recommendation for doses with DLT probabilities within $[\theta - \delta, \theta + \delta]$, and Figure 9.1 graphically displays this information. Assessing the overall performance of CRM-L across six practical situations, the average accuracy index measure is 0.628 for CRM-L and 0.684 for the optimal. The efficiency of the CRM-L designs in terms of average accuracy index can be computed by $0.628/0.684 = 0.918$, indicating that CRM-L is approximately 91.8% efficient in terms of its overall performance against the optimal for a sample size of 25 patients. Although here we have illustrated the efficiency of CRM-L against the optimal, any design can be assessed against the benchmark in a similar way.

TABLE 9.5

Compared proportion of recommendation for doses with DLT probabilities within $[\theta - \delta, \theta + \delta]$.

δ	0.05	0.10	0.15	0.20	0.25
CRM-L	0.46	0.74	0.90	0.99	0.99
Optimal	0.55	0.78	0.96	1.00	1.00

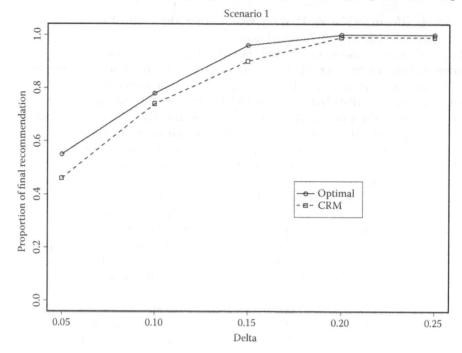

FIGURE 9.1

Compared proportion of recommendation for doses with DLT probabilities within $[\theta - \delta, \theta + \delta]$.

9.2.3.1   Super-optimality

Although not reflected in the scenarios in Table 9.4, it is possible for a dose-finding design to yield a higher PCS than the optimal [12]. In this case, it is important to keep in mind that the optimal design is nonparametric. Model-based designs, such as the CRM, utilize parametric assumptions, which could lead to information at one level providing information about all other levels. For instance, the working model and the true situation could be very similar or related by some power transformation, indicating that improving on the finite sample optimal design requires extraneous knowledge in the form of prior information or strong parametric assumptions that, in almost all practical cases, are unverifiable. It is also worth pointing out that super-optimality is almost certainly very specific to certain scenarios, and it cannot be broadened to a class of scenarios.

It may be the case that a particular skeleton encourages experimentation at some level. For instance, consider a CRM-L design in which a skeleton of (0.0001, 0.20, 0.85, 0.90, 0.95) is used, and suppose that the target DLT rate is 0.20. This seems to be a very poor design in that it heavily favors the selection of level 2 and will likely have poor operating characteristics if the true MTD is any dose other than level 2. If the true MTD is level 2, however, this design will probably do very well and, most likely, beat the optimal. As an example, consider the two scenarios in Table 9.6 with five dose levels and a target DLT rate of $\theta = 0.25$. In both scenarios, we ran 10,000 simulated trials of patients using the power model with two different skeletons. Skeleton 1 is (0.14, 0.30, 0.50, 0.66, 0.79), and Skeleton 2 is (0.10, 0.20, 0.30, 0.40, 0.50). The gap between the skeleton at level 1 (0.14) and level 2 (0.30) and the gap between 0.30 and the skeleton at level 3 (0.50) are sufficiently large to cause the method to home in on level 2, which is closest to the target rate of 0.25. Consequently, Skeleton 1 produces a super-optimal PCS of 48% in Scenario 1. Skeleton 2

TABLE 9.6

Compared proportions of MTD recommendation and accuracy measure for the optimal design and CRM-L after 10,000 simulated trials.

Scenario		Dose Level d_k					$\mathcal{A}_n$
		1	2	3	4	5	
1	$R(d_k)$	0.15	**0.25**	0.35	0.45	0.60	
	Skeleton 1	0.27	**0.42**	0.22	0.08	0.01	0.543
	Skeleton 2	0.28	**0.48**	0.20	0.04	0.00	0.627
	Optimal	0.25	**0.43**	0.24	0.07	0.00	0.580
2	$R(d_k)$	0.01	0.05	0.10	0.15	**0.25**	
	Skeleton 1	0.00	0.01	0.07	0.27	**0.66**	0.714
	Skeleton 2	0.00	0.02	0.16	0.37	**0.45**	0.529
	Optimal	0.00	0.01	0.07	0.23	**0.70**	0.743

Average $\mathcal{A}_n$: skeleton 1 = 0.578, skeleton 2 = 0.629, optimal = 0.662.

The true MTD is indicated in bold type. The target toxicity rate is 25% and the fixed sample size for each trial is 20 patients. First stage cohort size is 3.

possesses reasonable spacing between adjacent levels and produces a PCS of 42%. Scenario 2 in Table 9.6 illustrates the idea that a super-optimal result should be taken as a "red flag," rather than with the optimism of being a superior design. In Scenario 2, the MTD is now at the highest level, dose 5. Using the same two skeletons as Scenario 1, 10,000 simulated trials again produced a result close to that of the optimal (within 5%) with Skeleton 2, but performance significantly diminished with Skeleton 1. This result reiterates the fact that a super-optimal design in one scenario is not expected to be super-optimal across a range of scenarios. In fact, a design that is super-optimal will produce results well below what is optimal in other scenarios. This is again reflected in the average accuracy measure across the two scenarios. Although Skeleton 1 is super-optimal in Scenario 1, it possesses a lower overall mean accuracy index (0.578) than Skeleton 2 (0.629), with Skeleton 2 average index being close to optimal (0.662). Super-optimality is not an indication that the CRM-L design used in this scenario is a "better" design than the optimal. Rather, this should be considered an isolated case in which it is possible to beat the optimal.

9.3 Phase I–II Studies

There has been a recent increase in the interest of incorporating composite endpoints into the trial design, with the goal of finding a dose that is both safe and efficacious. To this end, many published phase I–II methods have extended dose-finding methodology to allow for the simultaneous consideration of information on toxicity and efficacy endpoints. As the dose increases, it is anticipated that the probability of both toxicity and efficacy will increase, although it is not difficult to construct a counterexample in which this may not be true, such as in molecularly targeted therapies [15]. Rather than identifying the MTD, the objective of the trial in this setting is to locate the most successful dose (MSD), defined as the dose that maximizes the overall probability of success (i.e., efficacy *and* no toxicity) [16]. The nonparametric optimal benchmark from the previous section was extended to MSD by Zohar and O'Quigley [8]. In studies attempting to locate the MSD, we have two binary random variables Y and Z, representing toxicity and efficacy, respectively. At dose level d_k, the probability of toxicity is denoted as $R(d_k)$, and the probability of efficacy is represented by $Q(d_k)$. The primary objective of the trial is to locate the dose d_ν that maximizes the probability of success $P(d_\nu) = Q(d_\nu) \times \{1 - R(d_\nu)\}$, in which case d_ν is termed the MSD.

9.3.1 Benchmark for most successful dose

As described above, the generation of complete information for the optimal design relies on the assumption of monotonicity of the dose–toxicity curve. This same assumption is leaned on to generate complete information for efficacy. It is assumed that a patient who experiences an efficacious response at a particular dose level would necessarily experience efficacy at any higher level. Similarly, if a patient does not have a response at a given dose level, he or she would also not respond to any lower level. For instance, complete information for both toxicity and efficacy could be represented as in Table 9.7.

As with toxicity, generating complete information for efficacy relies on latent outcomes. In the simulation of efficacy, the latent outcome, U_j, of each patient can be considered a uniformly distributed random variable $U_j \sim \text{Uniform}(0,1)$, which we term a patient's latent efficacy outcome and denote u_j for the jth entered patient [7, 10]. At the dose (d_k) assigned to patient j, if the latent outcome is less than or equal to its true efficacy probability (i.e., $u_j \leq Q(d_k)$), then patient j has an efficacious response; otherwise, the patient has a nonresponse outcome. Table 9.8 [8] presents the complete vectors of 15 simulated patients

TABLE 9.7

Example of complete information for both toxicity and efficacy.

Doses	d_1	d_2	d_3	d_4	d_5	d_6
Y	0	0	0	1	1	1
Z	0	0	1	1	1	1

TABLE 9.8

Simulated trial of complete information as shown in Zohar and O'Quigley [8].

Patient Number	Latent Toxicity	Toxicity at Dose Level d_k				Latent Efficacy	Efficacy at Dose Level d_k			
j	v_j	d_1	d_2	d_3	d_4	u_j	d_1	d_2	d_3	d_4
1	0.27	0	0	1	1	0.50	0	0	1	1
2	0.37	0	0	0	1	0.72	0	0	0	0
3	0.57	0	0	0	0	0.99	0	0	0	0
4	0.91	0	0	0	0	0.38	0	0	1	1
5	0.20	0	0	1	1	0.78	0	0	0	0
6	0.90	0	0	0	0	0.94	0	0	0	0
7	0.94	0	0	0	0	0.21	0	1	1	1
8	0.66	0	0	0	0	0.65	0	0	0	1
9	0.63	0	0	0	0	0.13	0	1	1	1
10	0.06	0	1	1	1	0.27	0	1	1	1
11	0.21	0	0	1	1	0.39	0	0	1	1
12	0.18	0	0	1	1	0.01	1	1	1	1
13	0.69	0	0	0	0	0.38	0	0	1	1
14	0.38	0	0	0	1	0.87	0	0	0	0
15	0.77	0	0	0	0	0.34	0	0	1	1
	$\widehat{R}(d_k)$	0.00	0.07	0.33	0.47	$\widehat{Q}(d_k)$	0.07	0.27	0.60	0.67

for true toxicity probabilities $R(d_1) = 0.06, R(d_2) = 0.17, R(d_3) = 0.30$, and $R(d_4) = 0.50$ and true efficacy probabilities $Q(d_1) = 0.10, Q(d_2) = 0.30, Q(d_3) = 0.60$, and $Q(d_4) = 0.70$. Patient 1, for instance, has a latent toxicity outcome of $v_1 = 0.270$ and a latent efficacy outcome of $u_1 = 0.50$. Therefore, he or she will experience a non-DLT at dose levels 1 and 2 because $v_1 > R(d_k)$ for $k = 1, 2$, and will suffer a DLT at levels 3 and 4 because $v_1 < R(d_k)$ for $k = 3, 4$. Similarly, he or she will experience a nonresponse at dose levels 1 and 2 because $u_1 > Q(d_k)$ for $k = 1, 2$, and will experience a response at levels 3 and 4 because $u_1 < Q(d_k)$ for $k = 3, 4$. We can use these simulated outcomes for both endpoints to estimate the toxicity probabilities by using the sample proportion of observed toxicities at each dose. That is, we can estimate $R(d_k)$ and $Q(d_k)$; $k = 1, ..., K$ from the sample proportions

$$\widehat{R}(d_k) = \frac{1}{n} \sum_{j=1}^{n} Y_j(d_k), \qquad \widehat{Q}(d_k) = \frac{1}{n} \sum_{j=1}^{n} Z_j(d_k),$$

and use them to select the MSD as the dose d_ν such that

$$d_\nu = \arg\max_k \widehat{Q}(d_k) \times \left(1 - \widehat{R}(d_k)\right).$$

The last row of Table 9.8 gives the sample proportions of the simulated trial. After 15 patients, the recommended dose is level 3, with an estimated toxicity probability of success $0.60 \times (1 - 0.33) = 0.40$, which is the maximum among all doses. Available **R** code for the optimal method for MSD is available for download at www.faculty.virginia.edu/model-based_dose-finding.

9.4 Conclusion

In this chapter, we have presented nonparametric optimal benchmark designs for adaptive dose-finding studies. Cheung [17] applied this benchmark to other complex dose-finding problems, such as those accounting for different types and grades of toxicities [18–20]. Contemporary dose-finding problems can be complex, depending on the design objective and the corresponding endpoints. Having a nonparametric benchmark for such cases can give statisticians a tool for evaluating properties of a design, serving as an upper limit of how well it is possible for a method to perform given a particular simulation scenario. The benchmark cannot be used in practice as a dose-escalation design because it requires knowledge of the true underlying dose–toxicity curve. But, it can be used in practice to compare designs, as it has been shown to be useful in investigating the efficiency of proposed designs relative to the benchmark.

References

1. B. Storer. Design and analysis of phase I clinical trials. *Biometrics*, 45(3):925–937, 1989.

2. J. O'Quigley, M. Pepe, and L. Fisher. Continual reassessment method: A practical design for phase I clinical trials in cancer. *Biometrics*, 46(1):33–48, 1990.

3. J. Babb, A. Rogatko, and S. Zacks. Cancer phase I clinical trials: Efficient dose escalation with overdose control. *Statistics in Medicine*, 17:1103–1120, 1998.

4. M. Stylianou and N. Flournoy. Dose finding using the biased coin up-and-down design and isotonic regression. *Biometrics*, 58(1):171–177, 2002.

5. Y. Ji, Y. Li, and B. Bekele. Dose-finding in phase I clinical trials based on toxicity probability intervals. *Clinical Trials*, 4:235–244, 2007.

6. A. Iasonos and J. O'Quigley. Adaptive dose-finding studies: A review of model-guided phase I clinical trials. *Journal of Clinical Oncology*, 32:2505–2511, 2014.

7. J. O'Quigley, X. Paoletti, and J. Maccario. Non-parametric optimal design in dose finding studies. *Biostatistics*, 3:51–56, 2002.

8. S. Zohar and J. O'Quigley. Optimal designs for estimating the most successful dose. *Statistics in Medicine*, 25:4311–4320, 2006.

9. X. Paoletti, J. O'Quigley, and J. Maccario. Design efficiency in dose finnding studies. *Computational Statistics and Data Analysis*, 45:197–214, 2004.

10. X. Paoletti. Comparative evaluation of phase I trial designs, Ph.D. Thesis, University of Paris VII Jussieu, 2001.

11. Y. K. Cheung. *Dose Finding by the Continual Reassessment Method.* Chapman and Hall/CRC Biostatistics Series, New York, 2011.

12. N. Wages, M. Conaway, and J. O'Quigley. Performance of two-stage continual reassessment method relative to an optimal benchmark. *Clinical Trials*, 10:862–875, 2013.

13. J. O'Quigley and L. Shen. Continual reassessment method: A likelihood approach. *Biometrics*, 52:673–684, 1996.

14. J. O'Quigley and S. Zohar. Retrospective robustness of the continual reassessment method. *Journal of Biopharmaceutical Statistics*, 25:903–920, 2010.

15. N. A. Wages and C. Tait. Seamless phase I/II adaptive design for oncology trials of molecularly targeted agents. *Journal of Biopharmaceutical Statistics*, 20:1013–1025, 2015.

16. J. O'Quigley, M. Hughes, and T. Fenton. Dose-finding design for HIV studies. *Biometrics*, 57:1018–1029, 2001.

17. Y. K. Cheung. Simple benchmark for complex dose finding studies. *Biometrics*, 70:389–397, 2014.

18. B. Bekele and P. Thall. Dose-finding based on multiple toxicities in a soft tissue sarcoma trial. *Journal of the American Statistical Association*, 99:26–35, 2004.

19. S. Lee, B. Cheng, and Y. K. Cheung. Continual reassessment method with mutliple toxicity constraints. *Biostatistics*, 12:386–398, 2011.

20. S. Lee, D. Hershman, P. Martin, J. Leonard, and Y. K. Cheung. Toxicity burden score: A novel approach to summarize multiple toxic effects. *Annals of Oncology*, 23:537–541, 2012.

10

Practical Implementation: Protocol Development

Alexia Iasonos

Memorial Sloan Kettering Cancer Center

John O'Quigley

University Pierre and Marie Curie

CONTENTS

10.1 Designing an Actual Trial

Traditionally, the design of phase I trials has been seen as a clinical objective in the sense of quantifying and understanding the safety profile of a new agent or combination of agents when given in a first-in-man trial or in a new patient population. The goal is to escalate and de-escalate until we find a safe and tolerable dose with the additional constraints that are present in any clinical trial that we have to accomplish as efficiently as possible. This means that we need to minimize the number of patients enrolled in order to answer the study's objective, minimize cost and resources by minimizing trial duration, while at the same time try to get the right dose which is the maximum tolerated dose (MTD) or the vicinity of the

MTD as fast as possible so that patients enrolled in this trial can be treated at and around the MTD. The initial questions that clinical investigators need to address are as follows:

1. How many dose levels will we explore?
2. What is the actual amount of dosage increase between adjacent dose levels?
3. How many patients are needed to complete the study?
4. How long will the trial take to complete?
5. What is the definition of dose-limiting toxicity (DLT)?

10.1.1   Dose levels and amount of dosage increase

The answers to questions 1 and 2 are often based on preclinical studies and other studies of similar agents in the class or different formulations of the drug. Preclinical data give them an estimate of MTD in other species that are extrapolated in humans as a guess estimate, although these estimates are often too rough and not applicable to human studies (Le Tourneau et al., 2010). Typically, five to six levels are explored; dose levels are often discrete and prespecified, and in some cases, the rationale is to add two levels below and two levels above the presumed MTD in humans. The amount of increase in actual dosage between consecutive dose levels often follows modified Fibonacci which means that the percent increase in actual dosage between adjacent dose levels is higher earlier on and diminishes later on in the trial (e.g., % increase is 100, 67, 50, 40, 33, and 33, between adjacent levels). The following example follows modified Fibonacci 50, 100, 167, 250, and 350 mg.

10.1.2   Number of patients and trial duration

When using simple designs with fixed cohort sizes such as the $3 + 3$, the total sample size varies depending on when the trial stops, but we know that the maximum sample size is $6k$ (k is the number of levels); for example, 30 patients when we test five levels. The sample size for designs such as $3 + 3$ depends on the number of levels. The continual reassessment method (CRM) has been studied extensively both in terms of fixed and variable sample sizes in the presence of early stopping rules (O'Quigley and Reiner, 1998). When using a fixed sample size, a sample size of 20–30 is adequate for CRM designs for single-agent studies when we test up to eight levels (Iasonos et al., 2008). Since we reach the MTD faster, we could test more dose levels without increasing the sample too much when using model-based designs such as CRM (refer to Section 10.4.1). Cheung (2013) developed a software that calculates the sample size that corresponds to a closed-form formula for sample size determination associated with the use of the Bayesian CRM.

Stopping rules are interesting from a mathematical and practical standpoint. O'Quigley and Reiner (1998) developed a stopping rule that estimates the probability that all remaining patients will be treated at the same level as the current estimate of the MTD and the final recommended MTD will be the same. Stopping rules based on confidence intervals are not practically useful when the sample size is small (<30) such as in single-agent trials. The simple *ad hoc* rule of stopping the trial when the last six consecutive patients have been treated at the same dose is an easy and practically useful rule, and in simulations it has been shown to perform well for recommending an accurate dose (Goodman et al., 1995). This rule basically indicates when the method appears to have settled at the recommended MTD. While this rule is useful in single-agent trials with six levels, caution should be exercised when using this in combination trials or trials with increased dimensionality.

Trial duration depends on an accrual rate of, say, one or three patients per month, who will be enrolled; on DLT time observation, which is typically cycle 1 for chemotherapy agents; and whether we include grouped inclusions of say one to three patients treated per dose level. Trial duration is not easily estimated by considering as the total number of patients divided by the accrual rate, as we often lack complete information on previously enrolled patients or cohorts of patients to complete the DLT observation time period before deciding on the assigned dose of the next patient. The definition of DLT is prespecified in any phase I protocol. It includes what type of adverse events (AEs) are considered DLT, taking into account the severity (grade) of the AE and attribution or causality to the drug. Assuming that these definitions are clearly specified, another aspect that determines DLT is the timing or onset of AEs. For chemotherapy agents, only DLTs observed in cycle 1 are considered in dose escalation, which typically amounts to the first 21–28 days from the start of treatment. Simulated trials can estimate trial duration as a function of accrual rate, DLT time observation, and size of grouped inclusions. Refer to Section 10.6 for details. Comparisons of model-based designs such as the CRM and 3 + 3 showed that CRM is faster than 3 + 3, as the number of levels increases or the location of the MTD is not among the first two levels (Iasonos et al., 2008).

10.2 Case Studies

10.2.1 General summary from a case studies review

A comprehensive review of recent dose-finding trials that were model based confirmed the safety and general utility of model-guided trials (Iasonos and O'Quigley, 2014). A review of model-based dose-escalation trials has shown that model-based designs can be used successfully and in practice yield the same results that have been previously reported based on simulated trials. Iasonos and O'Quigley (2014) reported case studies from the PUBMED database published between January 2003 and September 2013. The authors identified 64 potentially eligible articles published between January 2003 and September 2013 through a database search, plus 39 articles from other sources (pediatric brain tumor consortium, articles that cited EWOC-CRM, or CRM, or similar). Forty-nine articles were excluded, primarily because they were describing a methodology without a completed phase I trial. After these exclusions, 53 phase I trials in cancer patients were included in the final synthesis. This review described the study design and disease setting, safety, and treatment allocation as reported in each article. A qualitative review reported on the following:

- Disease setting, treatment type (agent type, single- or multiple-agent regimen), DLT definition, and time frame of DLT observation.

- Patient population, aim to identify MTD for one or more group(s) of patients, and evaluation of the safety for a single or multiple schedules.

A quantitative review reported the individual trial level and summaries of the following parameters:

- Overall DLT rate, the primary outcome (total number of DLTs divided by the number of evaluable patients), and toxicity above MTD (proportion of DLTs observed among patients treated above the MTD).

- Overdose, underdose, and treated at MTD (proportion of patients treated above, below, and at the MTD, respectively). The proportion of patients treated within the MTD plus or minus one level was reported.

- Trial duration and sample size.

- Design parameters and model specifications: acceptable toxicity rate, cohort size, planned sample size, and the number of dose levels.

The results of this review confirmed known parameters in the dose-finding field. On average, these trials enrolled 35 patients, with 25 patients evaluable for DLT. The trials were completed within approximately 25 months, tested five dose levels, and targeted an acceptable toxicity rate of 26% (range 10–33%). In general, model-based designs such as CRM can be used in settings where the acceptable DLT rate/threshold varies, as this is a design-tuning parameter and it can be specifically set to each protocol or type of drug. The acceptable DLT rate is prespecified in phase I protocols, and the design is called upon to find the dose level that is associated with that rate. The acceptable DLT rate set at the outset in different trials in this review varied from 10% to 33%.

Fifty-four percent (28/52) of the trials tested a single-agent regimen, and 46% (24/52) of the studies involved a combination regimen. The mean DLT time frame of observation was 38 days (median = 28 days), corresponding to about two 21-day cycles. Excluding radiation trials, the average DLT window of observation is 28 days, which is often cycle 1.

To account for late-onset AE as DLTs without slowing accrual, time-to-event CRM (TITE-CRM) was used in 8 out of 53 trials. CRM with continuous dosing was used in 9 out of 53 trials, 12 trials used CRM-EWOC (Tighiouart et al., 2005), and 1 trial used lower-grade toxicities. The remaining 23 (43%) out of the 53 trials used the original CRM as introduced by O'Quigley et al. (1990). These trials include two-stage designs where the model guides escalation only in the second stage after the occurrence of the first DLT, and/or use a design with varying cohort sizes (refer to Section 10.4.1 for two-stage designs).

The observed DLT rate in these trials was 18% (range 0–75%), which is much lower than the acceptable DLT rate of 26%. Among patients enrolled in dose levels above the MTD, 36% of the patients had DLTs. This is also consistent with the 3 + 3 design, which has a > 33% DLT rate in doses above the MTD. Nineteen percent of the patients were treated at levels above the MTD, and given a sample size of 25 patients, on average, we can expect 4.7 patients to have been treated above the MTD. Thirty-nine percent of the patients were treated at the MTD, 39% of the patients were treated at levels below the MTD, and 74% of the patients were treated at levels within one level from the MTD. These results confirm previous studies that showed that on average, 40% or more patients are treated at the MTD when model-based designs are used. All of the above results are consistent with the statistical literature that has shown identical summary measures through simulations (Goodman et al., 1995, Iasonos et al., 2008). Additional measures such as trial duration and accrual rates were also provided at the individual trial level and as summary measures (Iasonos and O'Quigley, 2014). The discussion of this review also focused on whether these designs provide recommendations that may be counterintuitive or clinically not acceptable in the context of specific trials. Three trials that had a high observed DLT rate (50% or higher) were described in detail, and problems that are present in any phase I trial, such as the choice of cohort size and DLT time frame, were discussed. We present one trial below to show problems with model and prior specifications and one trial in Section 10.4.3 that had challenges with fast accrual and a 9-week DLT observation window.

10.2.2   Specific case study

The greater accuracy of model-based designs is already known, but this review helped confirm the very important secondary point that the great majority of patients are treated either at the MTD itself or at an immediately adjacent level. Nonetheless, it is often the very few "failed" studies that are highlighted and that help contribute to a lack of confidence in these simple but effective approaches. Our purpose here is to highlight "problematic" studies so that the problems that were encountered will be understood and easily avoided in the future. We provide some very simple guidelines that will guarantee that the method behaves well in this setting.

TABLE 10.1
Patient sequence and dose levels for study.

Doses	1.0	2.5	5	10	15	20	25	30	40	50
# Patients	3	4	5	4	0	0	2	—	—	—
# DLTs	0	0	0	0	—	—	2	—	—	—

CRM recommendation for next patient = dose level 9 (40 mg).
Source: B. Neuenschwander, et al. *Stat. Med.*, 27, 2420–2439, 2008.

Neuenschwander et al. (2008) presented a failed phase I study where, following two DLTs on the first two patients treated at level 7, the model recommendation was to treat at level 9 (Table 10.1). This is clearly problematic and against all ethical principles in dose-escalation trials. Furthermore, these data contradict a considerable body of published work. Such behavior by clinicians was not observed in any other study, simulated or real, and indeed, mathematical arguments have proved such behavior to be impossible when dose recommendations have been based on the CRM model (Cheung and Chappell, 2002, O'Quigley, 2006). Cheung and Chappell (2002) show that both Bayesian and likelihood-based one-parameter CRMs have the property of coherence, which means that the method cannot recommend escalation from any level following an observed DLT at that level. The only possible recommendations are to remain at the same level or to de-escalate to one of the lower levels. Coherence is not guaranteed for two-stage CRM at the point of transition between stages (from a nonmodel to a model stage); however, if the design is set up correctly, then coherence also applies in this case (Jia et al., 2014).

Neuenschwander et al. (2008) described this phase I study based on the CRM (O'Quigley et al., 1990) in detail, and the authors argued that it had failed because of the rigidity of the one-parameter dose–toxicity model. The suggestion from the Neuenschwander et al. (2008) study was to use instead a design called Bayesian logistic regression model or BLRM, which is a CRM design with a two-parameter logistic model. This setup was first studied in the context of dose finding by O'Quigley et al. (1990), described as two-parameter CRM. Elsewhere, this setup has been called ADEPT (Whitehead and Brunier, 1995), LDRS (Murphy and Hall, 1997) and BLR (Neuenschwander et al., 2008). Neuenschwander et al. (2008) argued that using a two-parameter logistic model will avoid a lack of flexibility and, furthermore, that making patient allocation decisions based only on the distance between the target and the current estimated mean rate ignores important information that the whole posterior distribution of the rate would provide. The latter point is easily seen to be incorrect since the probability mass under the curve is in a one-to-one correspondence with the distance of the mean rate from the target; in other words, we have changed one distance measure for another, but such a change could only ever have a quite negligible impact on the sequential recommendations.

CRM design stipulates that we need to experiment at the level indicated by the method or, at least, at some nearby level. If we experiment at the same level indicated by the method, then coherency is guaranteed. If we are at a nearby level, then although there is no mathematical guarantee of coherency, it is likely to be respected in practice. If we experiment at a level very far removed from that recommended by the method, then, of course, the theory no longer holds. In the study by Neuenschwander et al. (2008), the recommended level before patient inclusion based on the prior, i.e., essentially the best prior guess of the MTD, was level 10, which was very far removed from level 1, at which experimentation began. The prior indicating level 10 as the MTD adhered to the Bayesian principle: "the prior should reflect the clinician's best prior guess." In fact, keeping the Bayesian structure, the method recommends level 11 after having observed 0 DLTs in 16 patients, because the current posterior, based on all of the data up to the 16th patient, has its mode at level 11. Of course, this very strong prior essentially drives the study so that the 0 toxicities out of a total of 16 patients, all treated very far below the supposed MTD, are entirely compatible with the prior. The method drops from level 11 to level 9 once two toxicities are observed out of two patients at level 7. Table 10.2 shows the probability mass before any patient is treated and after the inclusion of 18 patients. Iasonos and O'Quigley (2014) illustrate how this would have been a de-escalation had the CRM design been correctly implemented.

10.2.3   Solutions and correct model specification

Neunschwander et al. (2008) suggested that the design behavior was attributable to the lack of flexibility of the one-parameter model and that a more flexible two-parameter model would better fit the data and thereby provide more reliable predictions and dose recommendations. While the conclusion is sensible and would hold in a situation of simple random sampling, it does not hold in the case of a sequential design where, ultimately, and even in the median term, most of the patients are concentrated at a single level. In fact, a two-parameter model is not even consistent (Iasonos et al., 2016) and will behave more erratically than a one-parameter design. Iasonos et al. (2016) showed illustrative cases where the two-parameter model can get stuck and never move from a dose despite accumulating data supporting otherwise. Shu and O'Quigley (2008) point out the very questionable behavior of the two-parameter design, where following a DLT for the first entered patient at dose level 1, the subsequent recommendation is to treat at dose level 6. To correct this behavior, one can restrict the possible estimates of the parameters so that escalation is more severely dampened. Nonetheless, even though a fix can be found, it is worrisome that it is needed. Table 10.3 is presented from the original paper on the CRM (O'Quigley et al., 1990) that describes a situation in which the actual observed data are generated by a two-parameter logistic model. The true probabilities are given by $R(d_i)$, and the target was 0.2, meaning that the MTD was then level 4. Over a large number of simulations, accuracy of

TABLE 10.2
Probability mass at each level for prior and posterior after the inclusion of 18 patients.

Doses	1.0	2.5	5	10	15	20	25	30	40	50
Prior	0.17	0.02	0.01	0.01	0.01	0.02	0.04	0.07	0.09	**0.56**
Post	0.01	0.01	0.01	0.01	0.02	0.03	0.10	0.28	**0.37**	0.19

TABLE 10.3
Performance of two-parameter logistic (2-parm CRM) versus one-parameter power model (1-parm CRM) when the true underlying model is the two-parameter logistic.

Dose	1	2	3	4	5	6
$R(d_i)$	**0.06**	**0.08**	**0.12**	**0.18**	**0.40**	**0.71**
1-Parm CRM	0.00	0.04	0.23	0.57	0.15	0.00
2-Parm CRM	0.01	0.11	0.16	0.48	0.19	0.05

Entries represent proportion of trials recommending each dose (as shown in O'Quigley, Pepe, Fisher 1990). $R(d_I)$ denotes the true DLT rates at each dose level; the target was 0.2, and true MTD was level 4.

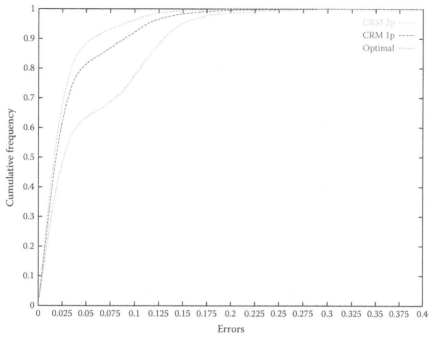

FIGURE 10.1
Cumulative distribution of errors. Optimal design, one-parameter CRM, and two-parameter CRM as shown in O'Quigley et al. (2002).

recommendation was clearly superior for the misspecified one-parameter CRM against the two-parameter CRM, even though the data were generated by this very same class of two-parameter models (57% versus 48%). Over a much wider class of situations, O'Quigley et al. (2002) compared the performance in terms of accuracy of recommendation of the correct MTD of the optimal design, one-parameter CRM, and two-parameter CRM. The superior performance of one-parameter CRM is very clear, and this is illustrated in Figure 10.1.

The solution to the problem is not to be found by adding more parameters to the model. There are three possible solutions, and indeed, only keeping to one of these approaches will ensure avoiding the poor behavior observed in this study:

1. Choose an appropriate prior so that the dose at which we carry out the experiment (e.g., dose level 1) is a dose indicated by the prior. This was the approach taken in O'Quigley et al. (1990).

2. Keep the prior chosen by the investigators, but then make sure to actually carry out the study in accordance with that prior. This may be a difficult solution in practice since, even when the clinicians are convinced that the MTD is level 10 before starting the study, the Institutional Review Board is likely to have trouble with the first entered patients being treated at a level so far removed from the lowest level. Evaluate the sensitivity of the dose allocation algorithm to the choice of model and prior. This was emphasized by Gatsonis and Greenhouse (1992), who showed that the marginal posterior distribution of the MTD was not sensitive to the form of the model, but it was sensitive to the choice of the prior distribution. Simulations showed that the two-parameter model cannot override the prior in certain cases, even as the sample size increased. We suggest the use of a noninformative prior making each dose equally likely to be the MTD, when reliable data cannot be the basis of an informative prior.

3. Abandon the use of any prior, and use a two-stage likelihood-based design. This requires that the first entered patients be treated according to some scheme decided upon by the clinical investigators. Such approaches can be very attractive and enable the investigators to make use of great flexibility. For instance, we can use intermediary grades to guide initial escalation whereby only one or two patients are included at any level in the presence of low-grade toxicities and more patients, say three, in the presence of intermediary toxicities. As soon as the first DLT is observed, then we switch to the second stage of the two-stage design and base escalation or de-escalation on our one-parameter working model. Refer to Section 10.4.1 for more details.

10.3   Formal and Informal Bayes in Phase I Clinical Trials

10.3.1   Choosing basic model structure

The influence of Bayesian methods in clinical trials has grown almost exponentially over the past two decades. Much of this is due to the now widespread availability of numerical computational techniques. Establishing priors is often guided more by facility and convenience than any firm considerations, and this is particularly so in phase I trials. Indeed, for underparameterized models, such as the one-parameter CRM, it is not at all clear how to proceed in a formal Bayesian way, and so, typically, some prior is chosen that is centered at the right place, i.e., the dose at which you wish to start the study, and is sufficiently imprecise to allow the model to respond in an acceptable way to the accumulating observations. Theory backs this up (Cheung and Chappell, 2002), and a broad range of simulations allow us to anticipate reasonably well how things will proceed in practice.

Bayes' formula, which is a simple incontrovertible formula of probability, is often appealed to, but, in most cases, the inferential steps that are taken may be quite far from what a rigorous Bayesian would recommend. More formal Bayes proceeds along much more established lines, and the place for improvisation is much more restricted. Inference is fairly straightforward and requires that the following two principles be respected:

- The prior distribution must be what you would genuinely use to predict in the absence of any data.

- No data of any form could cause you to change the prior once it is selected.

The second of the Bayesian principles might seem surprising but comes from the basic Bayesian school of thought whereby lack of knowledge, alongside any knowledge, is expressed via the prior. Even when subsequent observations violently contradict the prior, we should only allow the laws of probability, i.e., Bayes' theorem, to be used to obtain the correct posterior distribution. The idea is that any lack of knowledge, alongside any perception of knowledge, needs to be accurately described in the choice of prior distribution. Once we have accomplished this task to an acceptable degree of precision, then there remain only the actual data. The data can only influence our knowledge on any parameters through the likelihood function and subsequently the posterior distribution. The only allowable mechanism for doing this—i.e., for updating our prior concepts, speculations, or simply guesses on the possible values of the unknown parameters—is that of Bayes' theorem. This then necessarily rules out simulations as a way to assess the suitability of prior distributions. The advantage of this approach is that it is very easily formalized and, indeed, very easily computerized since every step can be well outlined in advance. For this reason, it is popular. However, in applied science, our initial guesses or assumptions can very often be so far away from what the data may describe that it would be asking far too much of Bayes' formula to retrieve the situation within any kind of reasonable time frame. We are therefore in favor of a much less formal approach to Bayesian modeling.

Simulations are almost routinely carried out in the context of clinical trial design, and, in view of the above, we must regard such analytical techniques as being no more than informally Bayesian. This is not where the case study described in Section 10.2.2 came unstuck, although simulations could certainly have helped. The problem in the study described previously was the desire to uncritically meet the first principle, i.e., to use the clinicians' input to obtain the best guess at the level that would end up being the MTD, the level at which, if the researchers had to place a bet, it would be there. It is not uncommon for clinicians to be optimistic about how high a level will be tolerated, and this is reflected in the constructed prior that puts nearly 60% of the total prior probability on level 10 out of 15 or more levels (Table 10.2). In some ways, the limitations of a pure Bayesian approach are well highlighted in this example. The formal approach would solicit information from the clinicians and then, in the light of these observations, update our estimates via Bayes' formula. However, the clinicians' own intuitive updating can be very far removed from that. A clinician might feel convinced that level 10 is the right level, and that the chances of seeing a DLT at level 7 are very close to zero. Both the clinician and the method (i.e., Bayes) will react to those unanticipated two DLTs out of two patients at level 7. The clinician will arguably disregard the prior. The prior will be updated through the data, but this will occur at a much slower pace. This is the reason why we evaluate different priors, i.e., see how the updating will react to unexpected information. This involves prior simulation, prior checking, and the acceptance of the procedure as more than just a statistical straight jacket but as a way to establish procedures whose behavior can be entirely anticipated.

Bayesians will often point out that the choice of the model alone is a way to supply prior information. If the model is very broad, covering a wide range of situations, then we might argue that such information is so weak that we can proceed as though none was so construed. For the problems in phase I studies, the models that we employ are anything but broad, and so it is worth recognizing from the outset that our choice of model is a more or less direct way of providing some prior information. Putting some distribution on the parameters of a model—the greater the dispersion, then usually the greater the uncertainty in the parameter value—is natural but is not at all orthogonal, or independent, of the choice of model. These two model features are intimately related and described in detail in Iasonos and O'Quigley (2012). CRM models usually make use of a so-called skeleton, a number, often interpreted as a probability of toxicity prior to experimentation, at each level. This skeleton will describe a strictly increasing function over the dose levels, and, in view of the model structure, any other skeleton obtained from the first by means of some positive power transformation will behave in an identical way. As a result, the actual values of the skeleton are not so important; more important is the spacing between adjacent dose levels on some suitable scale. Indeed, the model ought to reflect a spacing between the doses such that, on an appropriate scale, the spacing remains more or less constant over the dose range. The question of how large the spacing should be relates to the operating characteristics, i.e., how quickly we escalate or de-escalate as we make observations on the incoming patients. One desirable characteristic would be that if all of the observations were shifted up or down the dose scale by the same amount, then the recommended dose also ought to be shifted by the same amount. This is presented in more detail in the section below.

10.3.2   Priors and the use of pseudodata

Our goal is to fix any prior $g(a)$ for the working parameter a for the dose toxicity model $\psi(a)$ so that it is invariant, and at the same time, it is not heavily biased (refer to Chapter 1).

We would like the following invariance property to hold. Suppose that we have data on patients treated at dose levels 2 and 3 and no data elsewhere. Suppose that the observed rates are 0/4 at d_2 and 1/3 at d_3, and the recommendation is d_4. If these data are shifted so that the same patients are now treated at levels 3 and 4 with the same observed rates, i.e., 0/4 at d_3 and 1/3 at d_4, then we would like for the recommendation to be shifted in exactly the same way. That is, we would now recommend level d_{i+1} instead of d_i which here would be d_5. This property is not so important when the goal is to home in on a single level. Levels are not favored by the choice of a skeleton or a prior, unless of course that is a deliberate choice, and we look at this below. When we are also considering levels adjacent to that of the currently estimated MTD, then it is important that, in some sense, each level is given a fair chance. The idea is that if, for example, we consider level i to be the most likely candidate for being the MTD, then when considering levels $i-1$ and $i+1$ as potential MTD candidates, the evidence should be provided by the observations with minimal influence exerted by the choice of skeleton. In other words, the skeleton influence needs to be as weak as possible.

Indeed, in the paper of O'Quigley et al. (1990), the simple prior that appeared to be relatively noninformative at most of the levels became somewhat more informative at the highest level, making those few cases in which the highest level did correspond to the MTD to be quite difficult to attain. The problem can be overcome via the use of pseudodata. For this, we need the following proposition.

Proposition 10.1 *For any skeleton $\alpha_i, i = 1, \ldots, k$, and for any $w > 0$, then using likelihood alone, the models $\psi(d_i, a) = \alpha_i^{\exp(a)}$ and $\psi(d_i, a) = (\alpha_i^w)^{\exp(a)}$ are equivalent.*

By "equivalent" we mean that not only is the final recommendation the same but also that at every step all estimates coincide and, in particular, the running estimate of the MTD. The proof is trivial, following from an elementary property of likelihood estimators. One consequence of the proposition is that if we are in the likelihood framework, we are unable to interpret skeleton values as prior probabilities of toxicity since any arbitrary power transformation has no impact on estimates of toxicity rates. Note that, assuming the working model, then in light of the above proposition, there exists some a^* so that $\psi^{1/w}(d_i, a^*) = \alpha_i^{\exp(a^*)}$. If we represent any prior using pseudodata and this is written as $\tilde{R}(d_i), i = 1, \ldots, k$, it follows that

$$\delta_i = \log(-\log(\tilde{R}(d_i))) - \log(-\log(\tilde{R}(d_{i-1}))), \tag{10.1}$$

which can be compared with Equation 10.4. A constant $\delta = \delta_i$ for all i will satisfy the invariance property that we wish to have but will not of itself guarantee a single unique solution for α_i. As a result of the above proposition, there are an infinite number of skeletons that satisfy Equation 10.1. We lose no generality in allowing the prior pseudodata $\tilde{R}(d_i) = t_i^*/n_i^*, i = 1, \ldots, k$, to coincide with the skeleton, i.e., we fix $a = 0$, but, again, that does not determine our skeleton. It does nonetheless simplify our task, since we now only have one parameter to be concerned about rather than two. Finally, if we wish to start experimentation at level 2, then it makes sense to fix the skeleton value at level 2 to coincide exactly with the target rate, e.g., $\alpha_2 = \theta = 0.2$. This will also fix the prior data such that $\tilde{R}(d_i) = 2/10$, for example. If we have many levels, and we make use of a two-stage design, then it is better to hold off on fixing the skeleton (and prior) until we run into our first DLT (Iasonos and O'Quigley, 2012). Then, most likely, we would take the level below the level producing the first DLT to coincide with the target rate in order to be fairly conservative.

It is challenging to choose a parametric function, $g(a)$, that will have the properties that we require (Yuan and Yin, 2009). Such a function may be broadly "noninformative," but it will still, in general, favor certain levels over others. Table 10.4 shows the weights that

TABLE 10.4

Probability $\hat{p}_i$ at each dose level based on two approaches for given skeletons: Exponential prior (upper panel) and pseudodata (lower panel).

Skeleton	$d_i = 1$	2	3	4	5	6
Exponential prior						
s_1: 0.05, 0.10, 0.20, 0.30, 0.50, 0.70	0.46	0.11	0.12	0.15	0.13	0.03
s_2: 0.01, 0.07, 0.20, 0.38, 0.55, 0.70	0.38	0.17	0.18	0.15	0.09	0.03
s_3: 0.05, 0.11, 0.20, 0.30, 0.41, 0.52	0.47	0.11	0.11	0.10	0.09	0.12
s_4: 0.01, 0.07, 0.20, 0.38, 0.56, 0.71	0.37	0.17	0.19	0.16	0.09	0.02
s_5: 0.05, 0.11, 0.20, 0.31, 0.42, 0.53	0.47	0.11	0.12	0.11	0.09	0.11
Pseudodata						
s_1: 0.05, 0.10, 0.20, 0.30, 0.50, 0.70	0.11	0.07	0.09	0.18	0.36	0.18
s_2: 0.01, 0.07, 0.20, 0.38, 0.55, 0.70	0.07	0.08	0.14	0.22	0.28	0.21
s_3: 0.05, 0.11, 0.20, 0.30, 0.41, 0.52	0.12	0.07	0.09	0.13	0.16	0.43
s_4: 0.01, 0.07, 0.20, 0.38, 0.56, 0.71	0.07	0.08	0.14	0.22	0.29	0.19
s_5: 0.05, 0.11, 0.20, 0.31, 0.42, 0.53	0.12	0.07	0.10	0.13	0.17	0.40

s denotes different skeleton values for each dose level; $k = 6$, the number of levels.

correspond to each dose level prior to seeing any data under various prior distributions. The weights were calculated by first obtaining the partition $S_i, i = 1, \ldots, k$, of the parameter space of a to correspond to each level (O'Quigley, 2006). We then integrate the standardized likelihood at the respective interval to obtain, for $i = 1, \ldots, k$,

$$\hat{p}_i = \Pr\left(d_m = d_i\right) = H_j^{-1} \int_{\kappa_{i-1}}^{\kappa_i} \exp\{\mathcal{L}_j(u)\}g(u)\,du. \tag{10.2}$$

The approach becomes much simpler and more transparent when we make use of pseudodata, $\tilde{R}(d_i) = t_i^*/n_i^*$. We make sure that, up to any positive power transformation, $\tilde{R}(d_i)$ coincides with the skeleton rates. And, no generality is lost by choosing the power transformation to be one. This allows us to reduce the parameter dimensionality, and simulation studies confirm that the operating characteristics of such an approach are at least as good as established approaches (Iasonos and O'Quigley, 2016). For example for a skeleton given by $\alpha_i = (0.1, 0.2, 0.3, 0.5, 0.6, 0.7)$, if we have a total of 60 pseudopatients, the number of DLTs at each of the six dose levels will be $1/10, 2/10, 3/10, 5/10, 6/10$, and $7/10$. The data from the 60 pseudopatients should not be taken to have equal value as that from the real patients, but instead, the contribution to the likelihood from pseudodata should be small compared to that from data obtained from treated patients. We suggest dividing the sum of contributions from pseudodata to the log-likelihood function by the total number of pseudopatients, for example 60, which is equivalent to equating data from pseudopatients to that from one real patient. In other words, pseudopatients correspond to a single theoretical patient divided into 60 contributions spread across all levels. If we denote $\mathcal{L}_{n^*}(a)$ as the log likelihood from n^* pseudopatients, and $g(u)$ is defined in terms of pseudodata, i.e., $g(u) = \exp\{(1/n^*)\mathcal{L}_{n^*}(u)\}$, the probabilities given in Equation 10.2 are given by $\hat{p}_i = \Pr\left(d_m = d_i\right) = H_j^{-1} \int_{\kappa_{i-1}}^{\kappa_i} \exp\{\mathcal{L}_j(u) + (1/n^*)\mathcal{L}_{n^*}(u)\}\,du$, where $H_j = \sum_{\kappa_i} \int_{\kappa_{i-1}}^{\kappa_i} \exp\{\mathcal{L}_j(u) + (1/n^*)\mathcal{L}_{n^*}(u)\}\,du$.

In Table 10.4, we show these probabilities calculated for the exponential prior and for a prior based on pseudodata. The results show that the exponential prior is not as flat as we expected, as indicated by how far it is from an equal weight of $1/6$ for each dose level. The proposed skeleton and prior based on pseudodata have weights that are still not equal to $1/6$ at all levels but are closer to 0.2.

TABLE 10.5

Recommended skeleton values α_i when
experimentation starts at dose level 1 and $\theta = 0.25$.

k	$-\delta$	1	2	3	4	5	6	7
3	0.78	0.25	0.53	0.75				
4	0.50	0.25	0.43	0.60	0.73			
5	0.39	0.25	0.39	0.53	0.65	0.74		
6	0.30	0.25	0.35	0.47	0.57	0.66	0.73	
7	0.26	0.25	0.34	0.44	0.53	0.61	0.69	0.75

Refer to Equation 10.4 for δ and α_i values.

Here, we illustrate how to use pseudodata to form a prior and solve for the unknown dose–toxicity parameter a. Let us denote the pseudopatients at each level as n_i^*, with $n^* = \sum_i^k n_i^*$ and the pseudotoxicities at each level as t_i^*, then the score function based on the pseudo-observations alone is

$$\mathcal{U}_{n_*}(a) = \sum_{i=1}^{k} \left[t_i^* \frac{\psi'}{\psi}(d_i, a) + (n_i^* - t_i^*) \frac{-\psi'}{1-\psi}(d_i, a) \right], \qquad (10.3)$$

whereas the score function based on the data alone is $\mathcal{U}_j(a|\Omega_j) = \partial\mathcal{L}_j(a)/\partial a$. Our estimates are based on the equation $\mathcal{U}_j^+(a) = 0$, where $\mathcal{U}_j^+(a) = \mathcal{U}_j(a|\Omega_j) + (1/n^*)\mathcal{U}_{n_*}(a)$. In this way, the "weight" of the pseudo-observations corresponds to a single patient, so in a study with 25 patients, we can say that roughly (since it depends on an unknown reality) 4% (1/25) of the information has been "added in" by the prior (the existing data comes from 25 patients, and the added information is from one patient). This approach makes the prior contribution more explicit so that if 4% is deemed too strong, it can be readily reduced to a figure considered acceptable. It can equally well be made stronger by using a smaller value of n^*, and all of the prior data can be changed to mirror prior beliefs or simply to obtain some particular kind of operating behavior. Our purpose here is to fine-tune a design that can be used in most clinical situations. Table 10.5 provides general guidelines for skeletons and corresponding δ values that work well under different true scenarios as a function of k levels and for θ, target rate, within the interval of [0.2–0.3]. The skeleton in a particular clinical study should be chosen based on the review of the operating characteristics of a particular clinical scenario and other considerations such as use of single- or two-stage designs which we cover in Section 10.4.1. Operating characteristics over many simulated trials will evaluate the robustness of the design to the choice of these parameters.

10.4   Design Modifications

O'Quigley and Shen (1996) showed that, under certain conditions, the level to which a CRM design converges will be the MTD, i.e., the level closest to the target or acceptable DLT rate. Storer (1989) underlined the fact that large sample properties themselves will not be wholly convincing since, in practice, we are going to be working with small or moderate sample sizes. At the same time, if a scheme fails to meet such a basic statistical requirement as large-sample convergence, then we need to study closely whether this poor behavior is also reflected in its small-sample behavior. The tool to use here is mostly that of simulation, although for the standard up-and-down schemes, the theory of Markov chains enables us to carry out exact probabilistic calculations (Storer, 1993, O'Quigley and Reiner, 1998).

Whether Bayesian or likelihood based, once the scheme is under way, in the nonmonotone likelihood case, it is readily shown that a nontoxicity always points in the direction of higher levels and a toxicity in the direction of lower levels, the absolute value of the change diminishing with the number of included patients. For the case of nonmonotone likelihood, it is impossible to be at some level, observe a toxicity, and then for the model to recommend a higher level as claimed by some authors, unless pushed in such a direction by a strong prior. Furthermore, when targeting lower percentiles such as 0.2, it can be calculated, and follows our intuition, that a toxicity, occurring with a frequency a factor of 4 less than that for the nontoxicities, will have a much greater impact on the likelihood or posterior density. This translates directly into an operating characteristic whereby model-based escalation is relatively cautious and de-escalation more rapid, particularly early on when little information is available. In the model and examples of O'Quigley et al. (1990), dose levels would not be skipped when escalating. However, if the first patient treated at level 3 suffered a toxic side effect, the method skipped when de-escalating, recommending level 1 for the subsequent two entered patients before, assuming no further toxicities were seen, escalating to level 2.

Simulations in O'Quigley et al. (1990), O'Quigley and Chevret (1991), Goodman et al. (1995), Korn et al. (1994), and O'Quigley (1998) show the operating characteristics of CRM to be good in terms of the accuracy of final recommendation, while simultaneously minimizing the numbers of overtreated and undertreated patients. However, violation of the model requirements and allocation principle of CRM, described in the previous section, can have a negative, possibly disastrous, effect on operating characteristics.

10.4.1 Two-stage designs

There are clinical scenarios where we know so little before undertaking a given study that it is worthwhile splitting the design into two stages: an initial exploratory escalation followed by a more refined homing in on the target. Such an idea was first proposed by Storer (1989) in the context of the more classical up-and-down schemes. His idea was to enable more rapid escalation in the early part of the trial, where we might be quite far from a level at which treatment activity could be anticipated. Moller (1995) was the first to use this idea in the context of CRM designs. The idea presented by Moller was to allow the first stage to be based on some variant of the usual up-and-down procedures.

In the context of sequential likelihood estimation, the necessity of an initial stage was pointed out by O'Quigley and Shen (1996), since the likelihood equation fails to have a solution on the interior of the parameter space unless some heterogeneity in the responses has been observed. Their suggestion was to work with any initial scheme, Bayesian CRM or up-and-down, and, for any reasonable scheme, the operating characteristics appear relatively insensitive to this choice.

We believe that there is something very natural and desirable in two-stage designs and that currently they could be taken as the designs of choice. The reason is that early behavior of the method, in the absence of heterogeneity, appears to be rather arbitrary. A decision to escalate after inclusion of three patients tolerating some level, or after a single patient tolerating a level, or according to some Bayesian prior, corresponds to the simple desire to try a higher dose. This follows some kind of evidence of a low rate of toxicity at the current level. The use of a working model at this point, as occurs for Bayesian estimation, may be somewhat artificial, and the rate of escalation can be modified at will, albeit somewhat indirectly, by modifying our model parameters and/or our prior. Rather than leading the clinical team to think that something subtle and carefully analytic is taking place, our belief is that it is preferable that the clinical team be involved in the design of the initial phase. Operating characteristics that do not depend on data ought to be driven by clinical rather than statistical concerns. More importantly, the initial phase of the design, in which no toxicity has yet been observed, can be made much more efficient, from both the statistical and ethical angles, by allowing information on toxicity grade to determine the rapidity of escalation.

The simplest example of a two-stage design would be to include an initial escalation stage that exactly replicates the old standard design: starting at the lowest level, three patients are treated, and only if all of the three patients tolerate the dose do we escalate to a higher level. As soon as the first DLT is encountered, we close the first stage and open the second stage based on CRM modeling and using all of the available data. Such a scheme could be varied in many ways, for example, by including only a single patient at the lowest level, then two patients at the second lowest, and then continue as before. Another simple design, using information on toxicity severity (Table 10.6), enables rapid escalation through the lower levels. This is helpful when there are many dose levels, and the first included patient is treated at a low dose level. As long as we observe very low-grade toxicities, then we escalate quickly, including only a single patient at each level. As soon as we encounter more serious toxicities, then escalation is slowed down. Ultimately, we encounter DLTs, at which time the second stage, based on fitting a CRM model, comes fully into play. This is done by integrating this information and that obtained on all of the earlier non-DLTs to estimate the most appropriate dose level.

It is useful to use information on low-grade toxicities in the first stage of a two-stage design in order to allow rapid initial escalation, since it is possible that the starting dose is far below the target level. This can be accomplished by defining a grade severity variable $S(i)$ to be the average toxicity severity observed at dose level i, in this case the sum of the severities at that level divided by the number of patients treated at that level. The rule is to escalate, providing $S(i)$ is less than 2. Furthermore, once we have included three patients at some level, then escalation to higher levels only occurs if each cohort of three patients does not experience DLT. This scheme means that, in practice, as long as we see only toxicities of severities coded 0 or 1, then we escalate. The first severity, coded 2, necessitates a further inclusion at this same level and, anything other than a 0 severity for this inclusion, would require yet a further inclusion and a non-DLT before being able to escalate. This design also has the advantage that, should we be slowed down by a severe (severity 3), albeit non-DLT, we retain the capability of picking up speed (in escalation) should subsequent toxicities be of low degree (0 or 1). This can be helpful in avoiding being handicapped by an outlier or an unanticipated and possibly not drug-related toxicity. Once DLT is encountered, this phase of the study (the initial escalation scheme) comes to a close and we proceed on the basis of the CRM recommendation. Although the initial phase is closed, the information on both DLT and non-DLT thereby obtained is used in the second stage. Two-stage designs have been studied extensively both in the setting of drug combination studies (Wages et al., 2011a) and in single-agent studies (Iasonos and O'Quigley, 2012, Iasonos et al., 2011).

TABLE 10.6

Toxicity "grades" (severities) for trial.

Severity	Degree of Toxicity
0	No toxicity
1	Mild toxicity (non-dose-limiting)
2	Non-mild toxicity (non-dose-limiting)
3	Severe toxicity (non-dose-limiting)
4	Dose limiting toxicity (DLT)

A large number of studies, both theoretical and via simulations, show that CRM-based designs work well and perform close to the optimal design (O'Quigley et al., 2002, Paoletti and Kramar, 2009). This is particularly true when there is a fixed number of levels under study, preferably around six levels. For more than eight levels, it becomes difficult for any method, even the optimal, to locate the MTD with reasonable accuracy, given the sample sizes of phase I trials (20–30 patients). We often do not know how far away from the true MTD we start, and only by experimentation do we discover the answer. If there are more than eight levels, or there is a reasonable chance that there may be more than eight levels, then our suggestion is to use a two-stage design. An initial stage, in a two-stage design, will start off at a low, and usually the lowest, level and gradually escalate according to clinical rules prespecified in the protocol, not based on a model. The first DLT completes the first stage, and the second stage then kicks in as usual for a model-based design.

At the start of the second stage, the design and model parameters need to be defined. It may seem prudent to continue experimentation at one level below that at which the first DLT was observed. This seems reasonable whether the first observed DLT corresponds to one patient out of one, one out of two, or, indeed, one out of three. This level can be our first best guess at being the level corresponding to the target, typically 0.20, in which case both the skeleton and the prior data would correspond to 0.20. The skeleton can be centered around this level by calling this "level 3," leaving two available levels just below it. Once we have a prespecified number of levels, k, and we are also considering levels adjacent to that of the currently estimated MTD, then it is important that, in some sense, each level is allowed a fair try. In order to provide a recommendation that translates in the same way as the shift in the dose levels, we need for the skeleton spacing to not depend on the dose–toxicity model parameter a, i.e., the current level. Note that if

$$\delta_i = \log(-\log(\alpha_i)) - \log(-\log(\alpha_{i-1})) \tag{10.4}$$

and we choose $\delta_i = \delta$ for all i, then we achieve our objective, since it depends only on the spacing between the skeleton values and not the unknown parameter. We then calibrate the skeleton spacing so that from one value to the next, on the $\log(-\log)$ scale, the gaps are constant and equal to δ. The skeleton for the remaining levels is obtained from equal shifts in δ_i. The same procedure is applied to the levels above level 3. Information obtained at three levels or lower from the current best estimate of the MTD will be very small and, for practical purposes, negligible (Iasonos and O'Quigley, 2012). More details on these ideas can be found here (Iasonos and O'Quigley, 2016).

10.4.2 Grouped designs

O'Quigley et al. (1990) describe the situation of delayed response in which new patients become available to be included in the study, while we are still awaiting the toxicity results on already entered patients. The suggestion was, in the absence of information on such recently included patients, that the logical course to take was to treat at the last recommended level. This is the level indicated by all of the currently available information.

The likelihood for this situation is given by O'Quigley et al. (1990) and, apart from a constant term not involving the unknown parameter, is just the likelihood we obtain were the subjects to have been included one by one. There is therefore, operationally, no additional work required to deal with such situations.

The question does arise, however, as to the performance of CRM in such cases. The delayed response can lead to grouping, or we can simply decide on the grouping by design. Several authors (Goodman et al., 1995, O'Quigley and Shen, 1996) have studied the effects of grouping. The more thorough study was that of Goodman et al. (1995), in which cohorts of sizes 1, 2, and 3 were evaluated. Broadly speaking, the cohort size had little impact on operating characteristics and the accuracy of final recommendation. O'Quigley and Shen (1996) indicated that for groups of 3, and relatively few patients (16), when the correct level was the highest available level, and we start out at the lowest or a low level, then we might anticipate some marked drop in performance when contrasted with, say, one-by-one inclusion. Simple intuition would tell us this, and the differences disappeared for samples of size 25. Should we wish to increase stability, then extra stability can be achieved by grouped inclusions. The cost of this extra stability in terms of efficiency loss appears to be generally small. The findings of Goodman et al. (1995), O'Quigley and Shen (1996), and O'Quigley (1999) contradict the conjecture that any grouping would lead to substantial efficiency losses.

10.4.3   Designs for late-onset toxicities

While grouped inclusions allow for enrollment of new patients without waiting for the DLT outcome of previously enrolled patients and this can easily be achieved when we enroll a few patients at a time and accrual rate is slow, grouped inclusions can also be problematic if accrual is too fast. Treating patients in cohorts of six without updating the model is not beneficial with adaptive methods, as they lose their advantages of acting on the observed toxicities and reaching the MTD faster (Mathew et al., 2004). In cases where accrual rate is fast and/or when the DLT time frame is long, careful consideration should be made on what is allowed in terms of cohort size, grouped inclusions, and patients with delayed DLT outcomes when specifying the decision rules in the protocol, as this have an effect on trial duration and study design. This is a logistically complicated issue regardless of the design being used. The protocol needs to specify what is allowed when a new patient presents for enrollment while waiting for the DLT results of already included patients who have been observed for less than the DLT observation period. In the setting of late-onset DLTs, designs can either be aggressive and move through the levels quickly without waiting for the full observation follow-up of previous patients (use incomplete data), or be more cautious by waiting for late toxicities before enrolling new cohorts of patients (wait for complete data). In the trial by Muler et al. (2004), for example, TITE-CRM was followed, 19 patients were enrolled in 15 months, and the observation time frame for DLT was 9 weeks. In this trial, the accrual rate was much greater than the rate at which the DLTs can be observed, since 19 patients were enrolled in 15 months and the observation time frame for DLT was 9 weeks. This raises the question of what to do while waiting for the DLT results of already included patients who have been observed for less than 9 weeks when a new patient presents for enrollment. The standard CRM, in choosing the best current estimate of the MTD at which to treat, will only make use of patients for whom a DLT assessment can be made definitively. The TITE-CRM used in this trial uses information on all included patients, and those patients for whom the follow-up time is incomplete are treated as nontoxicities, albeit with a model weight to scale down their influence proportional to their total follow-up time. Once the follow-up time is complete for any individual, a DLT within that interval counts as a DLT. CRM and TITE-CRM react in the same way to this information. The same is true for a non-DLT if, at interval completion, it is still a non-DLT. However, CRM considers patients without a DLT and for whom follow-up is less than the entire 9-week interval as yet to provide information, whereas TITE-CRM counts it toward a non-DLT at that level. So many such patients, by summing, can count as a full or even several full non-DLTs at the levels at which they are treated. If one or more of these weighted non-DLTs turn out to be a late-onset DLT, then the method is behaving in an anticonservative fashion for at least some part of the trial, since an observed DLT has been counted as some percentage of a non-DLT (Iasonos and O'Quigley, 2014). The effect of this is to push toward more aggressive escalation in certain cases such as this trial. Late-onset DLTs were being counted for some period of the trial as partial non-DLTs with escalation proceeding accordingly. Subsequently, the model re-evaluated the recommended level and de-escalated based on the known DLTs when these late-onset DLTs occurred, which is why the final MTD is the correct dose. Given the fast accrual in this trial and the number of nonevaluable patients for DLT in the entire 9-week window, 8 out of 18 patients were treated at the level above the MTD, since the model could not react to late toxicities until they actually happened. In the setting of late-onset DLTs, designs can either be aggressive and move through the levels quickly or be more cautious by waiting for late toxicities first. If investigators waited for each cohort of three patients to be observed for a full 9-week period (i.e., 4.5 months per cohort), this trial could be completed in 27 months rather than 15 months. Attempts to balance the conflict of fast accrual and late-onset toxicities in methods such as TITE-CRM and the advantages of these methods have been discussed previously (Cheung and Chappell, 2000, Iasonos et al., 2008).

10.5 Protocol Scientific Review

Getting protocols approved in a timely manner is a priority of many institutions. Unlike rule-based designs that are simple to explain, often the statistical design of prospective protocols with Bayesian adaptive designs includes models, equations, or terms that are not easily understood by clinical investigators. Since research for the design of phase I trials has been so prolific, and many designs are novel, it is often not easy to understand the details behind model-based dose-escalation designs in a way that the operating characteristics are clear. The methodology of these complex adaptive dose-finding designs for early-phase studies can be difficult to understand. The lengthy, technical statistical language that accompanies these protocols often presents a challenge to the clinical investigators who participate in these trials or serve on institutional review boards (IRBs), leaving the responsibility for scientific review solely to the biostatistician. In addition, the methods in some protocols are technically incomplete or include techniques that have not been formally established through statistical methodological research. Navigating the statistical design complexities during the review process can, at a minimum, result in protocol activation delays or, more seriously, expose patients to unnecessary risk. Iasonos et al. (2015) discussed these challenges encountered in the review of phase I trials at Memorial Sloan Kettering Cancer Center and provided recommendations for essential statistical elements required to adequately review the validity and safety of novel dose-escalation designs.

The points below summarize some of the basic questions we should be asking when reviewing any phase I trial from a scientific perspective. Refer to Iasonos et al. (2015) for more detailed protocol assessment guidelines and a set of basic questions for investigators and reviewers to consider in assessing a design's performance. Investigators and scientific reviewers must consider how both patient safety and the trials objectives are met when a trial design is used.

- Describe design in words and with a model.
- What is the DLT observation window and do we wait until all treated patients complete DLT assessment?
- What is the cohort size and are there grouped inclusions?
- Provide operating characteristics of the design:
  - How accurate is the design in finding MTD?
  - At which levels will patients be treated?
  - Aggressive versus conservative dose escalation?

- Is there a fixed sample or stopping rules? What is the maximum sample size?

- What are the accrual rate and expected trial duration?

10.5.1   Scientific review of model-based dose-escalation designs

Tuning parameters: Phase I designs have several clinical parameters, such as a prespecified window of DLT observation; what type of adverse events define DLT; and design parameters that include cohort size, safety stopping rules, a predetermined safety threshold, e.g., 33% or below. Model-based dose-escalation designs generally rely on one or more tuning parameters to guide the dose escalation. One tuning parameter is the presumed dose–toxicity relationship, called the initial curve (the points correspond to the skeleton) for the experimental agent. As toxicity information becomes available, the presumed dose–toxicity relationship will be updated through the course of the trial (tuned) by combining it with actual data arising from the treatment of patients on the trial using an updating scheme, resulting in an updated curve. While each successive decision to escalate (or de-escalate) is based on the most recent data, the initial presumed dose–toxicity relationship continues to play a role in these decisions since it is included in the calculation of the update. Hence, the initial pretreatment choice influences subsequent decisions throughout the conduct of the study, although that influence diminishes over time as more data accumulate. Other tuning parameters include the prior information that could reflect information from historical data, such as completed studies. The prior informs the dose escalation early on in the trial in the absence of any safety data obtained from this ongoing study. Essential tuning parameters must be specified at the time the protocol is written and before any patients are enrolled, since their choice affects subsequent decisions (Iasonos and O'Quigley, 2016). Investigators can choose tuning parameters that lead to either conservative dose escalations and more treated patients or more aggressive dose escalations and fewer treated patients. Tuning parameters, on which the operating characteristics are dependent, allow the model to adapt more precisely to different clinical situations, provide flexibility to the investigators, and most importantly, protect patients. Many options exist, such as choosing to approach the MTD from a lower level, a conservative option known as escalation with overdose control (Tighiouart and Rogatko, 2010). Alternatively, they may allow cohorts of patients to skip dose levels in an attempt to reach the MTD faster, if the dose–toxicity curve is assumed to be nearly flat. There are many clinical parameters that are important, such as the starting dose level (Le Tourneau et al., 2010); the DLT evaluation period; the type of adverse events that are considered DLT per protocol; and how transparent the design is in terms of escalating, de-escalating, or maintaining the current level.

Operating characteristics: The operating characteristics of a trial are the statistical estimates of the expected number of DLTs at each dose level, the expected number of patients that may be overdosed, and the proportion of trials under which the MTD is correctly identified. The operating characteristics are dependent on the choice of the tuning parameters. Due to the nature of the adaptive design, operating characteristics can only be evaluated through simulations that predict how pretrial tuning parameters are influenced by accumulating clinical trial data. In the traditional 3 + 3 design, dose escalation depends only on the information gained from the treatment of the most recent three or six patients. In adaptive designs, only through simulations of hypothetical patients being treated at escalating doses under various assumed true dose–toxicity curves can one obtain the operating characteristics. The operating characteristics provide insight into how a particular design will perform in terms of safety and accuracy. Along with tuning parameters, a clear description of the trials operating characteristics is required for independent reviewers to assess the integrity of phase I trial designs. Some basic measures of operating characteristics include, but are not limited to, the following:

1. The accuracy of these designs is measured via the percent of trials out of many hypothetical trials, e.g., 1,000, that select the right MTD.

2. The safety is measured by the number of DLTs expected to be observed at each dose level.

3. Patient allocation is the percentage of patients treated at each level or the number of patients treated at each dose level.

These can be estimated by assuming a true dose–toxicity curve and simulate many hypothetical patients/trials. In such settings, we know where the true MTD is, and we can evaluate where the design is concentrating experimentation, how many patients are treated at each level (allocation), how many DLTs are observed (safety), and how often the design recommends the true MTD (accuracy). Operating characteristics enable investigators to also compare designs in terms of performance and in terms of how far their performance is relative to the optimal benchmark (refer to Chapter 9).

There is now an established class of adaptive models with known performance (Wages et al., 2011a, Iasonos et al., 2016, Wheeler, 2016), and for these models, most of the information is published. When using such designs, it is sufficient to cite the published work as long as the trial is following the published design exactly. However, this is not true for trials that follow novel dose-escalation designs or designs that include adaptations to existing designs without published research evaluating their performance. This field is moving fast, with new designs customized for specific phase I trials that involve multiple drugs, complicated schedules, expansion cohorts, and enriched patient populations. In trials of drug combinations with information borrowed from single-agent trials and assumptions made for drug interactions, synergy, and/or antagonism, investigators and reviewers need to be confident that the information borrowed or assumptions made are safe for patients. Overlapping toxicities, toxicity attribution, and dose–toxicity versus dose–efficacy effects in the setting of drug combinations are areas of active research (Wheeler et al., 2016, Iasonos and O'Quigley, 2017). Getting timely IRB approval from multiple sites is even more challenging, and the challenges involved in protocol scientific review in institutional committees have been described in Iasonos et al. (2015). Petroni et al. (2016) described the timeline and logistics involved in a timely dose assignment when using model-based designs and the responsibility for data quality in such studies.

10.6 Software

10.6.1 Available software

Different types of software is available that can help obtain the next dose given a set of data or simulate operating characteristics (refer to Chapter 1). Here, we describe just a few options, and this is not an exhaustive list. The Comprehensive R Archive Network (CRAN) (https://cran.r-project.org) provides open-source programs, and most of the software below is part of R.

Single-agent trials: The R package CRM (http://cran.r-project.org/web/packages/CRM/CRM.pdf) allows the use of two models for the dose–toxicity curve (one-parameter logistic and power model); assumes exponential prior; estimates the percentage of trials that select each dose levels, the expected number of patients, and the expected number of DLTs at each dose level; and estimates trial duration for a given accrual rate and cycle length. For a given set of data, it recommends the next dose based on the CRM as described by O'Quigley et al. (1990). BCRM (http://cran.r-project.org/web/packages/bcrm/bcrm.pdf)

allows the use of four models, has the option of four priors, and allows the user to use stopping rules.

Drug combinations: Available R functions for trials that involve drug combination are provided by Nolan Wages at http://www.faculty.virginia.edu/model-based_dose-finding/. The theory behind these models is based on the work presented by Wages et al. (2011b), and model and parameter specifications are discussed by Wages and Conaway (2013). The website and materials provided describe how to implement these methods and obtain the next dose in a phase I trial, and they also provide simulation functions to assess the method's operating characteristics. In addition, a function on how to estimate the nonparametric optimal benchmark is provided (refer to Chapter 9 for a more detailed description).

Retrospective analysis: Iasonos and Ostrovnaya (2011) provide R code on how to obtain a retrospective assessment (DLT rates per dose) of a completed phase I design regardless of the design that was followed in the dose escalation (http://onlinelibrary.wiley.com/doi/10.1002/sim4206/suppinfo).

More advanced problems: Cheung YK provided the R package dfcrm (http://cran.rproject.org/web/packages/dfcrm/) that can implement and study the TITE-CRM. In addition, other functions in this package make it possible to obtain a skeleton such that the method is calibrated (function "getprior"), check for coherence status of two-stage CRM design (function "cohere"), and evaluate model sensitivity via indifference intervals (function "crmsens").

Other software: Emory Cancer Institute: http://sisyphus.emory.edu/ewoc.html. The University of Texas MD Anderson Cancer Center: https://biostatistics.mdanderson.org/SoftwareDownload/Default.aspx.

The AplusB web application (Wheeler et al., 2016) can be used to obtain exact operating characteristics for A + B designs that can be compared to operating characteristics of model-based approaches.

10.6.2 Developing software

CRM is based on a binomial likelihood given in Equation 10.3. It is easy to write a function in R that can find the maximum likelihood estimate (MLE) of one-parameter dose–toxicity function. Available functions in R that can optimize a prespecified function and obtain the MLE are "optimize," or "optim," while "uniroot" finds the root of a function such as an estimating equation. To integrate a posterior density, the function "integrate" in R can be used. Once the model parameter space increases, or Bayesian models are involved, these functions are not the most efficient, and other software is often used such as Winbugs (http://www.mrc-bsu.cam.ac.uk/software/bugs/the-bugs-project-winbugs/; refer to Lunn et al. (2000).

10.7 Conclusion

Early fears about model-based designs such as the CRM being overly aggressive are seen to be not well founded, and clinical teams now use these designs with confidence. As with any study, care is always required to follow basic requirements. These are few, simple, clear, and in all cases, quite logical and intuitive. We have described the problems that can arise when the basic algorithmic structure is severely violated. When model-based guidance is broadly followed, then the large number of case studies shows that it works well, makes the best use of the available information, and keeps to a strict minimum the few patients treated at either a dose that may turn out to be unsafe or a dose that has almost no potential for therapeutic benefit.

Intuition can, to some degree, be a good guide. We are not suggesting that we can just have *ad hoc* designs, but, while the model-based approach will often be used with some hesitation by those concerned at its "black box" nature, we should emphasize that nothing mysterious is happening. Model-based algorithms help obtain the best possible statistical estimates we can from limited data that can potentially be contradictory. Even so, recommendations ought to always appear sensible. This is why it is reassuring to know that methods possess properties such as coherence whereby an observed DLT can never be followed by a recommendation to escalate from the level indicated by all of the observations prior to observing that DLT. Some problems have arisen, even in trials with healthy volunteers, where in a single go, all six subjects have been included simultaneously at a single previously untried level. Mathematical arguments can be found that would show this is not an efficient strategy if the goal is to find the MTD fast. Including all six subjects on a previously untested dose can be sensible only if accumulated data at a nearby level project the untested level to be safe, and even so, the uncertainty is so large that it is suggested to update the safety evaluation after three patients. There are cases where we need a minimum of six patients at a dose to evaluate the pharmacokinetic profile or the efficacy of the drug at that dose before testing a new dose level. The design of a trial needs to be specific to the objectives of the study. In other words, these studies are to be driven with the clinical aims in mind and with close supervision from clinical investigators. The model-based designs are there as an aid to decision making, and the statistician's role is to understand both the indications of the algorithm and the input from clinical colleagues. All of this information taken together can optimize our chances of finding an effective MTD. The dialog between different members of the clinical team and the statisticians can be enhanced by some of the software described above. It can be very helpful to sometimes project possible situations in which we see a run of non-DLTs, or some combination of non-DLTs and a DLT, in the light of which a recommendation can be obtained, and subsequently discussed.

There is now a very substantial body of study, as well as a large number of case studies, some of which we have recalled here, concerning the CRM, its properties, and behavior. This body of knowledge can help, in conjunction with several software options also recalled here, the reluctant phase I clinician to give up the standard 3 + 3 in favor of better procedures. At the same time, the very extent of study on the CRM can be intimidating, leaving the impression that this is not for general use but more for some highly specialized situations. That is not the case, and we make two suggestions for persuading reluctant clinicians away from the standard 3 + 3. The first is possible by virtue of the two-stage designs described in Section 10.4.1. The first stage of such a design can exactly mimic the standard 3 + 3; in other words, we escalate after every three patients as long as we see no toxicity. After observing the first DLT, this stage, that happens to coincide with the standard design, comes to a close, and we continue the trial using model-based recommendations. Certainly, this is not the most efficient, or effective, way to proceed, but it is certainly an improvement over the 3 + 3 design and involves nothing "radical" in order to get off the ground. It is a good way to build up confidence so that, for a second follow-up study, the clinical team may feel more ready to embrace in a less restrained sense the advantages of model-based designs.

The second suggestion is to make use of data-based priors. These appear simply as pseudodata, and it is a relatively straightforward exercise to make up data that can be more or less conservative, put some weighting on this with respect to the actual observations not yet seen, and then proceed (Iasonos and O'Quigley, 2016). In common to all of the model-based designs are technical features that are not immediately transparent to the clinical investigators, but transparency can be increased with the use of pseudodata and its relative weight to the real data obtained in the actual study. Essentially, before we even begin, we have some idea of where we want to be, and then all we are doing is using logical procedures to decide whether we remain at the level indicated by the prior data, we escalate, or we de-escalate. Building familiarity with how the algorithms make recommendations as a result of the incoming observations also helps build confidence and comfort in making full use of the powerful procedures that have become available in recent years.

References

Y. Cheung. Sample size formulae for the Bayesian continual reassessment method. *Clin Trials*, 10(6):852–861, 2013.

Y. Cheung and R. Chappell. Sequential designs for phase I clinical trials with late-onset toxicities. *Biometrics*, 56(4):1177–1182, 2000.

Y. Cheung and R. Chappell. A simple technique to evaluate model sensitivity in the continual reassessment method. *Biometrics*, 58(3):671–674, 2002.

C. Gatsonis and J. Greenhouse. Bayesian methods for phase I clinical trials. *Stat Med J Clin Oncol*, 11:1377–1389, 1992.

S. N. Goodman, M. L. Zahurak, and S. Piantadosi. Some practical improvements in the continual reassessment method for phase I studies. *Stat Med*, 14:1149–1161, 1995. doi:10.1002/sim.4780141102.

A. Iasonos, M. Gönen, and G. Bosl. Scientific review of phase I protocols with novel dose-escalation designs: How much information is needed? *J Clin Oncol*, 33(19):2221–2225, 2015.

A. Iasonos and J. O'Quigley. Adaptive dose-finding studies: A review of model-guided phase I clinical trials. *J Clin Oncol*, 32(23):2505–2511, 2014. doi:10.1200/JCO.2013.54.6051.

A. Iasonos and J. O'Quigley. Integrating the escalation and dose expansion studies into a unified phase I clinical trial. *Contemp Clin Trials*, 22(9):2114–2120, 2016.

A. Iasonos and J. O'Quigley. Interplay of priors and skeletons in two-stage continual reassessment method. *Stat Med*, 31:4321–4336, 2012. doi:10.1002/sim.5559.

A. Iasonos and J. O'Quigley. Phase I designs that allow for uncertainty in the attribution of adverse events. *J R Stat Soc: Ser C*, 2017. doi: 10.1111/rssc.12195.

A. Iasonos and I. Ostrovnaya. Estimating the dose-toxicity curve in completed phase I studies. *Stat Med*, 30(17):2117–2129, 2011.

A. Iasonos, N. A. Wages, M. R. Conaway, K. Cheung, Y. Yuan, and J. O'Quigley. Dimension of model parameter space and operating characteristics in adaptive dose-finding studies. *Stat Med*, 2016. doi:10.1002/sim.6966.

A. Iasonos, A. S. Wilton, E. R. Riedel, V. E. Seshan, and D. R. Spriggs. A comprehensive comparison of the continual reassessment method to the standard 3 + 3 dose escalation scheme in phase I dose-finding studies. *Clin Trials*, 5(5):465–477, 2008. doi:10.1177/1740774508096474.A.

A. Iasonos, S. Zohar, and J. O'Quigley. Incorporating lower grade toxicity information into dose finding designs. *Clin Trials*, 8(4):370–379, 2011. doi:10.1016/j.biotechadv.2011.08.021.Secreted.

X. Jia, L. Shing, and Y. Cheung. Characterization of the likelihood continual reassessment method. *Biometrika*, 101(3):599–612, 2014.

C. Le Tourneau, A. Stathis, L. Vidal, M. Moore, and L. Siu. Choice of starting dose for molecularly targeted agents evaluated in first-in-human phase I cancer clinical trials. *J Clin Oncol*, 28(8):1401–1407, 2010.

D. J. Lunn, A. Thomas, N. Best, and D. Spiegelhalter. WinBUGS—A Bayesian modelling framework: Concepts, structure, and extensibility. *Stat Comput*, 10:325–337, 2000.

P. Mathew, P. Thall, D. Jones, C. Perez, C. Bucana, P. Troncoso, S. Kim, I. Fidler, and C. Logothetis. Platelet-derived growth factor receptor inhibitor imatinib mesylate and docetaxel: A modular phase I trial in androgen-independent prostate cancer. *J Clin Oncol*, 22(16):3323–3329, 2004.

S. Møller. An extension of the continual reassessment methods using a preliminary up-and-down design in a dose finding study in cancer patients, in order to investigate a greater range of doses. *Stat Med* 14(9–10):911–922, 1995; discussion 923.

J. H. Muler, C. McGinn, D. Normolle, T. Lawrence, D. Brown, G. Hejna, and M. M. Zalupsk. Phase I trial using a time-to-event continual reassessment strategy for dose escalation of cisplatin combined with gemcitabine and radiation therapy in pancreatic cancer. *J Clin Oncol*, 22(2):238–243, 2004.

J. H. Murphy and D. Hall. A logistic dose-ranging method for phase I clinical investigations trial. *J Biopharm Stat*, 7(4):635–647, 1997.

B. Neuenschwander, M. Branson, and T. Gsponer. Critical aspects of the Bayesian approach to phase I cancer trials. *Stat Med*, 27:2420–2439, 2008.

J. O'Quigley. Another look at two phase I clinical trial designs. *Stat Med*, 18(20):2683–2690, 1999.

J. O'Quigley. Theoretical study of the continual reassessment method. *J Stat Plan Inference*, 136:1765–1780, 2006.

J. O'Quigley, X. Paoletti, and J. Maccario. Non-parametric optimal design in dose finding studies. *Biostatistics*, 3(1):51–6, 2002.

J. O'Quigley, M. Pepe, and L. Fisher. Continual reassessment method: A practical design for phase I clinical trials in cancer. *Biometrics*, 46(1):33–48, 1990.

J. O'Quigley and S. Chevret. Methods for dose finding studies in cancer clinical trials: a review and results of a Monte Carlo study. *Stat Med*, 10(11):1647–1664, 1991.

J. O'Quigley and E. Reiner. Miscellanea: A stopping rule for the continual reassessment method. *Biometrika*, 85(3):741–748, 1998.

J. O'Quigley and L. Z. Shen. Continual reassessment method: A likelihood approach. *Biometrics*, 52(2):673–684, 1996.

X. Paoletti and A. Kramar. A comparison of model choices for the continual reassessment method in phase I cancer trials. *Stat Med*, 28:3012–3028, 2009. doi:10.1002/sim.3682.

G. R. Petroni, N. A. Wages, G. Paux, and F. Dubois. Implementation of adaptive methods in early-phase clinical trials. *Stat Med*, 2016. doi:doi:10.1002/sim.6910.

J. Shu and J. O'Quigley. Dose-escalation designs in oncology: ADEPT and the CRM. *Stat Med*, 27(26):5345–5353, 2008.

B. E. Storer. Design and analysis of phase I clinical trials. *Biometrics*, 45(3):925–937, 1989.

B. Storer. Small-sample confidence sets for the MTD in a phase I clinical trial. *Biometrics*, 49(4):1117–1125, 1993.

M. Tighiouart and A. Rogatko. Dose finding with escalation with overdose control (EWOC) in cancer clinical trials. *Stat Sci*, 25(2):217–226, 2010.

M. Tighiouart, A. Rogatko, and J. Babb. Flexible Bayesian methods for cancer phase I clinical trials. Dose escalation with overdose control. *Stat Med*, 30(24):2183–2196, 2005.

N. A. Wages and M. R. Conaway. Specifications of a continual reassessment method design for phase I trials of combined drugs. *Pharm Stat*, 12(4):217–224, 2013. doi:10.1002/pst.1575.

N. Wages, M. Conaway, and J. O'Quigley. Dose-finding design for multi-drug combinations. *Clin Trials*, 8(4):380–389, 2011a.

N. A. Wages, M. R. Conaway, and J. O'Quigley. Continual reassessment method for partial ordering. *Biometrics*, 67(4):1555–1563, 2011. doi: 10.1111/j.1541-0420.2011.01560.x.

G. M. Wheeler. Incoherent dose-escalation in phase I trials using the escalation with overdose control approach. *Stat Papers*, 1–11, 2016. doi:10.1007/s00362-016-0790-7.

G. M. Wheeler, M. J. Sweeting, and A. P. Mander. AplusB: A Web Application for Investigating A + B Designs for Phase I Cancer Clinical Trials. *PLos One*, 11(7):e0159026, 2016. doi: 10.1371/journal.pone.0159026.

G. M. Wheeler, M. Sweeting, A. Mander, S. Lee, and Y. Cheung. Modelling semiattributable toxicity in dual-agent phase I trials with non-concurrent drug administration. *Stat Med*, 2016. doi:doi:10.1002/sim.6912.

J. Whitehead and H. Brunier. Bayesian decision procedures for dose determining experiments. *Stat Med*, 14:885–893, 1995.

Y. Yuan and G. Yin. Bayesian model averaging continual reassessment method in phase I clinical trials. *J Am Stat Assoc*, 104(487):954–968, 2009.

Part III

Phase II Dose-Finding Trials

11

Dose-Finding Studies in Phase II: Introduction and Overview

Björn Bornkamp

Novartis Pharma AG

CONTENTS

11.1 Introduction

Phase II dose-finding studies play an important role in drug development. They are the last study/studies before the confirmatory studies in Phase III start. By this, they have an important role not only in supporting the go/no-go decision to Phase III but also in terms of dose finding and dose selection for Phase III clinical trials. While the first two parts of this book primarily focused on dose finding in Phase I safety trials, this part considers situations where dose selection is determined primarily by efficacy studies as they are conducted in late Phase II. The purpose of Part III is to give a practical overview of model-based methods for analysis and design of dose-finding studies in Phase II. This chapter provides an overview of dose finding in Phase II in general and contains an outlook on the following chapters in this part. See also Table 11.1 for a summary.

TABLE 11.1
Chapters in Part III.

Chapter	Title
11	Dose-Finding Studies in Phase II: Introduction and Overview
12	The MCP-Mod Methodology: Practical Considerations and the DoseFinding R Package
13	Designing Phase II Dose-Finding Studies: Sample Size, Doses, and Dose Allocation Weights
14	Two-Stage Designs in Dose Finding
15	Longitudinal Dose–Response Models
16	Multiple Test Strategies for Comparing Several Doses with a Control in Confirmatory Trials
17	A Regulatory View on Dose-Finding Studies and on the Value of Dose–Exposure–Response Analysis

11.1.1 Regulatory setting

The primary regulatory guidance for dose finding is the ICH E4 document on "Dose–Response Information to Support Drug Registration" [1]. Despite the fact that this document is now more than 20 years old, dose finding and dose selection are still often inadequately performed. For example, Cross et al. [2] examined postapproval changes in dosages during the time period of 1980–1999. They concluded that around 20% of the drugs had their dosages changed. In 80% of those cases, the dose was reduced, indicating that patients were historically exposed to too high doses at the time of drug approval. More recently, Sacks et al. [3] provided an overview of the scientific reasons for delay or denial of approval of a drug by the U.S. Food and Drug Administration (FDA) during the time period of 2000–2012. Of those submissions that were not approved in the first-time application, uncertainties related to dose selection was one of the most common deficiencies. In December 2014, the European Medicines Agency (EMA) organized a dose-finding workshop [4] and published a report [5] reinforcing the importance of proper dose finding: "...Poor dose selection will [...] often lead to failed phase 3 trials, delayed/denials of regulatory submissions, [...], additional post-marketing commitments and further requirements for development ..." They also go further in pointing out one possible improvement by stressing the "...importance of rigorous, scientific dose finding (relying on model-based estimation, rather than hypothesis testing via pairwise comparisons)...." A regulatory openness and need for model-based approaches also becomes clear from the EMA qualification opinion provided on the multiple comparison and modeling (MCP-Mod) procedure for model-based dose–response testing and estimation [6], and the fit-for-purpose declaration received from the FDA [7].

11.1.2 Dose finding: overview and scope of Part III

> Alle Dinge sind Gift, und nichts ist ohne Gift; allein die dosis machts, dass ein Ding kein Gift sei.
>
> *Paracelsus (1493–1541), Septem Defensionsiones 1538*

Almost 500 years have passed since Paracelsus, a physician and one of the founding fathers of toxicology, noted the importance of dose: "Everything is poison, and nothing is without poison; only the dose determines, whether something is not poison." The insight that for every substance there will be a dose that will not cause harm, but also a dose that will be poisonous, was revolutionary. Even today, this insight is less trivial or uncontroversial than it sounds: a substance is not poisonous by itself; it depends on the dose of the substance.

The situation for dose finding in drug development is even more complicated: the drug is intended to have beneficial effects, but it will also have unwanted effects. Dose finding is the task of finding a dose (if any) with the right balance between these two effects. While this general statement holds for any dose-finding situation, the way dose finding is conducted can be very different. It depends among other things on the severity of the indication, the mode of action of the drug, and how quickly one can measure benefits and unwanted effects. To give a flavor of the considerations that play a role in how dose finding is performed, we go through a few example situations. We will start with the situations that will be considered in this part of the book, but we also outline more complex situations.

11.1.2.1 Situations where the efficacy dose–response curve is explored in Phase II dose-finding trials

For many indications in general medicine, such as for mild asthma or psoriasis, dose finding is driven primarily by the efficacy dose–response curve observed in Phase II, because safety is often difficult to quantify in Phase II trials (specific severe safety events might be very rare or might only occur after longer-term use). To keep the risk of unwanted effects as low as possible, one tries to find the smallest dose that provides almost maximal efficacy, i.e., the lowest dose that achieves the plateau of the efficacy dose–response curve, because it is reasonable to assume that the dose–response curve for unwanted effects continues to increase monotonically for higher doses.

This dose is then recommended for further use in larger, long-term Phase III trials, provided that the expected effect of the dose is sufficiently high. Establishing that a particular dose is the *lowest* dose that provides almost maximal efficacy requires the study of lower doses with submaximal efficacy, which is an important design consideration. Note that studying "low" doses and having a placebo control are ethically only possible in diseases where a lack of efficacy will not have direct severe consequences for the patient. In some situations, the most relevant safety endpoints are directly quantifiable in Phase II trials. In these situations, one could consider modeling the trade-off between wanted and unwanted effects directly by using a clinical utility index or by using a dose that provides an efficacy that is as high as possible, subject to having an acceptable safety profile.

11.1.2.2 Situations where the efficacy dose–response curve is not fully explored in Phase II dose-finding trials

One important consideration in dose finding in general is to consider the mode of action of the drug. Cytotoxic cancer drugs, for example, work by killing cells that divide rapidly, like cancer cells. But other cells are also killed, which causes side effects. So, the same mechanism leads to wanted and unwanted effects. If cancer cells survive, the tumor will recur, resulting in a treatment failure, which can be life-threatening. Ideally, the dose is as high as possible so that all cancer cells are killed, the upper limit in terms of dose being determined by the side effects caused by the drug. For this reason, dose-finding activities primarily happen in Phase I for these drugs with the aim of estimating the maximum tolerated dose (MTD), which is then used in subsequent trials. Limited further dose–response information is usually collected during drug development (i.e., no dedicated dose-finding trial is usually conducted in Phase II for cytotoxic drugs in oncology), and also the low dose range is not extensively investigated in this area, due to the fear of treatment failures. The situation is similar for drugs used in organ transplantation. These drugs not only suppress the immune system (the wanted effect) but also cause unwanted effects. A lack of efficacy has severe consequences (e.g., organ loss), so one also tries to find a dose that is as high as possible, subject to an acceptable level of unwanted effects. As an aside, note that for some of the newer oncology drugs, the mechanisms causing wanted and unwanted effects are less directly linked than for cytotoxic drugs, so that for many of these compounds dose finding should not be driven by safety alone.

Slightly different considerations apply for anti-infective drugs. Here, one can often find a drug concentration that stops the infection *in vitro*. Dose finding in humans and clinical practice then focuses on finding the dose that provides the adequate concentration at the target location *in vivo*. In addition, depending on the infectious disease, a lack of efficacy can be life-threatening, and there is also often fear of the development of drug resistances when bringing too low doses to the market. Also, in this case, the lower end of the dose–response curve is often not investigated in Phase II trials.

For some indications, it is difficult to perform dedicated efficacy dose-finding studies based on the efficacy measures that are most relevant, because these take too long to measure, for example, measuring the risk of cardiovascular death in heart failure patients. Assessing this efficacy–outcome measure may take several years, and it would be prohibitive to perform a dose-finding trial followed by another Phase III program. In these situations, preliminary dose finding is therefore often done on the most relevant short-term, measurable efficacy markers. Then, a more limited dose finding might be performed in Phase III, by assessing more than one dose in Phase III trials.

Part III of this book focuses solely on situations where a reliable efficacy marker exists that can be measured in a study of relatively short duration and where the complete efficacy dose–response curve can be investigated in dedicated Phase II studies.

It should be noted that in clinical development, the "dose" in "dose-finding" refers more generally to a treatment regimen, i.e., the combination of dose and dosing interval. Even more broadly speaking, aspects like the duration of therapy, the route of administration and dosage form (oral, injection, etc.), the time of dosing (after a meal, in the morning, etc.), finding partner drugs or drug–drug interactions, and the population (are there special populations requiring a different dose?) are closely related to the question of dose finding. Again, it depends on the indication and the type of drug, which in "dose-finding" considerations are the most important for a particular drug. For example, in transplantation, it is often more important to find an adequate combination of drugs rather than a particular dose, whereas for large molecules (like biologics) that are cleared slowly from the body, the dosing interval and treatment regimen (e.g., using a loading dose or not) are often at least as important as the amount of drug per administration. The focus of Part III is on dose–response testing and estimation when the primary objective is identifying the dose and not other aspects such as treatment frequency or route of administration. To address these more complex questions, more pharmacologically motivated models need to be utilized; see, for example, Refs. [8–10].

In the rest of this chapter, first the setting and notation for Phase II studies are described (Section 11.1.3), and then the objectives of typical Phase II studies and design aspects are discussed (Section 11.2). Section 11.3 then describes dose–response relationships that are commonly observed. In Section 11.4, a short overview of the pharmaceutical statistics literature on dose finding and an outlook on the following chapters are given.

11.1.3   Setting and notation

In Phase II dose-finding studies, patients are typically randomized to one of several dose levels $d_1, \ldots, d_k$, where k is around $4 - 7$ and d_1 is a placebo. The dose levels to use are specified before the start of the trial, although adaptive dose–response trials are becoming more common (see Chapter 14 for more details). The drug effect is then assessed at a specific time point after start of treatment, and often a model of the form

$$y_{ij} = \mu(d_i, \boldsymbol{\theta}) + \epsilon_{ij}, \ \epsilon_{ij} \overset{iid}{\sim} N(0, \sigma^2), i = 1, \ldots, k, j = 1, \ldots, n_i \qquad (11.1)$$

is employed. Here, y_{ij} denotes the response (clinical endpoint measurement) of the jth patient on dose d_i and $\mu(d_i, \boldsymbol{\theta})$ the mean response for the patients at dose d_i. Thus, $\mu(d_i, \boldsymbol{\theta})$ describes the dose–response curve that is typically nonlinear in the parameters $\boldsymbol{\theta}$. We discuss commonly used dose–response functions in Section 11.3. In practice, patient measurements over time are often available, so instead of focusing on the dose–response curve at a specific time point, one could perform dose–time–response modeling, a topic that is further discussed in Chapter 15.

In practice, extensions of model (11.1) to nonnormal endpoints (e.g., binary or count data) or nonparallel group designs (e.g., crossover designs) are necessary. In this chapter, the focus is on model (11.1), but most of the ideas discussed in this part of the book carry over to these more general situations with minor modifications.

11.2 Objectives and Design of Phase II Dose-Finding Studies

One way of thinking about the design of a trial is in terms of the input and output of the trial: what information is available to design a Phase II trial and what information needs to be generated in order to decide which trial to perform next?

In terms of input, in almost all situations the MTD has been determined in Phase I safety trials. In addition, a basic level of efficacy for a dose close to the MTD is often demonstrated in a Phase IIa (proof-of-concept) trial. In terms of output, at the end of the Phase II dose-finding trial, one typically would like to know the answer of the following questions:

1. Whether it makes sense to continue development of the drug in larger and more extensive Phase III trials?

2. If so, which dose (or doses) to use in the Phase III trials?

Figure 11.1 depicts a typical efficacy dose–response model, as it often holds for a variety of drugs in clinical practice. The response increases monotonically until it reaches a plateau, from where increasing the dose will no longer lead to a considerably larger effect. In order

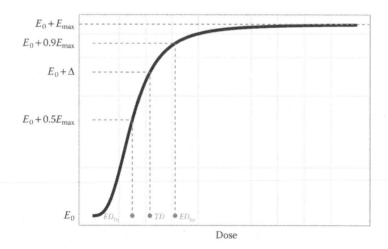

FIGURE 11.1
Typical dose–response curve. In this case, a sigmoid E_{max} function described in detail in Section 11.3.

to answer question (1) reliably, one has to determine the maximum effect one can achieve in the dose range and see whether this is a sufficiently high effect. Answering question (2) is more challenging in view of the trade-off between efficacy and tolerability/safety. In many situations, detailed information on safety, in particular on rare safety events, can only be studied in large Phase III trials, further complicating dose selection after Phase II.

Note that it is reasonable to assume that the tolerability/safety dose–response curve increases monotonically. That means among the doses on the plateau of the efficacy dose–response curve, the smallest dose will typically have the most favorable benefit–risk balance. Hence, dose-finding trials are typically designed to determine the efficacy dose–response curve well, i.e., characterizing the location of the increasing part and the plateau of the dose–response curve. Dose selection at the end of Phase II can then be based on information from the full efficacy dose–response curve as well as available safety markers.

11.2.1   Target doses

Dose–response curves are often described on the dose scale. For example, the dose achieving a specific percentage p of the asymptotic/plateau effect is often denoted by ED_p. For example, ED_{50} denotes the dose giving 50% of the plateau effect. More formally, for a monotonic dose–response function μ, for which the treatment difference $\mu(d) - \mu(0)$ converges to a plateau level $E_{\max}$ as d approaches infinity, ED_p solves

$$\frac{\mu(ED_p) - \mu(0)}{E_{\max}} = p \qquad (11.2)$$

for $p \in (0,1)$. Apart from the ED_{50}, the ED_{90} is often of interest as it describes the smallest dose achieving a large fraction of the maximum effect. Note that this definition of ED_p is only applicable to functions that are monotonically increasing and reaching a plateau level. Alternatively, the ED_p is also defined in terms of percentage of the maximum effect observed within the examined dose range (not the asymptotic plateau level). This approach is applicable to any dose-responsive curve μ. In what follows, this will be denoted as $\widetilde{ED}_p$ and defined as the smallest dose that solves

$$\frac{\mu(\widetilde{ED}_p) - \mu(0)}{\mu(d_{\max}) - \mu(0)} = p, \qquad (11.3)$$

where $d_{\max}$ denotes the dose that gives the maximum response in the utilized dose range $[d_1, d_k]$. For dose–response curves, where both definitions apply, $\widetilde{ED}_p \approx ED_p$ unless the effect at $d_{\max}$ ($\mu(d_{\max}) - \mu(0)$) is markedly different from the asymptotic maximum effect ($E_{\max}$).

Another dose of interest, here called target dose (TD), is the smallest dose that achieves a target effect of Δ over the placebo response level, i.e.,

$$\mu(TD) = \mu(0) + \Delta. \qquad (11.4)$$

The symbol Δ could have different meanings, e.g., it could be the effect size of a competitor drug or the effect judged to be clinically relevant or minimally clinically relevant. In the latter case, often the term "minimum effective dose" (MED) is used, as it is defined as the smallest dose giving a clinically relevant effect. Note that the TD does not exist if no dose fulfills Equation 11.4. For a monotonically increasing function with a plateau level, this could be the case, for example, if Δ is larger than the asymptotic plateau level $E_{\max}$.

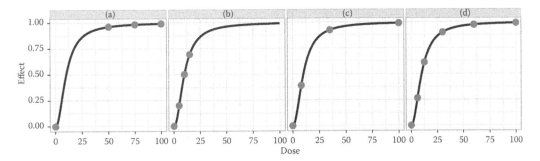

FIGURE 11.2
Different examples of dose designs.

11.2.2 Choosing doses to estimate the dose–response curve efficiently

To be able to gather sufficient information on the efficacy dose–response curve, one needs to place the doses adequately in the dose range $[d_1, d_k]$ used in the dose-finding trial. Figure 11.2 displays different dose allocations, together with example dose–response curves (which are in practice of course unknown at the design stage). Consider Figure 11.2a, where the lowest dose studied in Phase II is already on the plateau of the efficacy dose–response curve. If there is a safety concern for this lowest dose, further information on the dose–response relationship is needed. This would need to be obtained either by conducting another dose-finding trial or a confirmatory trial utilizing more than one dose to evaluate whether lower doses still have adequate efficacy but potentially less safety issues. A similar problem occurs if only the highest dose under investigation has a promising effect, and it is unclear whether the plateau of the efficacy dose–response curve has been reached (see Figure 11.2a). In particular, when there are no tolerability/safety concerns for this dose, it is unclear whether one can use even higher doses and achieve potentially better efficacy.

Determining the complete efficacy dose–response curve adequately (including the increasing part and the plateau of the curve) is hence a prerequisite for informed decision making. If one would know the true dose–response curve, doses could be identified rather easily in a reasonable way (see Figure 11.2c). In practice, information on the efficacy dose–response curve is limited at the design stage so that a reasonable dose allocation is difficult. One way to alleviate the problem is to use more doses and a wider dose range (larger ratio of the highest to lowest dose) to ensure that the dose–response curve is well captured. Basic rules of thumb suggest the use of 4–7 active doses over at least a 10-fold dose range; see, for example, Ref. [5]. Figure 11.2d shows a dense dose allocation that allows elucidating the dose–response curve. In terms of dose spacing, it often makes sense to place doses uniformly on the log-dose scale (i.e., the ratio of subsequent doses is a constant). The main argument for this is that drug-exposure summaries in the body are often log-normally distributed, i.e., higher doses will have a higher variability in exposure values. To cover the exposure range uniformly doses hence need to be further apart in the upper dose range. The problem of choosing adequate doses for a dose-finding trial is discussed more extensively in Chapter 13.

11.3 The $E_{\max}$ and Other Plausible Dose–Response Relationships

A very popular and useful dose–response function is the $E_{\max}$ curve. For a dose d, the hyberbolic $E_{\max}$ dose–response relationship $\mu(d, \boldsymbol{\theta})$ is given by

$$E_0 + E_{\max} \frac{d}{ED_{50} + d}, \tag{11.5}$$

where E_0 denotes the response at $d = 0$, and $E_{\max}$ and ED_{50} are as defined in Section 11.2.1 (see also Figure 11.3). The $E_{\max}$ function (11.5) is equal to the logistic function expressed in terms of log dose. This can be observed by rewriting the $E_{\max}$ curve by substituting log doses for doses (see Figure 11.3, right):

$$E_0 + E_{\max} \frac{1}{1 + \exp(-\log(d/ED_{50}))}.$$

A commonly used extension of the hyperbolic $E_{\max}$ function (11.5) is the sigmoid $E_{\max}$ function:

$$E_0 + E_{\max} \frac{d^h}{ED_{50}^h + d^h}, \tag{11.6}$$

where the Hill parameter $h > 0$ controls the steepness of the curve around ED_{50}. The curve now has an sigmoidal shape, see Figure 11.4. Large values of h lead to a steeper curve. The interpretation of the other parameters remains the same. In terms of log dose, one obtains the four-parameter logistic function:

$$E_0 + E_{\max} \frac{1}{1 + \exp(-h \log(d/ED_{50}))}.$$

11.3.1   Derivation from first principles

One of the reasons why the $E_{\max}$ dose–response function is popular might be that it can be derived from first pharmacological principles in specific simple situations. We give one such derivation as presented in Ref. [8, Chapter 16], to give a flavor of the type of argumentation.

Assume that the drug acts by binding to a receptor creating a drug–receptor complex, which then induces a beneficial response so that the drug is a simple agonist. $C_D(t)$ denotes the drug concentration in the target tissue and $C_R(t)$ the concentration of the receptor at time t. The concentration of the drug–receptor complex is $C_{DR}(t)$. The idea is then that the drug effect is given as a function of the concentration of the drug–receptor complex, $f(C_{DR}(t))$.

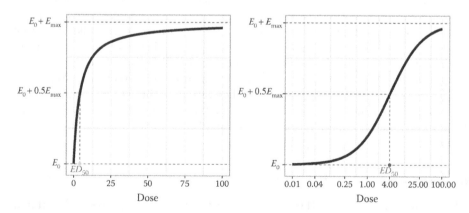

FIGURE 11.3

$E_{\max}$ dose–response shape plotted on dose and $\log_2$ dose scales.

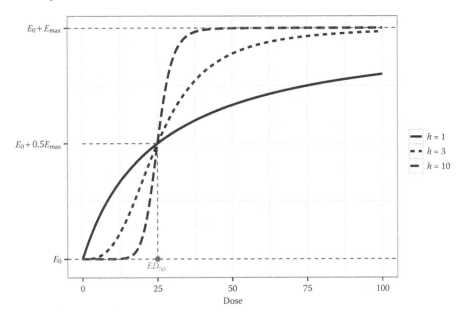

FIGURE 11.4
Sigmoid $E_{\max}$ function for different Hill parameters.

The law of mass action implies the following differential equation for the drug–receptor concentration:

$$C'_{DR}(t) = k_1 C_D(t) C_R(t) - k_{-1} C_{DR}(t), \qquad (11.7)$$

where k_1 and k_{-1} denote the rates of conversion from drug and receptor to the drug–receptor complex and back, respectively. The concentration of the receptor is assumed to be constant, i.e., $C_R(t) + C_{DR}(t) = c_R$. Plugging this into Equation 11.7 gives

$$C'_{DR}(t) = k_1 C_D(t) c_R - (k_{-1} + k_1 C_D(t)) C_{DR}(t). \qquad (11.8)$$

Furthermore, it is reasonable to assume that $C_D(t) = c_D$ is a constant as changes in concentration are often slower than the drug–receptor binding process. Then Equation 11.8 can be solved to give

$$C_{DR}(t) = \frac{k_1 c_R c_D}{k_{-1} + k_1 c_D} (1 - \exp(-(k_{-1} + k_1 c_D)t)). \qquad (11.9)$$

Because $\exp(-(k_{-1} + k_1 c_D)t)) \approx 0$ for large t, one obtains

$$C_{DR}(t) \approx \frac{c_R c_D}{K_d + c_D}, \quad \text{where} \quad K_d = k_{-1}/k_1. \qquad (11.10)$$

Assuming that the function f linking the drug–receptor complex concentration to the drug effect is linear, one obtains the $E_{\max}$ function in terms of concentrations. Then, K_d becomes the EC_{50}, the concentration that gives half of the maximum effect. In situations where dose proportionality of the concentrations holds (i.e., "linear PK"), concentrations c_D are just proportional to the dose of the drug (i.e., $c_D \propto d$). Plugging in the dose instead of concentrations then gives the $E_{\max}$ dose–response curve (11.5).

While the derivation here was only for a simplistic, specific situation, other more realistic derivations often lead to the same $E_{\max}$ dose–response curve or variations thereof. See Ref. [11] for further examples.

11.3.2   Empirical plausibility of the $E_{\max}$ function

In many situations, it seems plausible that the efficacy increases up to a plateau level and then stays on this level for the higher doses being studied. Empirically, this has been observed by Thomas et al. [12], who looked into a large number of efficacy dose–response relationships for small molecules of a big pharmaceutical company and concluded that in almost all of the situations, the $E_{\max}$ curve described the observed data adequately well.

The $E_{\max}$ function can be rewritten as $E_0 + E_{\max}F(\log(d)|\boldsymbol{\theta})$, where $F(\cdot|\boldsymbol{\theta})$ denotes the cumulative distribution function of the logistic distribution (see Equation 11.6). From an empirical viewpoint, many other cumulative distribution functions could be used, with F denoting the cumulative distribution function of a continuous random variable on $\mathbb{R}$ (e.g., the normal distribution). In most situations, these could provide a similar overall fit to the observed data as the $E_{\max}$ function so that the $E_{\max}$ function is by no means unique. This should be kept in mind for interpretation, in particular when it comes to interpretation of very specific aspects of the curve (which might be different between the different functions F above), not only the overall dose–response shape.

11.3.3   Beyond the $E_{\max}$ function

Even when the true underlying dose–response curve follows an $E_{\max}$ function, there are other functions available to adequately describe the data in the observed dose range. Consider, for example, the sigmoid $E_{\max}$ curve in Figure 11.5 on the left, and assume that we only observe data in the dose range $[0, ED_{30}]$ (e.g., for safety reasons). In this range, the response increases almost exponentially, and the exponential curve or the power curve (see Table 11.2) would adequately describe the data. When observing only data in the dose range $[0, ED_{70}]$ (on the right of Figure 11.5), one could use a linear dose–response function. One could imagine further constellations, where simpler functional forms can be an adequate as local approximation to an underlying truly sigmoidal $E_{\max}$ curve. In particular, when it is challenging to fit the sigmoid $E_{\max}$ function (e.g., if the number k of doses is small), it might be advisable to fit one (or several) of these simpler functions. Extrapolation beyond the observed range of doses with these more empirically derived functions should be done with care, or even avoided, when there is limited pharmacological background information

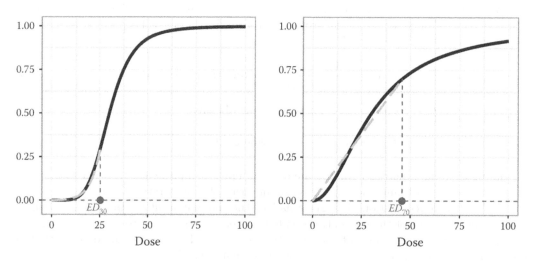

FIGURE 11.5
Two sigmoid $E_{\max}$ dose–response curves (black) and approximations by simpler functions (dashed grey lines) for a part of the dose range.

TABLE 11.2

Dose–response functions.

Name	Dose–Response Function	Parameter Constraints
Exponential	$E_0 + E_1(\exp(d/\delta) - 1)$	$\delta > 0$
Power	$E_0 + E_1 d^{\alpha}$	$\alpha > 0$
Linear	$E_0 + \delta d$	
Linlog	$E_0 + \delta \log(d + c)$	$c > 0$
Quadratic	$E_0 + \beta_1 d + \beta_2 d^2$	
Beta	$E_0 + E_{\max} B(\delta_1, \delta_2)(d/D)^{\delta_1}(1 - d/D)^{\delta_2}$	$\delta_1, \delta_2, D > 0$

For the beta, $B(\delta_1, \delta_2) = (\delta_1 + \delta_2)^{\delta_1 + \delta_2}/(\delta_1^{\delta_1} \delta_2^{\delta_2})$.

that supports the plausibility of the utilized dose–response function beyond the observed dose range.

Another reason to go beyond the $E_{\max}$ function is to be able to model nonmonotonic dose–response curves. Although not often observed in practice, just based on general plausibility, one would expect that safety issues will decrease efficacy at excessively high doses. There are also more formal pharmacological reasons for nonmonotonicity. For example, Lagarde et al. [13] cite receptor desensitization and negative feedback with increasing dose as two among other pharmacological reasons for nonmonotonicity for a particular class of drugs.

But even if the true underlying pharmacological dose–response function is monotonic in the studied dose range, the dose–response curve of interest might be nonmonotonic. Suppose that, for example, one is interested in the dose–response function as it would be observed in clinical practice, i.e., taking into account what happens after patients drop out of the trial. Patients on higher doses may more likely drop out due to safety or tolerability issues, and these patients might then continue on a placebo-like treatment through the rest of the trial with a reduced treatment effect. Due to the imbalance of dropouts for safety on the different doses, and because the observations of the dropouts are used for the final analysis, one might end up in a situation where the dose–response curve is nonmonotonic at higher doses. This clinical dose–response curve, which is, due to the way of handling the dropouts, a combination of efficacy and safety measures, might be the most relevant one for decision making as it might reflect clinical realities more adequately. Two dose–response functions that can accomodate nonmonotonicity are the quadratic or beta dose–response functions described in Table 11.2.

11.4 Review of the Statistical Literature on Dose Finding in Phase II Trials and Overview of the Remaining Chapters

A basic introduction to dose finding in clinical development is given in the book by Ting [14], who focuses not only on statistical but also on general drug development considerations. A review focusing on statistical methods for dose finding is given in Ref. [15]. Hemmings [16] provides an overview of dose finding from a regulatory perspective. Chapter 17 contains another regulatory overview from a more pharmacological perspective. Furthermore, Burman et al. [17] provide a review from a pharmaceutical development perspective.

When it comes to specific methodologies for estimating dose–response curves, one can distinguish between approaches trying to model the dose–response curve using a parametric function and methods trying to employ a semi- or nonparametric model for the curve. Another distinction is whether Bayesian or non-Bayesian methods are used. An extensive overview and simulation-based comparison of different methods is provided in the white papers of the PhRMA (Pharmaceutical Research and Manufacturers of America) group on adaptive dose-ranging studies [18, 19], studying parametric and nonparametric as well as Bayesian and non-Bayesian methods.

Bayesian parametric methods for estimating the dose–response curve have been proposed, for example, in Ref. [20], and the specification of prior distributions for parametric dose–response functions has been considered in Ref. [21]. Nonparametric Bayesian methods for estimating the dose–response curve have been considered, for example, in Refs [22–25], often coupled with the use of adaptive designs [26]. When it comes to nonparametric estimation, shape constraints such as monotonicity [27] or unimodality [28] are utilized. Completely nonparametric estimation of the dose–response curve would be challenging due to the usually rather small number of doses and relatively high residual variability. The MCP-Mod method introduced in Ref. [29] provides an approach somewhere between parametric and nonparametric modeling, because a candidate set of parametric dose–response curves is used to model the dose–response curve. Depending on the diversity of the candidate models, this approach can be rather flexible in terms of estimating the dose–response curve while still relying on parametric models. See Chapter 12 for more detail.

The use of optimal designs in nonadaptive studies is considered, for example, in Refs. [30, 31]. Useful additional information on optimal designs that are not specifically dedicated to dose-finding problems are found in Refs [32, 33]. Chapter 13 looks into design aspects for dose-finding studies, not only for choosing dose levels but also in terms of sample size calculation.

Bayesian [22, 25, 26] and non-Bayesian [34–36] approaches exist for adaptive designs. Case studies for completed adaptive dose-finding studies are reported in Refs [37–41]. Furthermore, authors in Refs [42–44] looked into factors that possibly impact the performance of an adaptive design compared to a fixed designs. Chapter 14 of this book provides an overview of different adaptation rules that can be used in two-stage adaptive designs.

Modeling the relationship of dose, exposure, and response over time is at the core of pharmacometric modeling, and Refs [8–10] provide introductions. It can also be useful to model dose, time, and response (see Ref. [45]), where the E_{max} function is employed over time and the parameters in the E_{max} function themselves evolve as parametric functions over time. Chapter 15 gives an overview of a specific class of longitudinal dose–response models.

In the confirmatory phase of clinical development, when performing comparisons between multiple active doses and a control group, strong control of the familywise error rate is relevant. An overview of multiple testing methods with focus on dose finding is given in Ref. [10], and a general overview of multiple testing is given in Ref. [46]. Chapter 16 provides an overview and comparison of different multiple testing strategies when multiple doses are compared to a control.

A recent stream of literature focuses on the design not only of single studies but also of entire development programs, factoring in, for example, time and financial aspects in a decision-theoretic approach. This work focuses, for example, on the question of the sample size of a Phase II trial versus that of the Phase III trials; see, for example, Refs [47–49].

11.5   Acknowledgments

As a co-editor of this book, the author would like to acknowledge the great help of Frank Bretz, Loïc Darchy, Vivian Lanius, Tobias Mielke, David Ohlssen, José Pinheiro, Oliver Sander, and Marc Vandemeulebroecke in the review process of the different chapters in Part III.

References

1. ICH. ICH Topic E4: Dose-response information to support drug registration, E4, 1994. http://www.ema.europa.eu/docs/en_GB/document_library/Scientific_guideline/2009/09/WC500002834.pdf.

2. J. Cross, H. Lee, A. Westelinck, J. Nelson, C. Grudzinskas, and C. Peck. Postmarketing drug dosage changes of 499 FDA-approved new molecular entities, 1980–1999. *Pharmacoepidemiology and Drug Safety*, 11(6):439–446, 2002.

3. L. V. Sacks, H. H. Shamsuddin, Y. I. Yasinskaya, K. Bouri, M. L. Lanthier, and R. E. Sherman. Scientific and regulatory reasons for delay and denial of FDA approval of initial applications for new drugs, 2000–2012. *Journal of the American Medical Association*, 311(4):378–384, 2014.

4. A. Mullard. Regulators and industry tackle dose finding issues. *Nature Reviews Drug Discovery*, 14:371–372, 2015.

5. European Medicines Agency. Report from dose finding workshop, 2015. http://www.ema.europa.eu/docs/en_GB/document_library/Report/2015/04/WC500185864.pdf.

6. European Medicines Agency. Qualification opinion of MCP-Mod as an efficient statistical methodology for model-based design and analysis of Phase II dose finding studies under model uncertainty, 2014. http://goo.gl/imT7IT.

7. Food and Drug Administration. Determination letter, 2016. http://www.fda.gov/downloads/Drugs/DevelopmentApprovalProcess/UCM508700.pdf.

8. A. Källén. *Computational Pharmacokinetics*. Chapman and Hall, Boca Raton, FL, 2007.

9. M. Lavielle. *Mixed Effects Models for the Population Approach: Models, Tasks, Methods and Tools*. CRC Press, Boca Raton, FL, 2014.

10. J. Gabrielsson and D. Weiner. *Pharmacokinetic and Pharmacodynamic Data Analysis: Concepts and Applications*, 4th edition. Swedish Pharmaceutical Press, Stockholm, 2007.

11. T. P. Kenakin. *A Pharmacology Primer: Theory, Applications, and Methods*, 3rd edition. Elsevier Academic Press, London, UK, 2009.

12. N. Thomas, K. Sweeney, and V. Somayaji. Meta-analysis of clinical dose–response in a large drug development portfolio. *Statistics in Biopharmaceutical Research*, 6:302–317, 2014.

13. F. Lagarde, C. Beausoleil, S. M. Belcher, L. P. Belzunces, C. Emond, M. Gueret, and C. Rousselle. Non-monotonic dose–response relationships and endocrine disruptors: A qualitative method of assessment. *Environmental Health*, 14:13, 2015.

14. N. Ting. *Dose Finding in Drug Development*. Springer, New York, 2006.

15. F. Bretz, J. C. Hsu, J. C. Pinheiro, and Y. Liu. Dose finding—A challenge in statistics. *Biometrical Journal*, 50:480–504, 2008.

16. R. Hemmings. Philosophy and methodology of dose finding—A regulatory perspective. In S. Chevret, Ed., *Statistical Methods for Dose-Finding Experiments*, pp. 19–57. John Wiley & Sons, Hoboken, NJ, 2006.

17. C.-F. Burman, F. Miller, and K. W. Wong. Improving dose finding: A philosophic view. In A. Ping and S.-C. Chow, Eds, *Handbook of Adaptive Designs in Pharmaceutical and Clinical Development*, p. 10. CRC Press, Boca Raton, FL, 2011.

18. B. Bornkamp, F. Bretz, A. Dmitrienko, G. Enas, B. Gaydos, C.-H. Hsu, F. König, M. Krams, Q. Liu, B. Neuenschwander, T. Parke, J. C. Pinheiro, A. Roy, R. Sax, and F. Shen. Innovative approaches for designing and analyzing adaptive dose-ranging trials. *Journal of Biopharmaceutical Statistics*, 17:965–995, 2007.

19. V. Dragalin, B. Bornkamp, F. Bretz, F. Miller, S. Padmanabhan, N. Patel, I. Perevozskaya, J. Pinheiro, and J. Smith. A simulation study to compare new adaptive dose-ranging designs. *Statistics in Biopharmaceutical Research*, 487–512, 2010. doi:10.1198/sbr.2010.09045.

20. N. Thomas. Hypothesis testing and Bayesian estimation using a sigmoid E_{max} model applied to sparse dose designs. *Journal of Biopharmaceutical Statistics*, 16:657–677, 2006.

21. B. Bornkamp. Practical considerations for using functional uniform prior distributions for dose–response estimation in clinical trials. *Biometrical Journal*, 56:947–962, 2014.

22. A. P. Grieve and M. Krams. ASTIN: A Bayesian adaptive dose–response trial in acute stroke. *Clinical Trials*, 2:340–351, 2005.

23. B. Bornkamp and K. Ickstadt. Bayesian nonparametric estimation of continuous monotone functions with applications to dose–response analysis. *Biometrics*, 65:198–205, 2009.

24. R. Prado and M. West. *Time Series Modeling, Computation and Inference*. Chapman and Hall, Boca Raton, FL, 2010.

25. S. M. Berry, B. P. Carlin, J. J. Lee, and P. Müller. *Bayesian Adaptive Methods for Clinical Trials*. CRC Press, Boca Raton, FL, 2011.

26. P. Müller, D. A. Berry, A. P. Grieve, and M. Krams. A Bayesian decision-theoretic dose finding trial. *Decision Analysis*, 3:197–207, 2006.

27. C. Kelly and J. Rice. Monotone smoothing and its applications to dose–response curves and the assessment of synergy. *Biometrics*, 46:1071–1085, 1990.

28. C. Köllmann, B. Bornkamp, and K. Ickstadt. Unimodal regression using Bernstein-Schoenberg splines and penalties. *Biometrics*, 70:783–793, 2014.

29. F. Bretz, J. C. Pinheiro, and M. Branson. Combining multiple comparisons and modeling techniques in dose–response studies. *Biometrics*, 61:738–748, 2005.

30. H. Dette, F. Bretz, A. Pepelyshev, and J. C. Pinheiro. Optimal designs for dose finding studies. *Journal of the American Statisical Association*, 103:1225–1237, 2008.

31. F. Bretz, H. Dette, and J. Pinheiro. Practical considerations for optimal designs in clinical dose finding studies. *Statistics in Medicine*, 29:731–742, 2010.

32. A. C. Atkinson, A. N. Donev, and R. D. Tobias. *Optimum Experimental Design, with SAS*. Oxford University Press, Oxford, UK, 2007.

33. V. V. Fedorov and S. L. Leonov. *Optimal Design for Nonlinear Response Models*. Chapman and Hall, Boca Raton, FL, 2014.

34. V. Dragalin, F. Hsuan, and S. K. Padmanabhan. Adaptive designs for dose finding studies based on the sigmoid $E_{\max}$ model. *Journal of Biopharmaceutical Statistics*, 17:1051–1070, 2007.

35. A. Ivanova, J. Bolognese, and I. Perevozskaya. Adaptive design based on t-statistic for dose–response trials. *Statistics in Medicine*, 27:1581–1592, 2008.

36. V. Dragalin, V. V. Fedorov, and Y. Wu. Two-stage design for dose finding that accounts for both efficacy and safety. *Statistics in Medicine*, 27:5156–5176, 2008.

37. S. Berry, W. Spinelli, G. S. Littman, J. Z. Liang, P. Fardipour, D. A. Berry, R. J. Lewis, and M. Krams. A Bayesian dose finding trial with adaptive dose expansion to flexibly assess efficacy and safety of an investigational drug. *Clinical Trials*, 7:121–135, 2010.

38. M. Vandemeulebroecke, F. Bretz, J. Pinheiro, and B. Bornkamp. Adaptive dose-ranging studies. In A. Ping and S.-C. Chow, Eds, *Handbook of Adaptive Designs in Pharmaceutical and Clinical Development*, p. 11. CRC Press, Boca Raton, FL, 2011.

39. B. Jones, G. Layton, H. Richardson, and N. Thomas. Model-based Bayesian adaptive dose finding designs for a phase II trial. *Statistics in Biopharmaceutical Research*, 3:276–287, 2011.

40. A. T. Cohen, R. Boyd, J. Mandema, L. DiCarlo, and R. Pak. An adaptive-design dose-ranging study of PD 0348292, an oral factor Xa inhibitor, for thromboprophylaxis after total knee replacement surgery. *Journal of Thrombosis and Haemostasis*, 11:1503–1510, 2013.

41. F. Mercier, B. Bornkamp, D. Ohlssen, and E. Wallstroem. Characterization of dose–response for count data using a generalized MCP-Mod approach in an adaptive dose-ranging trial. *Pharmaceutical Statistics*, 14(4):359–367.

42. H. Dette, B. Bornkamp, and F. Bretz. On the efficiency of two-stage response-adaptive designs. *Statistics in Medicine*, 32:1646–1660, 2013.

43. E. McCallum and B. Bornkamp. Accounting for parameter uncertainty in two-stage designs for phase II dose–response studies. In O. Sverdlov, Ed., *Modern Adaptive Randomized Clinical Trials: Statistical and Practical Aspects*, pp. 427–449. CRC Press, Boca Raton, FL, 2015.

44. F. Miller. When is an adaptive design useful in clinical dose finding trials? In E. Fackle-Fornius, Ed. *Festschrift in Honor of Hans Nyquist on the Occasion of His 65th Birthday*, pp. 28–43. Department of Statistics, Stockholm University, Stockholm, 2015. https://su.diva-portal.org/smash/get/diva2:881610/FULLTEXT01.pdf.

45. H. Tan, D. Gruben, J. French, and N. Thomas. A case study of model-based Bayesian dose response estimation. *Statistics in Medicine*, 30:2622–2633, 2011.

46. F. Bretz, T. Hothorn, and P. Westfall. *Multiple Comparisons Using R*. CRC Press, Boca Raton, FL, 2011.

47. Z. Antonijevic, J. Pinheiro, P. Fardipour, and R. J. Lewis. Impact of dose selection strategies used in phase II on the probability of success in phase III. *Statistics in Biopharmaceutical Research*, 2:469–486, 2010.

48. N. Patel, J. Bolognese, C. Chuang-Stein, D. Hewitt, A. Gammaitoni, and J. Pinheiro. Designing phase II trials based on program-level considerations a case study for neuropathic pain. *Therapeutic Innovation and Regulatory Science*, 46:439–454, 2012.

49. Z. Antonijevic, Ed. *Optimization of Pharmaceutical R&D Programs and Portfolios.* Springer, Heidelberg, Germany, 2015.

12

The MCP-Mod Methodology: Practical Considerations and the DoseFinding R Package

Xiaolei Xun

Novartis Pharma

Frank Bretz

Novartis Pharma AG

CONTENTS

12.1 Introduction to MCP-Mod

In this chapter, we describe MCP-Mod, a structured approach for dose–response testing and estimation that is intended to enable more informative Phase II trial designs and provide a more solid basis for subsequent dose-selection strategies and decisions.

Compared to traditional approaches for Phase II dose-finding trials based on naive pairwise dose-versus-placebo comparisons, MCP-Mod has the advantage of enabling the use of more doses in the design without requiring a much larger number of patients. A naive approach using pairwise comparison uses only the information from the respective dose to estimate the dose response, which means that the required sample size depends strongly on the doses studied when a fixed precision is required at each dose. By using modeling techniques, MCP-Mod allows us to interpolate information across dose levels, and the total sample size will depend less on the number of doses studied. The possibility of using more doses will typically result in information-richer dose-finding designs and a better basis for decision making at the end of Phase II. In this sense, the MCP-Mod approach is efficient, as it uses the available data better than the traditional pairwise comparisons [1].

The original MCP-Mod procedure was motivated by the work of Tukey et al. [2], who proposed to simultaneously use several trend tests based on different functional dose–response descriptions and to subsequently adjust the resulting p-values for multiplicity. These ideas were extended in Ref. [3] by combining the advantages of multiple comparison and modeling approaches for a single, normally distributed efficacy endpoint in a parallel-group design. Since then, the methodology has been subject to several investigations, most notably the extension to general parametric models described in Ref. [4]. Their framework is quite broad and can be utilized in situations involving, for example, generalized nonlinear models, linear and nonlinear mixed-effects models, and Cox proportional hazards models, with the main restriction being that a univariate dose–response relationship is modeled, that is, both dose and response correspond to univariate measurements.

This chapter is organized as follows. In Section 12.2, we introduce the original MCP-Mod approach for normally distributed data as well as its generalization for general parametric models. In Section 12.3, we describe practical considerations related to the use of MCP-Mod. Finally, we illustrate in Section 12.4 the `DoseFinding R` package [5], which provides a convenient interface to the general approach adopted here.

12.2　MCP-Mod Methodology

The MCP-Mod approach is a multistage procedure that combines the advantages of the multiple comparisons and modeling approaches.

At the trial design stage, a suitable set of candidate models is identified through clinical team discussions and statistical considerations, which also impacts decisions on the number doses, required sample sizes, patient allocations, etc. The trial analysis stage consists of the MCP and the Mod steps. The MCP step focuses on detecting the existence of any dose–response signal. It is tested using suitable contrast tests deduced from the candidate model set, adjusting for the fact that multiple candidate models are considered. Once a dose–response signal is established, one proceeds to the Mod step, where the best model out of the prespecified candidate model set or a model averaging approach is used for dose–response and target dose estimation.

The findings of the dose–response analysis may then form the quantitative basis for selecting the dose for the Phase III program. In the following, we first describe the individual steps of the MCP-Mod approach for normally distributed data, and then an extension to more general distributions.

12.2.1　MCP-Mod for normally distributed data

The original MCP-Mod approach for a single, normally distributed endpoint was proposed in Ref. [3]. Consider the comparison of a new drug against a placebo in a dose–response trial. Assume that patients are randomized to receive either placebo d_1 or one of the active doses $d_2, \ldots, d_k$, with n_i patients allocated to dose d_i. We consider the model, for $i = 1, \ldots, k$, $j = 1, \ldots, n_i$,

$$y_{ij} = \mu(d_i) + \varepsilon_{ij}, \quad \varepsilon_{ij} \overset{i.i.d.}{\sim} N(0, \sigma^2), \tag{12.1}$$

where the observed response y_{ij} for patient j at dose d_i is assumed to be normally distributed with homogeneous variance across the doses, the mean response at dose d_i can be represented by a dose–response model parameterized by a parameter vector $\boldsymbol{\theta}$ as $\mu(d_i) = f(d_i, \boldsymbol{\theta})$, and ε_{ij} are the independent error terms.

TABLE 12.1

Dose–response functions and their standardized versions.

Model	$f(d, \boldsymbol{\theta})$	$f^0(d, \boldsymbol{\theta}^0)$
$E_{\max}$	$E_0 + E_{\max}d/(ED_{50} + d)$	$d/(ED_{50} + d)$
Sigmoid $E_{\max}$	$E_0 + E_{\max}d^h/(ED_{50}^h + d^h)$	$d^h/(ED_{50}^h + d^h)$
Exponential	$E_0 + E_1[\exp(d/\delta) - 1]$	$\exp(d/\delta) - 1$
Power	$E_0 + E_1 d^\alpha$	d^α
Linear	$E_0 + \delta d$	d
Linear logdose	$E_0 + \delta \log(d + c)$	$\log(d + c)$
Quadratic	$E_0 + \beta_1 d + \beta_2 d^2$	$d + (\beta_2/|\beta_1|)d^2$
Beta	$E_0 + E_{\max}B(\delta_1, \delta_2)(d/D)^{\delta_1}(1 - d/D)^{\delta_2}$	$(d/D)^{\delta_1}(1 - d/D)^{\delta_2}$

For the beta model $B(\delta_1, \delta_2) = (\delta_1 + \delta_2)^{\delta_1 + \delta_2}/(\delta_1^{\delta_1}\delta_2^{\delta_2})$.

At the trial design stage, a set of M candidate shapes need to be identified. Recall some commonly used dose–response models from Table 11.2. These models can be expressed in the form

$$f(d, \boldsymbol{\theta}) = \theta_0 + \theta_1 f^0(d, \boldsymbol{\theta}^0),$$

where $f^0(d, \boldsymbol{\theta}^0)$ is the standardized version of $f(d, \boldsymbol{\theta})$; see Table 12.1 for examples. We will see below that the optimal contrast for model selection is invariant to any shift and scale change on the mean response vector, thus independent of intercept and slope of the dose–response model $f(d, \boldsymbol{\theta})$. As a result, we only need to consider standardized dose–response models when choosing candidate shapes. Besides choosing an expression for $f^0(d, \boldsymbol{\theta}^0)$, we also need some initial guesses for the parameter vector $\boldsymbol{\theta}^0$, called guesstimates. For example, they can be derived from some initial knowledge of the expected percentage of the maximum response for a given dose. Each of these candidate shapes thus produces a mean response vector $\boldsymbol{\mu}_m = (\mu_{m1}, ..., \mu_{mk})'$, where μ_{mi} depends on both dose d_i and the parameter vector $\boldsymbol{\theta}^0$ of the standardized model, for $m = 1, ..., M$. The specification of guesstimates is important for the MCP step. See Section 12.3.2.2 for further discussion.

To test for any dose–response signal given a candidate shape, we use single-contrast tests, which were first introduced in Refs [6, 7] in the context of dose–response testing. These are powerful methods to detect an overall dose–response trend and can be applied to a variety of different statistical models, including general linear models allowing for covariates and/or factorial treatment structures. Later, in Ref. [8], multiple contrast tests were introduced to achieve more robustness against the misspecification of the contrast coefficients.

In the following introduction of a single-contrast test, we drop the index m to keep the notation simple in this paragraph. The test for a dose response trend is formulated in terms of a linear contrast test on $\mathbf{c}'\boldsymbol{\mu}$, where $\mathbf{c}$ is a vector of contrast coefficients such that $\sum_{i=1}^k c_i = 0$ and $\boldsymbol{\mu} = (\mu_1, ..., \mu_k)'$ is the vector of mean responses across the dose levels. The null hypothesis of no dose–response effect, i.e., $\mu_1 = \cdots = \mu_k$, is therefore $H : \mathbf{c}'\boldsymbol{\mu} = 0$. Given an alternative shape $\boldsymbol{\mu}$, optimal contrast coefficients that maximize the power to detect this true underlying shape are proportional to

$$c_i = n_i(\mu_i - \overline{\mu}), \text{ for } i = 1, ..., k,$$

where $\overline{\mu} = \sum_{i=1}^k n_i \mu_i / \sum_{i=1}^k n_i$ is the overall mean [3]. After normalization, the unique solution is given by $\mathbf{c}/\|\mathbf{c}\|$, where $\|\mathbf{c}\| = \sqrt{\sum_{i=1}^k c_i^2}$. For example, a linear contrast test for equally spaced doses and balanced patient allocation is defined such that the difference between any two adjacent contrast coefficients is a constant.

In the MCP-Mod approach, each candidate shape $\boldsymbol{\mu}_m$ can therefore be represented by an optimal contrast $\mathbf{c}_m = (c_{m1}, \ldots, c_{mk})'$ such that the power of the test when the true underlying mean response equals $\boldsymbol{\mu}_m$ is maximized. For example, if the linear model has been included in the candidate set, the linear contrast test introduced above is then a powerful test to detect the linear trend. Since contrast tests are shift and scale invariant, it is sufficient to work with the standardized versions of the dose–response models.

The test statistics of the single contrast tests are

$$T_m = \frac{\sum_{i=1}^{k} c_{mi}\overline{y}_i}{S\sqrt{\sum_{i=1}^{k} c_{mi}^2/n_i}}, \text{ for } m = 1, \ldots, M,$$

where $\overline{y}_i$ is the observed mean at dose d_i, $S^2 = \sum_{i=1}^{k}\sum_{j=1}^{n_i}(y_{ij} - \overline{y}_i)^2/(N - k)$ denotes the mean squared error, and $N = \sum_{i=1}^{k} n_i$ is the total sample size. Under model (12.1) and under the null hypothesis $H : \mathbf{c}'\boldsymbol{\mu} = 0$, the test statistics $T_1, \ldots, T_M$ jointly follow a central multivariate t distribution with $N - k$ degrees of freedom and a correlation matrix depending on the sample sizes and the contrast coefficients.

A multiple contrast test then uses the maximum test statistic to account for multiplicity. The final test statistic $T_{\max}$ for testing an overall dose–response signal using multiple shapes is then $T_{\max} = \max_m T_m$. Let $q_{1-\alpha}$ denote the multiplicity-adjusted critical value. A dose–response signal is established if $T_{\max} \geq q_{1-\alpha}$. Any dose–response model with a test statistic larger than $q_{1-\alpha}$ can be declared statistically significant at level α, which forms a reference set $\{M_1, \ldots, M_L\}$ of L significant models.

At the analysis stage, every single-contrast test thus translates into a decision procedure for whether a candidate dose–response curve is significant given the observed data, while controlling the Type I error rate of incorrectly declaring a significant dose–response signal at prespecified level α. If no candidate shape is statistically significant, then the MCP-Mod procedure stops and indicates that a dose–response signal cannot be established from the observed data. But notice that such a result does not necessarily mean that the compound has no effect at all, and we may still desire to estimate the dose–response relationship.

Once the overall dose–response signal is established, we can select one model out of the reference set of L significant models. This model could be the one with the most significant contrast test statistic, or based on other model selection criteria such as the Akaike Information Criterion (AIC) or the Bayesian Information Criterion (BIC). Alternatively, multiple significant models can be selected if model averaging is preferred [9]. Furthermore, fitting the selected model to the data and estimating adequately the target dose(s) of interest can be achieved using standard inverse nonlinear regression techniques.

Finally, we conclude this section by emphasizing that the inclusion of several candidate models in the MCP-Mod procedure addresses the issue of possible model misspecifications in contrast to a direct application of a model-based approach and includes the associated statistical uncertainty in a hypothesis-testing framework.

12.2.2　General parametric models

Practical problems often involve nonnormal response variables, e.g., a count, binary, or time-to-event variable, or multidimensional variables when modeling longitudinal measurements. In this section, we describe the generalized MCP-Mod procedure for general parametric models, where the core idea of MCP-Mod remains applicable. More details can be found in Ref. [4].

Let $\mathbf{y}$ denote the response (vector) of a patient receiving dose d. We consider the model

$$\mathbf{y} \sim F(\mu(d), \mathbf{z}, \boldsymbol{\eta}), \tag{12.2}$$

where $\mu(d)$ is the dose–response parameter, $\mathbf{z}$ are possible covariates, and $\boldsymbol{\eta}$ contains the nuisance parameters. This formulation generalizes the notation for a normally distributed endpoint to any parametric distribution (if F is a normal distribution, $\mu(d)$ is then the mean response at dose d, and $\boldsymbol{\eta} = \sigma^2$ is a nuisance parameter). The main idea is to extract dose–response parameters $\mu(d)$ from model (12.2) and perform contrast test and dose–response model fitting on these parameters.

Because all dose–response information is contained in $\mu(d)$, this parameter should be easily interpretable in order to communicate with clinical teams, to choose candidate dose–response shapes, to specify clinically relevant effects, etc. As an example, consider the Weibull distribution. It is typically parameterized by a scale parameter λ and shape parameter α, neither of which is easily interpretable. For the purpose of interpretability, the model could be re-parameterized in terms of the median time to event $\mu = \log(2)^{1/\alpha}/\lambda$ and α and then use μ as an interpretable dose–response parameter. See Table 12.2 for recommended dose–response parameters for common distributions.

At the design stage, same as for normal endpoints, we will specify a set of candidate dose–response shapes $\boldsymbol{\mu}_1, \dots, \boldsymbol{\mu}_M$, and each of the candidate shapes determines an optimal contrast to evaluate the associated dose–response signal. Consider a dose–response mean vector $\boldsymbol{\mu}_m = (\mu(d_1), \dots, \mu(d_k))'$, for k doses $d_1, \dots, d_k$ including placebo. The optimal contrast for this shape satisfies

$$\mathbf{c}_m^{\text{opt}} \propto \mathbf{S}^{-1}\left(\boldsymbol{\mu}_m - \frac{\boldsymbol{\mu}_m \mathbf{S}^{-1}\mathbf{1}}{\mathbf{1}'\mathbf{S}^{-1}\mathbf{1}}\right), \text{ for } m = 1, \dots M,$$

where $\mathbf{1}$ is a vector of 1's of proper length and $\mathbf{S}$ is the covariance matrix of the estimated dose–response parameters $\widehat{\boldsymbol{\mu}}$ [10].

At the analysis stage, we will fit an ANCOVA-type model with dose as a factor, for any distribution $F(\cdot)$, and extract estimated dose–response parameter $\widehat{\boldsymbol{\mu}}$ and estimated covariance matrix $\widehat{\mathbf{S}}$ using appropriate estimation methods such as maximum likelihood, generalized estimating equations, and partial likelihood. The contrast test statistics is then

$$z_m = (\mathbf{c}_m^{\text{opt}})'\widehat{\boldsymbol{\mu}}/\sqrt{(\mathbf{c}_m^{\text{opt}})'\widehat{\mathbf{S}}(\mathbf{c}_m^{\text{opt}})}, \text{ for } m = 1, \dots, M.$$

In many parametric estimation problems, $\widehat{\boldsymbol{\mu}}$ is asymptotically multivariate normally distributed with covariance matrix $\mathbf{S}$, such as in generalized linear models, parametric time-to-event models, and mixed-effects models. When this condition is met, the joint distribution of the contrast statistics $(z_1, \dots, z_M)$ is also multivariate normal. p-Values are then calculated via the joint distribution of $z_1, \dots, z_m$ under the null hypothesis of no dose–response, while controlling the overall Type I error rate at prespecified level α.

Once a dose–response signal is established, one proceeds to the Mod step, fitting the dose–response profile and estimating target doses based on all models with significant contrast test statistics in the MCP step. There are many ways to fit the dose–response models to the observed data, including approaches based on maximizing the likelihood or the

TABLE 12.2

Recommended dose–response parameters for common distributions.

Distribution	Example $\mu(d)$
Bernoulli	Probability or logit(probability)
Poisson	log (mean)
Negative binomial	log (mean)
Weibull	Median of the survival distribution

restricted likelihood. An alternative two-stage approach was suggested in Ref. [4], which is based on generalized least squares $[\widehat{\boldsymbol{\mu}} - \boldsymbol{\mu}(d)]'\widehat{\mathbf{S}}^{-1}[\widehat{\boldsymbol{\mu}} - \boldsymbol{\mu}(d)]$ and has some computational advantages. Although this approach relies on asymptotic results, it has the appeal of being a general-purpose application, as it depends only on $\widehat{\boldsymbol{\mu}}$ and $\widehat{\mathbf{S}}$.

12.3　Practical Considerations

In this section, we discuss practical considerations when implementing MCP-Mod. These are grouped into three sets of topics: general considerations on when to apply MCP-Mod, considerations at the trial-design stage, and considerations at the trial-analysis stage. Given the nature of this section, we present the individual considerations as bullet points, each being preceded by a key word for ease of use.

12.3.1　When to (or not to) apply MCP-Mod

MCP-Mod is best used in trials satisfying certain characteristics.

- *Therapeutic area.* There are no limitations on using MCP-Mod in a specific indication or therapeutic area because it uses empirical dose–response models; see Section 3 in Ref. [11] for an extensive list of trials that employed MCP-Mod. In certain indications (like cancer, transplantation, or infectious diseases), it is often unethical to administer placebo or doses with potentially suboptimal efficacy, and hence it may not be of interest to characterize the full efficacy dose–response profile. In such cases, MCP-Mod cannot be directly applied, and its usage has to be tailored to the specific trial objectives. For example, if the number of dose levels is insufficient for dose–response modeling (e.g., with two active doses), then MCP-Mod could be reduced to the MCP part to test for a dose–response signal.

- *Drug development stage.* MCP-Mod, as described in Section 12.2, is primarily intended for Phase II dose-finding trials to support dose selection for Phase III. If MCP-Mod is considered as primary analysis in a confirmatory Phase III trial, a suitable extension of the methodology is necessary [12]; see also Chapter 16.

- *Trial design.* It is possible to use MCP-Mod in parallel group or crossover designs. Titration or dose-escalation designs are out of scope, because the administered dose levels depend on the observed responses for the same patients, thereby making any naive dose–response modeling inappropriate.

   Response-adaptive extensions of MCP-Mod with one or multiple interim analyses are possible and often advisable, as they may result in, for example, power gains to detect a dose–response signal or in higher precision to estimate the dose–response curve or a target dose of interest [13–16]; see also Chapter 14. Adaptive designs in confirmatory Phase III trials using MCP-Mod, with dose selection at interim, have recently been described in Ref. [17], extending the work described in Ref. [12].

- *Response.* The original MCP-Mod approach described in Section 12.2.1 was derived for a normally distributed response variable assuming homoscedasticity across doses. The generalized MCP-Mod approach discussed in Section 12.2.2 allows the response to be a binary, count, continuous, or time-to-event variable, either measured at a fixed time point (cross-sectional analysis) or repeatedly over time (longitudinal analysis). Specific extensions of MCP-Mod to binary data were considered in Refs. [18, 19].

It is generally recommended that MCP-Mod is performed when the drug response is at steady state, i.e., when its effect has stabilized over time. Otherwise, the time course of the onset of action as well as the covariance over time also needs to be taken into account, using, for example, pharmacokinetic/pharmacodynamic models.

- *Dose.* Typically, the actual dose levels employed in a given trial are used in MCP-Mod. However, in a broader sense, "dose" can be any univariate, continuous, quantitative measurement, as long as an ordering of the measurements is possible and the differences between measurements are interpretable; see the discussion on concentration–response analyses below.

- *Regimen.* According to the previous definition of "dose," MCP-Mod can be applied to trials with multiple regimens under certain circumstances. One possibility is to "concatenate" the regimens and to assign, for example, model contrasts as described in Section 12.2, but filling up the coefficients with 0 for the nontargeted regimens. Another possibility is to first convert the regimens to a common univariate scale (e.g., total daily dose in the case of b.i.d. and o.d. applications). One could then model the dose–response for the different regimens on that common scale and introduce an additional multiplier $r > 0$ to adjust for regimen (e.g., using the administered dose d for the o.d. regimen but rd for the b.i.d. regimen with the same total daily dose d). For the MCP step, one could assume a fixed multiplier ($r = 1$) and work with the total daily dose, thereby not distinguishing between the regimen. One could then assess the sensitivity to misspecifications of r at the design stage. For the Mod step, one would estimate the parameter r from the data.

  Out of scope are situations when the primary trial objective is the regimen and not the dose, where multiple regimens are employed but each with only one or two doses. Out of scope are also situations when the different regimens differ substantially, such as where some treatment groups include a loading dose and others do not. In this case, a naive dose–response modeling approach can only account for differences in the maintenance dose and is therefore inappropriate.

- *Concentration–response analyses.* According to the previous definition of "dose," MCP-Mod can be applied to concentration–response trials, where concentration is measured by an adequately chosen exposure metric. However, there are a few additional complications in setting up such an analysis and interpreting the results. For example, it is not immediately clear how to categorize the concentrations in deriving an optimal contrast or how to derive an alternative trend test. Another issue is the lack of randomization to concentrations, which could lead to bias in estimating the concentration–response relationship due to unobserved confounders [20, 21]. Limited practical experience exists with these types of analyses as prespecified primary analyses.

12.3.2 Considerations for MCP-Mod at the design stage

In the following, we give considerations on dose and candidate model selection at the trial design stage, as well as various miscellaneous topics.

12.3.2.1 Considerations on dose selection

- *Number of doses.* When using two active doses, it is technically possible to perform the MCP and Mod steps, but in particular for the Mod step, only a very limited set of dose–response models can then be fitted. For a sensible implementation of MCP-Mod, at least three active doses and placebo should be available, with the general recommendation being the use of four to seven active doses. When these doses cover the effective range well (i.e., increasing part and plateau of the dose–response curve), a larger number of active doses are unlikely to produce a benefit [22]. As a general rule of thumb, the recommendation is to use a dose range that is at least 10-fold, i.e., the ratio of the highest versus the lowest dose should be at least 10 [23]; see also Chapter 13.

- *Dose spacing.* A heuristic approach to select the individual doses at the trial design stage is to cover the exposure range efficiently. As outlined in Chapter 13, the exposure values per patient and dose often follow a log-normal distribution, i.e., they are right-skewed, with the variance increasing in the mean response. Thus, the interval between consecutive doses can increase at higher doses. Log spacing of doses is often used in practice by maintaining a constant ratio of consecutive doses. The nonparametric binary dose-spacing method proposed in Ref. [24] is based on dividing dose intervals into halves.

  An alternative approach is to apply optimal design theory with the aim of producing the information needed to efficiently and reliably characterize the benefit of a drug over a dose range of interest; see Chapter 13. Given a fixed total number of patients, optimal designs determine the necessary number of dose levels, their location within the dose range under investigation, and the proportion of patients allocated to each dose level, such that the variance of the dose–response and/or target dose estimate is minimized. While standard optimal designs calculated under a misspecified dose–response model can be inefficient, robust designs can be constructed instead that take into account a set of candidate dose–response profiles within classes of models commonly used in drug development practice [25]. Such designs can be used as benchmarks by calculating relative efficiencies for practically feasible designs [26]. Clinical teams can then balance any additional financial and logistical challenges resulting from an optimal design (larger total number of dose levels, need for producing additional dose levels not considered in previous trials, etc.) against the benefit of an increased information value resulting from larger precision in dose–response estimation.

- *Choice of control group.* In general, the use of a control group, such as a placebo or an active control, is highly recommended to enable more informative dose-finding trials. In certain situations, however, a placebo group cannot be used due to ethical reasons, e.g., if effective treatments already exist on the market or the condition is very severe. If placebo cannot be used, the MCP part of MCP-Mod focuses on establishing a dose–response trend among the active doses, whereas the Mod step could still be conducted to model the dose–response relationship among the active doses.

  If no placebo is used, the extrapolation of the dose–response from the lowest dose to the zero dose (i.e., placebo) becomes problematic, and the use of an active control could facilitate the assessment of the overall level of efficacy of the dose–response curve. The statistical analysis for an active controlled dose-finding trial can be formulated in terms of a mixture of two regression models [27], and the aim of the dose-finding trial could be to estimate the smallest dose of the new compound achieving the same treatment effect as the active control; see also Refs. [28–30].

12.3.2.2   Considerations on candidate model set

- *Selection of candidate models.* As a rule of thumb, a set of three to seven dose–response shapes corresponding to two to four dose–response models are appropriate. Note that multiple dose–response shapes might be used for each dose–response model, where the shapes define the contrasts to be used in the MCP step and the models are those to be fitted in the Mod step. For large uncertainty, a broad candidate set should be used, while in other situations, a narrow candidate set may be appropriate. Below we list some considerations to be taken into account when setting up a candidate model set:

- *Existing information.* In many situations, limited information about the shape of the dose–response curve is available at the trial design stage. For example, information might be available about the dose–response curve for a similar compound in the same indication or the same compound in a different indication. Also, dose–exposure–response models might have been developed based on earlier data (e.g., from a proof-of-concept trial). Such information can be used to predict the dose–response curve at a specific time point. Note that if substantial prior knowledge about the dose–response model is available and there are a sufficient number of doses, the candidate set could consist of only one, single dose–response model (such as the four-parameter sigmoid $E_{\max}$ model) that is flexible enough to cover a variety of different dose–response shapes [31].

- *General experience.* An $E_{\max}$-type model should always be included in the candidate model set. A meta-analysis of the dose–response curves for small molecules conducted in Ref. [32] showed that in many situations, the monotonic $E_{\max}$ model or the sigmoid $E_{\max}$ model is applicable.

- *Statistical considerations.* If only a few active doses are available, it is difficult to fit complex models, such as the sigmoid $E_{\max}$ with four parameters, in a trial with three active doses. Such models would thus have to be excluded from the candidate model set, and one would rather rely on parsimonious dose–response models with fewer parameters to obtain an adequate breadth of the candidate set.

  Another consideration is the evaluation of the performance of MCP-Mod under model misspecification. For example, the impact of omitting the true dose–response model from the candidate model set can be small if other models in the candidate set can pick up the omitted model. This can be evaluated for the MCP part (impact on power) using explicit calculations [33] and for the Mod part (impact on precision for dose–response and dose estimation) using simulations [25].

  Using a broad candidate model set may have an impact on the degree of multiplicity adjustment for the MCP part and increase the critical value. At the same time, the more candidate models are used, the higher the correlation between the contrast test statistics will be. Therefore, the required sample size to achieve a designated power will increase with a broader candidate model set, but the actual impact will have to be investigated on a case-by-case basis. A similar trade-off is in terms of dose–response model fitting, because a broader candidate set will decrease potential bias (in case of model misspecification) but increase the variance of the estimates.

- *Umbrella profiles.* A recurrent consideration is the inclusion (or not) of an umbrella-shaped dose–response model in the candidate set. While biological exposure–response relationships are often monotonic, downturns of the clinical dose–response relationship at higher doses have been observed. Such effects are attributable to, for example, treatment discontinuation at high doses due to patients experiencing adverse events or generally being less compliant regarding drug intake. We recommend routinely considering the inclusion of an umbrella-shaped dose–response model in the candidate set, unless umbrella profiles can be excluded with certainty at the trial design stage.

- *Choice of guesstimates.* The specification of guesstimates for the parameters in the standardized version of the models in the candidate set is critical for the MCP step. These prior parameter values are used to obtain the model contrasts and critical values for the MCP step, which in turn determine the effective power to detect a dose–response signal. The guesstimates need to be obtained from experts in the clinical team, along with statistical input as described above, and translated into model parameters. Possible strategies and examples for successfully achieving such translation are described in Ref. [33].

In practice, the determination of guesstimates should be accompanied by a sensitivity analysis to assess the misspecification of the parameters in the standardized models and, in particular, the impact it has on the effective power to detect a dose–response signal in the MCP step. In many regards, the derivation of guesstimates for the candidate model parameters, as well as the choice of the candidate models themselves, is closely related to the ideas used in elicitation of prior distributions in Bayesian inference [34]. Note that the guesstimates are not used at the Mod step, and all of the parameters will be estimated from the observed data [35]. Several authors have extended MCP-Mod using likelihood ratio tests [36–38] or resampling-based approaches [39] that do not require the specification of guesstimates.

- *Model selection versus model averaging.* The Mod step can be performed using either a single model selected from the initial candidate set or a weighted average of the candidate models that are significant at the MCP step. The main advantage of the former is that a single model is provided for future inference, which might be simpler to interpret by clinicians. However, selecting a single model discards model uncertainty, which may lead to confidence intervals with a coverage probability smaller than the nominal level [40, 41] even if it is selected from the set of significant models rather than the initial set of candidate models. While model averaging does not provide a complete solution to this problem, simulations indicate rather consistently a slightly better performance on average in terms of dose–response and dose estimation over a wide range of scenarios. Model averaging can be done by weighting the models proportional to a suitable information criterion [9]. Alternatively, bagging can be used where one takes bootstrap samples, performs model selection on each bootstrap sample using a suitable information criterion, and then uses the mean over all predictions as the overall estimate [42]. For more details on model selection versus model averaging in dose–response trials, we refer to [43, 44].

- *Model selection criteria.* Whether MCP-Mod is implemented using model selection or model averaging, a suitable model selection criterion needs to be specified. See Ref. [43] for a brief review of the mathematical background of different selection criteria based on either the AIC or the BIC, and comparison with respect to their asymptotic properties. They noted that the BIC-type criteria as well the AIC are consistent (i.e., they pick the best approximating model out of the candidate set with a probability converging to 1 with increasing sample size). However, only the BIC asymptotically picks the best approximating model with fewest parameters (if there is more than one best approximating model in the case of nested models) although in the simulation scenarios with finites sample sizes investigated by the authors the BIC-type criteria selected too simplistic models. In contrast, AIC-type criteria asymptotically tend to prefer too complex models. On the other hand, the BIC-type criteria select too simplistic models when the sample size is small. They also observed that BIC-type criteria select different models for different total sample sizes, even when the estimated dose–response curves and the uncertainty around each dose–response curve are the same (i.e., the confidence intervals width around the curve). This is different from other situations in clinical trials, where only the standard error is important, not the total sample size itself, and is an important point to consider at the trial design stage when using BIC-type criteria.

The use of alternative approaches that are not based on a penalized log-likelihood function of the model has to be assessed carefully. For example, using MCP-Mod, it is natural to base the model selection on the contrast tests from the MCP step [3, 45]. The limitation is that such model selection approaches may not be compatible with the necessary model-fitting step afterward. For example, fitting the model with the highest test statistics may not be possible because of numerical convergence problems. Such problems occur, for example, when the model to be fitted contains many parameters in comparison to the number of doses, or when the doses are not spread appropriately across the dose range under investigation.

12.3.2.3 Miscellaneous considerations

- *Choice of α.* The choice of the significance level α depends on the specific trial and its context. While it is common to set $\alpha = 0.025$ (one sided) for confirmatory trials in Phase III, there is more flexibility in the choice of α for dose-finding trials in Phase II. It is important to understand the consequences of false-positive decisions and balance them with the degree of uncertainty that a sponsor is willing to accept in moving forward. If we incorrectly reject the null hypothesis of no dose–response at the MCP step of MCP-Mod, we would incorrectly conclude in favor of significant dose–response signal, complete the Mod step, and plan the Phase III program accordingly. A more stringent choice of α would reduce this risk but at the same time inflate the false-negative error rate. Because it is primarily the sponsor's risk of moving into Phase III with an inefficacious drug, setting $\alpha = 0.05$ or even 0.1 (one sided) seems to be acceptable. Note that we recommend one-sided tests for the MCP step as we are only interested in detecting a significant trend for improving the disease condition.

- *Sample size calculations.* As discussed more broadly in Chapter 13, sample size calculations at the trial design stage could be based either on power considerations to achieve a prespecified probability of establishing a true dose–response signal or on a prespecified precision for dose–response and dose estimation. Using MCP-Mod, sample size calculations based on power considerations can be performed such that the MCP part has a desired (average or minimum) probability under an assumed set of dose–response curves [33]. ADDPLAN-DF as well as the sampSizeMCT function from the DoseFinding R package can be used for sample size calculations for that purpose. It is known, however, that the sample sizes sufficient for establishing a dose–response trend may not be sufficient for estimating precisely the dose–response curve or a target dose of interest. In practice, one may therefore justify the sample size using power calculations for the MCP part, with simulations performed to ensure adequate performance in terms of dose and dose–response estimation. This will typically result in an increased sample size for the MCP part but provide more precise dose and dose–response estimates.

- *Safety data analyses.* In general, safety dose–response modeling is less common, but MCP-Mod remains applicable in its usual form; see Ref. [46] for an application to longitudinal toxicological data. The key is to identify one (or more) relevant safety variable(s) as opposed to current *post hoc* safety signal detection practices based on extensive frequency tables analyses. A related and equally relevant problem is to synthesize two univariate models, one for a key efficacy marker or parameter and the other for safety. One possibility is to derive a clinical utility index (CUI) that combines safety and efficacy information in one variable. Although the derivation of a CUI is hard in practice, MCP-Mod could then be applied again and benefit from its flexibility of including nonmonotonic shapes because CUIs are likely to follow an umbrella shape as a function of dose. An extension of MCP-Mod was proposed in Ref. [47] to select the best joint model based on two continuous correlated efficacy and safety outcomes and to get the final optimum dose(s) from the best joint model for the Phase III study; see also Ref. [48].

- *Multiregional trials.* Assessing the efficacy and safety profiles in relevant patient populations (such as different gender, age classes, and grades of disease severity) is becoming increasingly important. Multiregional trials are particularly important as they are conducted in different regions and potentially serve different submissions. If, for example, a multiregional dose-finding trial includes Japanese patients, we could be interested in assessing the similarity of the two dose–response curves for the Japanese and non-Japanese patients, respectively; that is, whether the maximum difference in response between two (potentially different) nonlinear parametric regression models is smaller than a prespecified equivalence margin [49]. Alternatively, we could be interested in assessing whether the target doses from the two patient populations differ relevantly. If we succeed in demonstrating either of these two objectives using a suitable equivalence test, evidence is provided that the difference in response over the entire dose range under investigation or between the two target doses is clinically irrelevant. In the multiregional trial example above, such a result may provide sufficient evidence that the same dose can be administered both in Japanese and non-Japanese patients. To be feasible, this approach requires an adequate number of doses per patient population to be able to detect a dose–response signal and to estimate the dose–response curve in each population. In practice, the requirements for demonstrating similarity of target doses or dose–response curves are more relaxed, not least because we typically do not have enough patients in the regional subgroups.

12.3.3   Considerations for MCP-Mod at the analysis stage

In the following, we give considerations on various topics related to the use of MCP-Mod at the trial analysis stage.

- *Recalculation of contrast coefficients.* Often, the contrast coefficients and the critical value required for the MCP step cannot be taken over from the design stage due to dropouts, covariate effects, etc. Therefore, these values have to be recalculated at the trial analysis stage. For the Mod step, the model-fitting process uses only the observed data and does not depend on, for example, the guesstimates.

- *Non-significant models.* In its original version, MCP-Mod stops if the MCP step fails to declare a significant dose–response signal. However, failing to reject the null hypothesis of no dose–response does not necessarily imply that the compound under investigation has no effect. Possible reasons for a nonsignificant result could include small sample sizes or high variance so that in practice one would still like to obtain a response estimate for each of the investigated doses. An exploratory analysis at the Mod step, based on the initial candidate model set, seems therefore reasonable, although the results have to be interpreted with great care, keeping in mind that no dose–response signal had been established at the MCP step.

  A related consideration arises whether the model selection or averaging should be based on the set of significant models (as suggested in the original Refs [3, 50]) or the initial set of candidate models, after a significant dose–response signal. At this point, we suggest following the original recommendation, with the understanding that deviations from it could be justified on a case-by-case basis. For example, one could argue that even if a particular contrast test was not significant, the associated model could still be true and the nonsignificance may only have been due to a particularly bad choice of the contrast coefficients at the design stage.

- *Nonconvergent models.* Most of the common dose–response models are nonlinear in their parameters. This means that iterative algorithms have to be used to calculate the model parameter estimates. In some situations, convergence might fail, which is often due to the fact that the best fitting model shape corresponds to the case, where one of the model parameters is infinite or 0. One approach to overcome this problem is to use bounds on the nonlinear model parameters, which ensures the existence of an estimate. In many situations, the assumed bounds can be justified in terms of requiring that the shape space underlying the corresponding model is covered almost exhaustively. The `defBnds` function from the `DoseFinding` package proposes reasonable default boundaries. A complication arises when the estimate is exactly equal to one of the selected bounds. The standard asymptotic approximations based on the Fisher information matrix can then become very unreliable (or perhaps cannot be even computed). Boostrapping provides a robust way of calculating confidence intervals in this case.

- *Interpolation and extrapolation.* This consideration is often raised as to what extent MCP-Mod can support the selection of a dose for Phase III that has not been directly studied in a Phase II trial. Interpolation is making a prediction within the dose range under investigation, generally safe and therefore encouraged. We recommend that as with any statistical inference, the prediction uncertainty should be reported, either on the "y-axis" (i.e., the mean response estimates) or on the "x-axis" (i.e., dose estimate). One may consider using simultaneous confidence bands around the dose–response estimate instead of marginal confidence intervals at each dose to provide a more accurate quantification of the uncertainty [51, 52]. Extrapolation is making a prediction outside the dose range under investigation and generally discouraged.

- *Dose justification for Phase III.* At the end of Phase II, one would ideally like to select a dose with a favorable benefit–risk balance and carry it forward into the Phase III program. However, in case of insufficient information (e.g., due to small sample sizes in Phase II), one may consider selecting more than one dose to increase the likelihood of a successful Phase III program [53]. In other cases, using interpolation (see "Interpolation and extrapolation"), one may select a dose for Phase III that had not been investigated previously but for which a promising benefit–risk balance could be expected. As a general principle, one should provide a strong justification of the dose(s) being selected for Phase III based on the available information, which includes available efficacy and safety profiles, PK/PD modeling, meta-analysis of similar trials, etc. [23].

- *Missing data.* The handling of missing data in Phase II dose-finding trials is often of less emphasis, despite its importance in view of informing the subsequent Phase III program. Thus, inadequate handling of missing data may result in disagreements with regulatory agencies regarding the readiness to initiate Phase III or Phase III dose selection. Occasionally, issues around dose selection due to missing data handling have jeopardized, delayed, or even prevented drug approval.

    In case of normally distributed endpoints, one possibility is to fit a longitudinal multivariate normal model ("MMRM" analysis, see Ref. [54]). From this model, one could then extract the estimates of efficacy for each dose at the time points of interest and the associated covariance matrix, and then apply the generalized MCP-Mod approach from Section 12.2.2. This approach would imply the same assumption on the missing data process as MMRM and requires the joint normality of the estimates. Similarly, multiple imputation methods followed by an analysis of the imputed data can be used as well to obtain the estimates for each dose and their covariance matrix as inputs for MCP-Mod. Going beyond continuous endpoints, the impact of dropouts on the analysis with recurrent event data was investigated by Ref. [55].

- *Supportive analyses.* Standard diagnostic checks can be conducted to assess, for example, whether the distributional assumptions are justified (e.g., residual plots in case of a normal distribution). One can also perform a sensitivity analysis with respect to the used candidate set of models. If, for example, a nonmonotonic model is excluded from the initial candidate model set of models, one might perform a sensitivity analysis to assess the robustness of conclusions.

- *Software.* There are several software solutions for planning and analyzing MCP-Mod. The `DoseFinding` R package is publicly available on the CRAN servers [5]. It contains numerous functions that are of interest for MCP-Mod at the trial design stage. This includes functions for power and sample size calculation for the MCP part (`powMCT`, `sampSizeMCT`) as well as for the calculation of optimal designs and other features for the Mod part (`optDesign`, `planMod`). A detailed introduction of the `DoseFinding` package is given in Section 12.4; see also Chapter 3 for its use at the trial design stage.

  `ADDPLAN-DF` is a stand-alone application maintained by ADDPLAN, Inc., an Aptiv Solutions Company. It enables the calculation of power and sample size for the MCP part of MCP-Mod. It also allows the calculation of optimal designs for estimating dose–response models for the Mod part. In addition, `ADDPLAN-DF` allows users to evaluate the operating characteristics of the chosen analysis and design methods using a built-in simulation engine.

  `PROC MCPMOD` is a procedure developed by Cytel for SAS users that focuses on the analysis of dose-finding trials using MCP-Mod. It supports responses for normal, binary, count, and survival endpoints using either raw or summarized data. Furthermore, a suite of SAS macros developed by [56] implements and performs MCP-Mod in many situations of practical relevance.

12.4   DoseFinding R Package

The `DoseFinding` R package implements the design and analysis of dose-finding trials [5]. In the following, we will illustrate the application of MCP-Mod with two examples. The first example illustrates MCP-Mod for normally distributed data as described in Section 12.2.1, using model selection. The second example illustrates a more complex application of the generalized MCP-Mod approach from Section 12.2.2 for a linear mixed-effects model, using model averaging.

12.4.1   MCP-Mod with normally distributed data and model selection

Consider a randomized, double-blind, balanced, parallel-group trial in which a total of 100 subjects were randomized to either placebo or one of four active doses coded as 0.05, 0.20, 0.60, and 1. The response variable was assumed to be normally distributed and a larger value indicated better outcome, and had homogeneous variance across the dose levels. The data are available in `biom` dataset in the `DoseFinding` R package, with two variables `dose` and `resp`.

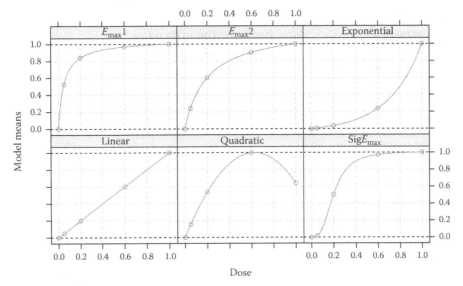

FIGURE 12.1
Candidate dose–response shapes.

Assume that at the trial design stage, six shapes (Figure 12.1) are chosen into the candidate model set. Using the standardized versions of dose–response models, these shapes are as follows: an $E_{\max}$ model with $ED_{50} = 0.05$, an $E_{\max}$ model with $ED_{50} = 0.2$, an exponential model with $\delta = 0.3$, a linear model, a quadratic model with $\delta = -0.8$, and a sigmoid $E_{\max}$ model with $ED_{50} = 0.2$ and the Hill parameter $h = 3$.

These candidate shapes are defined using the function `Mods` and visualized using `plot`. The output object `candMod` will be used as input object for other functions to extract the mean response or target doses, etc.

```
candMod <- Mods(emax=c(0.05, 0.2), exponential=0.3,
        linear=NULL, quadratic=-0.8, sigEmax=c(0.2, 3),
        doses=c(0,0.05,0.2,0.6,1))
plot(candMod)
```

For the MCP step at the analysis stage, the multiple contrast test is performed using function `MCTtest`. By specifying `models=candMod`, optimal contrasts are derived automatically (Table 12.3). In this example, all models result in small p-values indicating a strong evidence for the existence of a dose–response relationship (Table 12.4).

```
MCTtest(dose, resp, data=biom, models=candMod)
```

For the Mod step, we can fit the individual models using `fitMod` and select the best model using the AIC criterion. For example, we use the following to fit an $E_{\max}$ model and calculate corresponding AIC. Other models can be fit similarly. The AIC values for these different models are given in Table 12.5. The $E_{\max}$ model has the smallest AIC, and therefore it is selected as the final model for further analyses.

```
fitEmax   <- fitMod(dose, resp, data=biom, model="emax",
        bnds=c(0.001, 1.5))
AIC(fitEmax)
```

TABLE 12.3

Optimal contrasts for the candidate shapes for the `biom` data.

Dose	E_{max} $ED_{50} = 0.05$	E_{max} $ED_{50} = 0.2$	Exponential $\delta = 0.3$	Linear	Quadratic $\delta = -0.8$	Sigmoid E_{max} $ED_{50} = 0.2,$ $h = 3$
0	−0.8	−0.64	−0.3	−0.44	−0.59	−0.51
0.05	−0.17	−0.36	−0.29	−0.38	−0.39	−0.49
0.2	0.21	0.06	−0.26	−0.2	0.09	0.01
0.6	0.36	0.41	−0.02	0.27	0.67	0.48
1	0.4	0.53	0.87	0.74	0.22	0.51

TABLE 12.4

Results of the contrast test for the `biom` data.

Model	Test Statistics	Adjusted p-Values
E_{max}, $ED_{50} = 0.05$	3.339	0.0015
E_{max}, $ED_{50} = 0.2$	3.464	0.0011
Exponential, $\delta = 0.3$	2.260	0.0321
Linear	2.972	0.0050
Quadratic, $\delta = -0.8$	3.292	0.0021
Sigmoid E_{max}, $ED_{50} = 0.2, h = 3$	3.406	0.0018

TABLE 12.5

AIC values of the fitted models for the `biom` data.

Model	AIC
E_{max}	219.14
Exponential	223.13
Linear	220.50
Quadratic	219.72
Sigmoid E_{max}	220.82

To find a dose that achieves the target effect over placebo based on a fitted model, we use function TD. In the `biom` example where increasing response is beneficial, the dose achieving an effect of 0.4 over placebo is 0.16, calculated by the code below.

```
TD(fitEmax, Delta=0.4, direction="increasing")
```

Alternatively, we use function ED to find a dose that achieves a certain percentage of the full effect size within the observed dose range over placebo.

To generate a plot of the estimated dose–response curve as shown in Figure 12.2, which could be useful in reporting of the analysis results, we simply use the `plot` function as below.

```
plot(fitEmax, plotData="meansCI", CI=TRUE, level=0.95)
```

The fitted model is shown as difference to placebo, imposed with 95% confidence intervals. And to predict the effect of more doses, we can use the generic function `predict`. For example, dose levels 0.1 and 0.5 achieve an effect of 0.63 and 0.9, respectively, obtained using the code below.

```
pred <- predict(fitEmax, doseSeq=c(0.1,0.5),
          predType="ls", se.fit=TRUE)
```

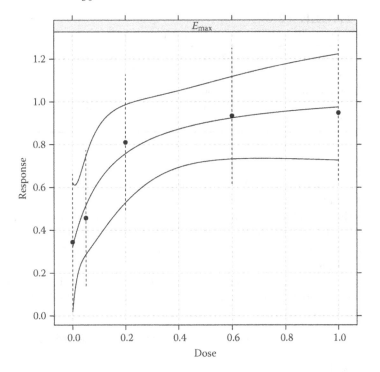

FIGURE 12.2

Estimated dose–response curve for the `biom` data.

12.4.2 Generalized MCP-Mod and model averaging

Consider a Phase II clinical trial conducted for a neurodegenerative disease. The disease status was measured through a functional scale, with smaller values indicating more severe neurodegeneration. The drug was intended to reduce the rate of disease progression, measured by the linear slope of the functional scale over time. The objectives of the trial were to estimate the dose–response, if any, and to select a dose to be brought into the confirmatory stage of the development program.

The example data are available in `neurodeg` in the `DoseFinding` R package, originally simulated in Ref. [4] to illustrate the use of the generalized MCP-Mod approach. A total of 250 patients were allocated equally to either placebo or four doses at 1, 3, 10, and 30 mg. Patients were followed up for 1 year, with measurements of the functional scale taken at baseline and every 3 months thereafter.

In the following, we will first fit a longitudinal model to extract the information on the rate of disease progression and then apply the generalized MCP-Mod approach.

Based on historical data, we can assume that the functional scale response is normally distributed, and its decreases over 1-year follow-up period can be modeled by a simple linear trend. Let y_{ij} denote the measurement of patient i at time j. A linear mixed-effects model for y_{ij} is

$$y_{ij} = \beta_0 + b_{0i} + [\mu(d) + b_{1i}]t_{ij} + \varepsilon_{ij},$$
$$b_i = (b_{0i}, b_{1i})' \sim N(0, \Omega) \text{ and } \varepsilon_{ij} \sim N(0, \sigma^2),$$

where the slope $\mu(d)$ associated with dose d contains the dose–response relationship. The `lme` function in the `nlme` package is used to fit the above model. The estimated slopes associated

TABLE 12.6

Results of the contrast test for the `neurodeg` data.

Model	Test Statistics	Adjusted p-Values
E_{max}	4.561	< 0.001
Quadratic	3.680	< 0.001
Exponential	1.277	0.1822
Linear	2.274	0.0246

with the doses are $\hat{\mu} = (-5.099, -4.581, -3.220, -2.879, -3.520)'$. The corresponding estimated variance–covariance matrix $\hat{\Sigma}$ has a compound symmetry structure with 0.149 on diagonal and 0.0094 off-diagonal.

Assume that the candidate shapes chosen at the design stage are as follows: an E_{max} model with $ED_{50} = 1.11$, a quadratic model with $\delta = -0.022$, an exponential model with $\delta = 8.867$, and a linear model. We can set up candidate shapes, derive the optimal contrast, and perform a multiple contrast test similarly as in the previous example. The complete code is given below. The results of the contrast test are shown in Table 12.6. All models except the exponential model give a small p-value, which provides evidence for the existence of a dose–response effect.

```
fm      <- lme(resp~as.factor(dose):time, neurodeg, ~time|id)
muH     <- fixef(fm)[-1]
covH    <- vcov(fm)[-1,-1]
doses <- c(0, 1, 3, 10, 30)
mod     <- Mods(emax=1.11, quadratic=-0.022, exponential=8.867,
                linear=NULL, doses=doses)
contMat <- optContr(mod, S=covH)
MCTtest (doses, muH, S=covH, type="general", critV=TRUE,
         contMat=contMat)
```

We can use an extension of the AIC criterion, which is suitable for the two-stage model-fitting approach, to select the best model for the Mod step [4]. In the following, instead, we illustrate a bootstrap model averaging approach. The basic idea is to simulate a large number of dose–response parameter $\mu^{(b)}$, for $b = 1, \ldots, B$, from the sampling distribution of $\hat{\mu}$, i.e., a five-dimensional normal distribution with mean $\hat{\mu}$ and covariance matrix $\hat{\Sigma}$ introduced earlier. For each of the generated $\mu^{(b)}$, fit all four candidate models to this summary data using generalized least squares and select the best model using an AIC-type criterion [4]. Finally, these B best models selected from each replication can be used to predict quantities of interest like target doses or effect estimate at given doses. An example code is provided below. It generates 5,000 bootstrap samples and for each replication returns the index of the model selected, predicted response at doses 0, 1, 3, 10, and 30 mg and the effect of doses 1, 3, 10, and 30 mg.

```
set.seed(10000)
nSim <- 5000
sims <- rmvnorm(nSim, muH, covH)
results <- apply(sims, 1, function(x){
  fit <- vector("list", 4)
  fit[[1]] <- fitMod(doses, x, type="general", model="emax",
                bnds=defBnds(30)$emax, S=covH)
  fit[[2]] <- fitMod(doses, x, type="general", model="quadratic",
                S=covH)
```

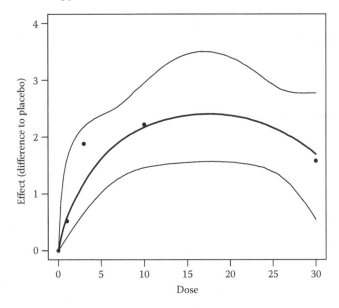

FIGURE 12.3
Bootstrapped dose–response curve for the `neurodeg` data.

```
fit[[3]] <- fitMod(doses, x, type="general", model="exponential",
                   bnds=defBnds(30)$exponential, S=covH)
fit[[4]] <- fitMod(doses, x, type="general", model="linear",
                   S=covH)
aics    <- sapply(fit, gAIC)
sel     <- which.min(aics)
fitsel  <- fit[[sel]]
pred    <- predict(fitsel, doseSeq=c(0,1,3,10,30),
                   predType="ls-means")
c(sel, pred, pred-pred[1])
})
```

It turns out that the exponential model is never selected; the linear model is selected 6 out of 5,000 times; and the E_{max} and quadratic models are each selected 52% and 48% times, respectively. The bootstrapped dose–response curve based on 5,000 bootstrap samples is shown in Figure 12.3. One can see that the estimated curve shows a slight unimodality, which is introduced because the point estimate for the slope at dose 30 mg is slightly smaller than for 10 and 3 mg. For the `neurodeg` dataset, the linear and exponential models can clearly be ruled out, but both the E_{max} and the quadratic models seem to describe the data adequately. Selecting one model over another model in such a situation is potentially problematic, as it does not represent the underlying uncertainty adequately. Using a model averaging approach seems more realistic in this example.

Acknowledgments

The authors would like to acknowledge the contribution of Georgina Bermann, Björn Bornkamp, Ekkehard Glimm, Björn Holzhauer, Byron Jones, Baldur Magnusson, David

Ohlssen, Oliver Sander, Marc Vandemeulebroecke, and Melanie Wright, who provided comments and ideas for additions to an earlier version of Section 12.3 ("Practical Considerations") of this chapter.

References

1. European Medicines Agency. Qualification opinion of MCP-Mod as an efficient statistical methodology for model-based design and analysis of phase II dose finding studies under model uncertainty, 2014. http://goo.gl/imT7IT.

2. J. W. Tukey, J. L. Ciminera, and J. F. Heyse. Testing the statistical certainty of a response to increasing doses of a drug. *Biometrics*, 41:295–301, 1985.

3. F. Bretz, J. C. Pinheiro, and M. Branson. Combining multiple comparisons and modeling techniques in dose–response studies. *Biometrics*, 61:738–748, 2005.

4. J. C. Pinheiro, B. Bornkamp, E. Glimm, and F. Bretz. Model-based dose finding under model uncertainty using general parametric models. *Statistics in Medicine*, 33:1646–1661, 2014.

5. B. Bornkamp, J. C. Pinheiro, and F. Bretz. *DoseFinding: Planning and Analyzing Dose Finding Experiments*. R Package Version 0.9-13, 2015.

6. R. P. Abelson and J. W. Tukey. Efficient utilisation of non-numerical information in quantitative analysis: General theory and the case of simple order. *Annals of Mathematical Statistics*, 34:1347–1369, 1963.

7. W. Schaafsma and L. J. Smid. Most stringent somewhere most powerful tests against alternatives restricted by a number of linear inequalities. *Annals of Mathematical Statistics*, 37:1161–1172, 1966.

8. H. Mukerjee, T. Roberston, and F. T. Wright. Comparison of several treatments with a control using multiple contrasts. *Journal of the American Statistical Association*, 82:902–910, 1987.

9. S. T. Buckland, K. P. Burnham, and N. H. Augustin. Model selection: An integral part of inference. *Biometrics*, 53:603–618, 1997.

10. B. Bornkamp. Comparison of model-based and model-free approaches for the analysis of dose–response studies, Diploma thesis, Fachbereich Statistik, Universität Dortmund, Germany, 2006.

11. B. Bornkamp, F. Bretz, and J. C. Pinheiro. Request for CHMP qualification opinion, 2013. http://www.ema.europa.eu/docs/en_GB/document_library/Other/2014/02/WC500161026.pdf.

12. F. König. Confirmatory testing for a beneficial treatment effect in dose-response studies using MCP-Mod and an adaptive interim analysis, July 9, 2015. Isaac Newton Institute, http://www.turing-gateway.cam.ac.uk/sites/default/files/asset/doc/1606/Franz%20Konig.pdf.

13. B. Bornkamp, F. Bretz, H. Dette, and J. C. Pinheiro. Response-adaptive dose-finding under model uncertainty. *Annals of Applied Statistics*, 5:1611–1631, 2011.

14. V. Dragalin, B. Bornkamp, F. Bretz, F. Miller, S. K. Padmanabhan, N. Patel, I. Perevozskaya, J. C. Pinheiro, and J. R. Smith. A simulation study to compare new adaptive dose-ranging designs. *Statistics in Biopharmaceutical Research*, 2:487–512, 2010.

15. Y. Franchetti, S. J. Anderson, and A. R. Sampson. An adaptive two-stage dose–response design method for establishing proof of concept. *Journal of Biopharmceutical Statistics*, 23:1124–1154, 2013.

16. F. Miller. Adaptive dose-finding: Proof of concept with type I error control. *Biometrical Journal*, 52:577–589, 2010.

17. S. Krasnozhon, A. Graf, B. Bornkamp, F. Bretz, G. Wassmer, and F. König. Adaptive designs for confirmatory model based decisions using MCP-Mod. *Poster presented at the 35th Annual Conference of the International Society for Clinical Biostatistics*, Vienna, Austria, 2014.

18. N. Benda. Model-based approaches for time-dependent dose finding with repeated binary data. *Statistics in Medicine*, 29:1096–1106, 2010.

19. B. Klingenberg. Proof of concept and dose estimation with binary responses under model uncertainty. *Statistics in Medicine*, 28:274–292, 2009.

20. Food and Drug Administration. Guidance for industry: Exposure-response relationships—Study design, data analysis, and regulatory applications, 2003. http://www.fda.gov/downloads/drugs/guidance complianceregulatoryinformation/ guidances/ucm072109.pdf.

21. J. R. Nedelman, D. B. Rubin, and L. B. Sheiner. Diagnostics for confounding in PK/PD models for oxcarbazepine. *Statistics in Medicine*, 26(2):290–308, 2007.

22. B. Bornkamp, F. Bretz, A. Dmitrienko, G. Enas, B. Gaydos, C. H. Hsu, F. König, M. Krams, Q. Liu, B. Neuenschwander, T. Parke, J. C. Pinheiro, A. Roy, R. Sax, and F. Shen. Innovative approaches for designing and analyzing adaptive dose-ranging trials (with discussion). *Journal of Biopharmaceutical Statistics*, 17:965–995, 2007.

23. European Medicines Agency. Report from dose finding workshop, 2014. http://www. ema.europa.eu/docs/en_GB/document_library/Report/ 2015/04/WC500185864.pdf.

24. A. Hamlett, N. Ting, R. C. Hanumara, and J. S. Finman. Dose spacing in early dose response clinical trial designs. *Drug Information Journal*, 36:855–864, 2002.

25. H. Dette, F. Bretz, A. Pepelyshev, and J. C. Pinheiro. Optimal designs for dose finding studies. *Journal of the American Statisical Association*, 103:1225–1237, 2008.

26. F. Bretz, H. Dette, and J. C. Pinheiro. Practical considerations for optimal designs in clinical dose finding studies. *Statistics in Medicine*, 29:731–742, 2010.

27. H. Dette, C. Kiss, N. Benda, and F. Bretz. Optimal designs for dose finding studies with an active control. *Journal of the Royal Statistical Society, Series B*, 76:265–295, 2014.

28. H. Dette, K. Kettelhake, and F. Bretz. Designing dose finding studies with an active control for exponential families. *Biometrika*, 102(4):937–950, 2015.

29. H. Helms, N. Benda, and T. Friede. Point and interval estimators of the target dose in clinical dose-finding studies with active control. *Journal of Biopharmaceutical Statistics*, 25:939–957, 2015.

30. H. Helms, N. Benda, P. Zinserling, T. Kneib, and T. Friede. Spline-based procedures for dose-finding studies with active control. *Statistics in Medicine*, 34:232–248, 2015.

31. N. Thomas. Hypothesis testing and Bayesian estimation using a sigmoid E_{max} model applied to sparse dose designs. *Journal of Biopharmaceutical Statistics*, 16:657–677, 2006.

32. N. Thomas, K. Sweeney, and V. Somayaji. Meta-analysis of clinical dose–response in a large drug development portfolio. *Statistics in Biopharmaceutical Research*, 6:302–317, 2014.

33. J. C. Pinheiro, B. Bornkamp, and F. Bretz. Design and analysis of dose finding studies combining multiple comparisons and modeling procedures. *Journal of Biopharmaceutical Statistics*, 16:639–656, 2006.

34. J. Bernardo and A. Smith. *Bayesian Theory*. John Wiley & Sons, Chichester, UK, 1994.

35. J. C. Pinheiro, F. Bretz, and M. Branson. Analysis of dose–response studies—modeling approaches. In N. Ting, editor, *Dose Finding in Drug Development*, pp. 146–171. Springer, New York, 2006.

36. C. Baayen, P. Hougaard, and C. B. Pipper. Testing effect of a drug using multiple nested models for the dose-response. *Biometrics*, 71:417–427, 2015.

37. H. Dette, S. Titoff, S. Volgushev, and F. Bretz. Dose response signal detection under model uncertainty. *Biometrics*, 71:996–1008, 2015.

38. G. Gutjahr and B. Bornkamp. Likelihood ratio tests for a dose–response effect using multiple nonlinear regression models. *Biometrics*, 2016. doi:10.1111/biom.12563.

39. M. Fu. A resampling based approach in evaluation of dose–response models. Doctoral dissertation, Temple University, 2014.

40. C. Chatfield. Model uncertainty, data mining and statistical inference (with discussion). *Journal of the Royal Statistical Society Series A*, 158:419–466, 1995.

41. H. Leeb and B. M. Poetscher. Model selection and inference: Facts and fiction. *Econometric Theory*, 21:21–59, 2005.

42. L. Breiman. Bagging predictors. *Machine Learning*, 24:123–140, 1996.

43. K. Schorning, B. Bornkamp, F. Bretz, and H. Dette. Model selection versus model averaging in dose finding studies. *Statistics in Medicine*, 2016. doi:10.1002/sim.6991.

44. D. Verrier, S. Sivapregassam, and A. C. Solente. Dose-finding studies, MCP-Mod, model selection, and model averaging: Two applications in the real world. *Clinical Trials*, 11:476–484, 2014.

45. A. Wakana, I. Yoshimura, and C. Hamada. A method for therapeutic dose selection in a phase II clinical trial using contrast statistics. *Statistics in Medicine*, 26:498–511, 2007.

46. W. Wouter. The power and type I error of statistical analysis approaches for longitudinal toxicological data. M.Sc. thesis, University of Ghent, 2012.

47. A. Tao, Y. Lin, J. C. Pinheiro, and W. J. Shih. Dose finding method in joint modeling of efficacy and safety endpoints in phase II studies. *International Journal of Statistics and Probability*, 4:33–45, 2015.

48. H. Dette, K. Kettelhake, K. Schorning, W. K. Wong, and F. Bretz. Optimal designs for active controlled dose finding trials with efficacy-toxicity outcomes, 2016. Available at https://arXiv:1601.00797v1.

49. H. Dette, K. Moelenhoff, S. Volgushev, and F. Bretz. Equivalence of dose response curves, 2015. Available at https://arxiv.org/abs/1505.05266.

50. F. Bretz, J. C. Pinheiro, and M. Branson. On a hybrid method in dose finding studies. *Methods of Information in Medicine*, 43:457–461, 2004.

51. S. Gsteiger, F. Bretz, and W. Liu. Simultaneous confidence bands for non-linear regression models with application to population pharmacokinetic analyses. *Journal of Biopharmaceutical Statistics*, 21:708–725, 2011.

52. W. Liu. *Simultaneous Inference for Regression*. Taylor & Francis, Boca Raton, FL, 2010.

53. Z. Antonijevic, J. Pinheiro, P. Fardipour, and R. J. Lewis. Impact of dose selection strategies used in phase II on the probability of success in phase III. *Statistics in Biopharmaceutical Research*, 2(4):469–486, 2010.

54. O. Siddiqui, H. M. J. Hung, and R. O'Neill. MMRM vs. LOCF: A comprehensive comparison based on simulation study and 25 NDA datasets. *Journal of Biopharmaceutical Statistics*, 19(2):227–246, 2009.

55. M. Akacha and N. Benda. The impact of dropouts on the analysis of dose-finding studies with recurrent event data. *Statistics in Medicine*, 29:1635–1646, 2010.

56. B. Bornkamp, V. Bezlyak, and F. Bretz. Implementing the MCP-Mod procedure for dose–response testing and estimation. In S. Menon and R. C. Zink editors *Modern Approaches to Clinical Trials Using SAS: Classical, Adaptive, and Bayesian Methods*, pp. 193–224. SAS Institute Inc., Cary, NC, 2015.

13

Designing Phase II Dose-Finding Studies: Sample Size, Doses, and Dose Allocation Weights

José Pinheiro

Janssen Research & Development

Björn Bornkamp

Novartis Pharma AG

CONTENTS

13.1 Introduction

This chapter focuses on the design of Phase II dose-finding studies and addresses the question on how to choose the total sample size, doses, and dose allocations.

At the end of a Phase II dose-finding study, one would like to be able to decide whether it makes sense to continue development of the drug in larger and more extensive Phase III trials, and if so, which dose (or doses) to use in these trials. There are thus two aspects of interest: (1) the magnitude of the treatment effect and (2) the nature of the dose–response curve to be able to perform dose selection for Phase III adequately. One can formulate (and simplify) this into more concrete statistical objectives:

1. Is there a dose-related effect of the drug?

2. What is the nature of the dose–response curve, and where are doses of interest located in the dose range?

The first objective is a testing problem, while the second is an estimation problem. Both objectives considered separately would result in rather different study designs. For detecting a dose–response effect would not be necessary to study more than one dose if a monotonicity assumption on the dose–response curve could be made. The best design in terms of optimizing the power to detect a dose–response signal would only use a placebo group and a high dose (as this maximizes the treatment effect) with equal allocation. However, this would not lead to information on the nature of the dose response curve. So, the selection of study doses is primarily driven by objective (2) in what follows. For calculation of the total sample size, both objectives (1) and (2) will be considered.

The selection of doses and the total sample size for the trial are interrelated so that the total sample size may differ for a different selection of doses. Here, we focus on answering the two questions separately, assuming in each situation that the other question has already been answered. In practice, these two steps might be iterated.

The outline of this chapter is as follows: after introducing the notation in the next section, we will introduce an example study. Then, the selection of doses and dose allocation weights will be discussed in Section 13.2. Finally, the selection of the total sample size will be discussed in Section 13.3. In all cases, the example study will be used to illustrate the methods using the `DoseFinding` R package [1]. All methods presented in this chapter are also available via the ADDPLAN DF software [2].

13.1.1   Notation

We assume the same setting as in Chapter 11: patients are assumed to be randomized to one of the dose levels $d_1, \ldots, d_k$, where $d_1 = 0$ is the placebo group and the assumed stochastic model is of the form

$$y_{ij} = \mu(d_i, \boldsymbol{\theta}) + \epsilon_{ij}, \ \epsilon_{ij} \overset{iid}{\sim} N(0, \sigma^2), i = 1, \ldots, k, j = 1, \ldots, n_i, \qquad (13.1)$$

where y_{ij} denotes the response (clinical endpoint measurement) of the jth patient on dose d_i and $\mu(d_i, \boldsymbol{\theta})$ describes the dose–response curve and thus the mean response for the patients on dose d_i. The dose–response curve $\mu(d_i, \boldsymbol{\theta})$ is typically nonlinear in at least one of the parameters $\boldsymbol{\theta}$. See Chapter 11 for examples of dose–response functions.

13.1.2   Example study

To illustrate the methods introduced in this chapter, an example motivated by a real clinical dose-finding study in chronic obstructive pulmonary disease (COPD) will be used. The purpose of this study was to characterize the dose–response curve for once-daily dosing of a compound in terms of a lung function measurement called FEV1 (forced expiratory volume within 1 s, measured in liters). The measurement was assessed after 7 days of treatment. We assume the FEV1 measurement to be normally distributed with a standard deviation of 0.34 L. The considered doses are 12.5, 25, 50, and 100 mg. Based on earlier data, the dose–response functions shown in Figure 13.1 and in Table 13.1 were considered plausible for the dose–response relationship at the design stage. It was also assumed that the maximum effect in the range up to 100 mg was approximately 0.15 L for all dose–response functions. In addition, a difference of 0.12 L was considered to be the minimum difference of clinical relevance. The true placebo response is assumed to be 0 here. This does not change any of the following design calculations.

13.2   Doses and Dose Allocation Weights

We will now consider the determination of doses as well as allocation weights for the doses, assuming that the total sample size is fixed. First, a way to come up with dose spacings based

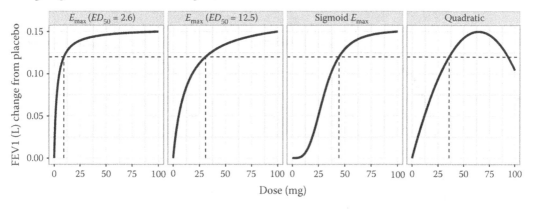

FIGURE 13.1
Candidate dose–response functions for the example study, shown with the minimally clinically relevant difference of 0.12 L and the doses giving an effect of 0.12 L for each dose–response function.

TABLE 13.1
Candidate dose–response functions for the example study.

Function	$\mu(d, \theta)$
E_{max}	$0.1539d/(d + 2.6)$
E_{max}	$0.1688d/(d + 12.5)$
Sigmoid E_{max}	$0.1524d^{3.5}/(d^{3.5} + 30.5^{3.5})$
Quadratic	$(4.656 \times 10^{-3})d - (3.613056 \times 10^{-5})d^2$

on general drug exposure considerations is discussed in Section 13.2.1. Then, in Section 13.2.2, doses and dose allocations will be derived based on optimal design considerations.

13.2.1   Some general principles

Before discussing the choice of doses from a formal mathematical perspective, we give some general rules of thumb for the dose range, the number of doses, and the dose spacing to study.

A common problem in dose-finding designs is that the dose range selected is too narrow to identify the complete dose–response curve [3, 4]. Figure 13.2 shows the selection of three active doses for two designs with a hypothetical true dose–response curve, which is in practice of course not known at the design stage. Both designs would not be adequate to determine the dose–response curve. For design (a), one would not know the location of the increasing part of the dose–response curve and where the plateau starts, i.e., one would not know whether there are lower doses that are also on the plateau of the efficacy dose–response curve but that might have a better safety profile. For design (b), one would not know how much to increase the dose while still gaining efficacy.

To minimize the risk of these situations occurring in practice, one should try to study a wide dose range in Phase II, i.e., the ratio of the highest to the lowest dose should be adequately large. In a recent publication [4], it is recommended to study a dose range of >10-fold as a rule of thumb. The highest dose is often determined by safety considerations based on earlier trials, but there is usually some flexibility in choosing the lowest dose. It is also recommended to choose around four to seven active doses to determine the curve. In the

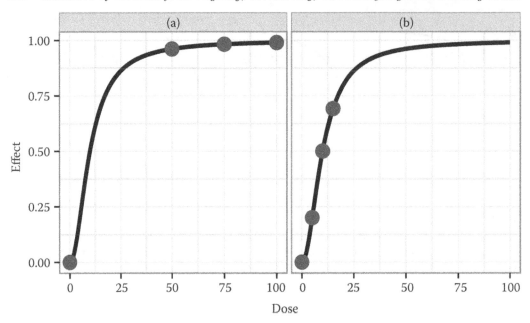

FIGURE 13.2
Examples for too narrow selections of the dose range.

simulations described in Ref. [5], four active doses already lead to satisfactory performance in situations where the dose range is adequate to characterize the dose–response curve and parametric dose–response models are used for estimation.

In terms of the spacing of doses, it is often adequate to use doses such that the ratio between two sequential dose levels is constant (log dose spacing). Exposure summaries for a given dose, like the area under the curve (AUC) or the maximum concentration ($C_{\max}$), are in many situations log-normally distributed: The variance grows with the mean exposure. To cover the exposure range efficiently, doses thus have to be denser in the lower dose range and have to be farther apart in the higher dose range. This approach will avoid having the exposure distributions highly overlapping between the doses. Given that the drug exposure (e.g., drug concentration in plasma) is usually an important predictor for the drug effect, this is an important, often applicable, consideration.

Figure 13.3 illustrates hypothetical log-normal exposure distributions of doses that are equally spaced on the $\log_2$ scale and on the original dose scale. One can see that for equal spacing, the exposure range of 50–100 is sampled very densely, because the doses lead to highly overlapping exposure ranges, and a few doses produce exposure values in this range. The lower dose range is not sampled densely enough or not at all. Log dose spacing covers the exposure range more efficiently, as it covers the lower range better than equally spaced doses, but also covers the mid and upper exposure ranges. This is important as the increasing part of the response curve might be anywhere in the studied exposure range.

The actual spacing of doses can also be chosen based on considerations of exploring the exposure range efficiently: If there is large variability in the exposure values per dose, larger spaces between doses (and thus potentially less doses) are sufficient to cover the exposure range of interest, while for small exposure variability, a smaller spacing (and more doses) might be necessary to cover the whole exposure range.

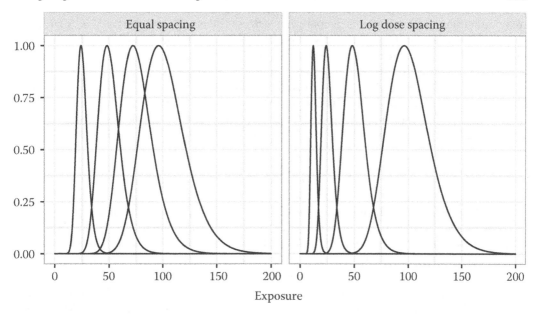

FIGURE 13.3
Hypothetical exposure probability densities (scaled to have a maximum of 1) for log-dose spacing (doses: 12.5, 25, 50, and 100) and equal spacing (doses: 25, 50, 75, and 100). The densities are log-normal distributions with mean on log scale equal to the log dose and standard deviation 0.2.

13.2.2 Optimal design theory

A more formal idea is to base the choice of doses on the expected dose–response shapes. In many situations, some information is available on the shape of the dose–response curve before the start of the trial. This is the idea underlying, for example, the MCP-Mod methodology. This information can also be used to come up with a design of the study, i.e., the dose levels to use as well as the allocation weights.

The idea underlying optimal design theory is to select a design so that a specific performance metric (design criterion) is optimized (see Refs [6, 7] for an overview or Refs [8, 9] for a discussion in the context of dose-finding studies). Most performance metrics are a function of the asymptotic covariance matrix $\mathbf{V}$ (the inverse of the Fisher information of the parameter $\boldsymbol{\theta}$) in model (13.1):

$$\mathbf{V} = \mathbf{V}(\mathbf{d}, \mathbf{w}, \boldsymbol{\theta}) = \frac{\sigma^2}{N} \left(\sum_{i=1}^{k} w_i g(d_i, \boldsymbol{\theta}) g(d_i, \boldsymbol{\theta})^\top \right)^{-1}, \qquad (13.2)$$

where $g(d_i, \boldsymbol{\theta})$ denotes the gradient of the dose–response function $\mu(\cdot, \boldsymbol{\theta})$ with respect to $\boldsymbol{\theta}$ evaluated at d_i, and $\mathbf{w} = (w_1, \dots, w_k)^\top$ denotes a vector of allocation weights (subject to $w_i \geq 0$ and $\sum_{i=1}^{k} w_i = 1$) for the doses $\mathbf{d} = (d_1, \dots, d_k)^\top$. A commonly used performance metric is the D-optimality criterion. Its motivation stems from the fact that an asymptotic confidence set for $\boldsymbol{\theta}$ is given by

$$\{\boldsymbol{\theta} | (\widehat{\boldsymbol{\theta}} - \boldsymbol{\theta})^\top \mathbf{V}^{-1} (\widehat{\boldsymbol{\theta}} - \boldsymbol{\theta}) < c\}$$

for some $c > 0$ (depending on the desired coverage probability). The volume of this confidence set is proportional to $\sqrt{\det(\mathbf{V})}$. That means if we can minimize $\det(\mathbf{V})$, we can create maximum information on the parameter $\boldsymbol{\theta}$. As the covariance matrix $\mathbf{V} = \mathbf{V}(\mathbf{d}, \mathbf{w}, \boldsymbol{\theta})$ depends on the design through $\mathbf{d}$ and $\mathbf{w}$, one can search over these quantities to find a design that leads to good performance. The design minimizing the determinant of the asymptotic covariance matrix will also minimize the maximum prediction variance on the considered dose range (see Ref. [6, Chapter 11]). This makes the D-criterion attractive to use when the main purpose of the study is to estimate the dose–response curve.

Alternatively, designs may be optimized to minimize the asymptotic variance associated with estimating a particular parameter function $h(\boldsymbol{\theta})$. Using the delta method, this variance can be approximated by

$$\mathbf{c}(\boldsymbol{\theta})^{\top} \mathbf{V} \mathbf{c}(\boldsymbol{\theta}), \tag{13.3}$$

where $\mathbf{c}(\boldsymbol{\theta}) = \frac{\partial h(\boldsymbol{\theta})}{\partial \boldsymbol{\theta}}$. Again, this expression can be used to compare different designs $(\mathbf{d}, \mathbf{w})$ in terms of the variance they imply on estimating $h(\boldsymbol{\theta})$. The related optimality criterion is called the c-optimality criterion. An example for the function $h(\cdot)$ is the doses of interest, such as the TD, $\widehat{ED}_p$ (see Refs [8, 9]), or the dose–response function μ itself evaluated at a specific dose.

All of the above considerations require knowledge of the true dose–response function $\mu(d, \boldsymbol{\theta})$, and the model parameter $\boldsymbol{\theta}$ as the asymptotic covariance matrix $\mathbf{V}(\mathbf{d}, \mathbf{w}, \boldsymbol{\theta})$ depends on the assumed dose–response function and the parameter value $\boldsymbol{\theta}$. As this information is not available at the design stage, uncertainty on the dose–response function and parameters should be taken into account. One way of doing so is to set up a candidate set of dose–response functions μ_m with given parameter values $\boldsymbol{\theta}_m$ and design the study taking into account this set of models. Note that here some of the candidate dose–response functions might come from the same model function class and only differ in terms of the parameter value $\boldsymbol{\theta}_m$. One can then define a model-averaged (compound) design criterion:

$$\sum_{m=1}^{M} \frac{\alpha_m}{p_m} \log(\det(\mathbf{V}_m(\mathbf{d}, \mathbf{w}, \boldsymbol{\theta}))), \tag{13.4}$$

where $\alpha_1, \dots, \alpha_M$ are prior model weights, p_m is the number of parameters in dose–response function m, and $\mathbf{V}_m$ is the covariance matrix associated with model M_m. Note that the division by p_m is necessary as the matrices $\mathbf{V}_m$ might be of different dimensions. In essence, the weighted geometric mean of the individual design criteria is used (see Ref. [8] for further design criteria taking into account model uncertainty). Similarly, also c-optimal design criteria can be averaged.

13.2.3 Illustration of COPD example

We will now illustrate the described theory using the `DoseFinding` R package and the example discussed in Section 13.1.2. The main purpose of this study was to determine the dose–response curve; hence, the D-optimality criterion would be an adequate approach for study design. Candidate dose–response functions for that purpose are given in Table 13.1. Designs will be optimized with respect to the compound D-optimality criterion (13.4) with equal prior weights $\alpha_m = 1/4$.

In principle, one could calculate "optimal" doses and allocation weights using optimal design theory. However, in practice, there are usually practical limitations on the doses that can be utilized, e.g., only specific dose strengths might have been pre-produced for the study.

As a hypothetical example, we assume here for our purposes that placebo and two dose strengths (12.5 and 50 mg) are available from production. We assume that a total of three pills can be taken by the patients and that a maximum dose of 100 mg can be taken per day due to other considerations.

This gives the following actual dose levels that can be offered to patients by taking three pills at a time in a blinded fashion: 0, 12.5, 25, 37.5, 50, 62.5, 75, and 100. Given these candidate doses, we can now calculate the model-averaged D-optimal design using the `optDesign` function from the `DoseFinding` package.

```
## define candidate set of models
mods <- Mods(emax = c(2.6, 12.5),
             sigEmax = c(30.5, 3.5),
             quadratic = -0.00776,
             placEff = 0, maxEff = 0.15,
             doses = c(0,100))
## calculate optimal design
doses <- c(0,12.5,25,37.5,50,62.5,75,100)
optD <- optDesign(mods, doses=doses,
                  probs=rep(1/4,4))
optD
#Calculated D - optimal design:
#      0    12.5      25    37.5      50     100
#0.28614 0.18311 0.09688 0.08018 0.08045 0.27325
```

From the output above, one can see that the optimal design would put approximately half of the patients on the placebo and the maximum dose to be able to determine the boundaries of the curve well, and then put further patients on 12.5, 25, 37.5, and 50 mg, with unbalanced allocations. Now assume that we are interested in designs with balanced allocations (to simplify the trial logistics) and four active doses only. Also assume that we want to force the placebo and a 100 mg dose to be part of the design. These constraints give a set of candidate designs, for which we can calculate the D-criterion value using the `calcCrit` function from the `DoseFinding` package and compare it to the optimal design calculated above. Assume that $\lambda_{\min}$ is the compound criterion value—calculated as in Equation 13.4—for the optimal design, and $\lambda_p, p = 1, \ldots, P$ are the corresponding values of the compound design criterion for the P different candidate designs, and that the efficiency of a design is defined as $\mathrm{Eff}_p = \frac{\exp(\lambda_{\min})}{\exp(\lambda_p)}$. From the way the optimal design was calculated and from the additional constraints on the candidate designs, it follows that $\lambda_p > \lambda_{\min}$ and $\mathrm{Eff}_p \in [0, 1]$. The function $\exp(\cdot)$ is applied to the criterion values so that the the efficiency values are interpretable on the sample size scale (see Equations 13.2 and 13.4). The efficiency can be interpreted as follows: the total sample size would need to be multiplied by $1/\mathrm{Eff}_p$ as compared to the optimal design to reach the same design criterion value as the optimal design.

```
## all balanced designs with placebo and 4 active doses
doses3 <- t(rbind(0,
                  combn(doses[-c(1,8)], 3),
                  100))
## function to calculate criterion of balanced design on the given doses
bal <- rep(1/5,5) # balanced allocations
calcC <- function(doseVec){
  cc <- calcCrit(bal,
                 doses=doseVec,
                 models=mods,
                 probs=rep(1/4,4))
  exp(optD$crit)/exp(cc) # efficiencies
}
```

```
## calculate efficiencies
effs <- apply(doses3, 1, calcC)
## sort according to the best
ord <- rev(order(effs))
doses3[ord[1],] # best design
#[1]    0.0  12.5  25.0  50.0 100.0
max(effs)
#[1] 0.9538424
doses3[ord[2],] # second best design
#[1]    0.0  12.5  25.0  37.5 100.0
doses3[ord[length(ord)],] # worst design
#[1]    0.0  50.0  62.5  75.0 100.0
```

It can be seen that the balanced design utilizing placebo, 12.5, 25, 50, and 100 mg gives a similarly high criterion value as the optimal design above that allowed for unbalanced allocations and did not have a restriction on the number of active doses. The efficiency of ≈95% means that the total sample size would only need to be increased by 5% ($1/0.95 - 1$) as compared to the optimal design to reach the same performance metric. The next best design would use placebo, 12.5, 25, 37.5, and 100 mg. The worst candidate design would allocate patients to placebo, 50, 62.5, 75, and 100 mg. It has an efficiency of only ≈ 0.43. Intuitively, it is clear that this design is inadequate for the description of the dose–response curve as the increasing part of the curve is completely missed for all considered candidate models (see Figure 13.1).

Note that optimal design theory traditionally uses asymptotic approximations of the performance metrics as it is based on the asymptotic covariance matrix. It is known that these approximations are sometimes not very reliable for the type of nonlinear models and data situations considered here. The alternative would be to evaluate the different candidate designs by simulations; however, this will often get computationally prohibitive. So, the approximations used here are useful for a rapid comparison of a relatively large number of candidate designs. A simulation-based comparison would become more appropriate when the list of candidate designs has been narrowed down to a manageable size. Note also that the purpose here is not to obtain absolute values for performance measures but a relative comparison of different candidate designs. In the next section, we will rely on simulation to calculate the total sample size using similar performance metrics, although asymptotics would also be applicable in this situation.

13.3   Sample Size Calculation

As discussed in Section 13.1, both power considerations for a dose–response signal detection test as well as estimation precision can be used to perform sample size calculations. In practice, of course, both questions are always important, although the prioritization might be different between different studies. In what follows, first sample size calculations based on testing will be considered in Section 13.3.1 and then based on estimation precision in Section 13.3.2. In this section, we will assume that the doses and dose allocation weights are given. For simplicity, we restrict ourselves to the balanced sample size allocation case in what follows, though the generalization to unbalanced designs with fixed allocation weights is straightforward.

13.3.1 Detection of a dose–response signal

The traditional approach for the design and analysis of clinical studies with multiple doses is to use pairwise comparisons between the different doses and the control (often a placebo). In this context, sample size calculation is determined by a prespecified minimum power to obtain at least one dose significantly different from the control under an assumed clinically relevant effect, typically accounting for multiplicity. In exploratory Phase II dose-finding studies, this "testing" approach has been criticized as inappropriate by regulators and industry trialists alike (see Chapter 11 and Ref. [5]).

A more efficient approach for evaluating the presence of a dose–response signal is to use trend tests that leverage information from all doses used in the study. In this section, we will use the model-based trend tests in the MCP-Mod approach (described in Chapter 12) to illustrate the key ideas of sample size calculation for identifying a dose–response signal. These ideas can be readily extended to other methods for dose–response trend tests. The material in this section is based on Ref. [10].

We initially consider the power calculation assuming a single *true* dose–response curve, later generalizing it to multiple models. Denote the common sample size per group by n, and assume that M candidate model shapes are used for MCP-Mod, with corresponding model functions μ_m and parameter vectors $\boldsymbol{\theta}_m$, $m = 1, \ldots, M$. First consider power calculation under a given specific model m in the candidate set for MCP-Mod. The power to detect a dose–response signal, that is, to achieve statistical significance in the MCP step of MCP-Mod, is determined by the distribution of the maximum of the model contrast test statistics $T_1, \ldots, T_M$ in MCP-Mod, under the alternative hypothesis that the dose–response mean vector is $\boldsymbol{\mu}_m = (\mu_m(d_1, \boldsymbol{\theta}_m), \ldots, \mu_m(d_k, \boldsymbol{\theta}_m))'$.

Let $q_{1-\alpha}$ denote the multiplicity-adjusted critical value for the MCP step in MCP-Mod. The power to detect the presence of a dose–response signal under $\boldsymbol{\mu}_m$ is then given by

$$
\begin{aligned}
\pi_m(n) &= P(\max_l T_l \geq q_{1-\alpha} | \boldsymbol{\mu} = \boldsymbol{\mu}_m) \\
&= 1 - P(T_1 < q_{1-\alpha}, \ldots, T_M < q_{1-\alpha} | \boldsymbol{\mu} = \boldsymbol{\mu}_m).
\end{aligned}
\tag{13.5}
$$

Under the distributional assumptions (13.1), and balanced allocation $T_1, \ldots, T_M$ jointly follow a noncentral multivariate t distribution [11] under the alternative with correlation matrix $\boldsymbol{R}$, noncentrality parameter $\boldsymbol{\delta}_m$, and $k(n-1)$ degrees of freedom. Here, $\boldsymbol{R} = (\rho_{ij}) = (\boldsymbol{c}_i'\boldsymbol{c}_j)$, where $\boldsymbol{c}_i$ represents the contrast vector corresponding to model i in the candidate set (standardized to have $||\boldsymbol{c}_i|| = 1$), and $\boldsymbol{\delta}_m = (\delta_{m,1}, \ldots, \delta_{m,M})'$, where $\delta_{m,i} = \sqrt{n}\boldsymbol{c}_i'\boldsymbol{\mu}_m/\sigma$, $i = 1, \ldots, M$. Numerical integration methods [12] are available to calculate the integral in Equation 13.5 in practice, being implemented, for example, in the mvtnorm R package [13].

We illustrate power calculation under a single-candidate model with the COPD example introduced in Section 13.1 and using the powMCT function available in the DoseFinding package [1].

```
## load library
library(DoseFinding)
```

```
## candidate set of models and assumed placebo and max effects
mods <- Mods(emax = c(2.6, 12.5),
             sigEmax = c(30.5, 3.5),
             quadratic = -0.00776,
             doses = c(0,12.5, 25, 50, 100))
```

```
## matrix of model contrasts
```

```
contMat <- optContr(mods, w = 1)

## use first emax model as alternative only with max. effect = 0.15
mod1 <- Mods(emax = 2.6, placEff = 0, maxEff = 0.15,
         doses = c(0,12.5,25,50,100))

## power under Model 1, one-sided alpha=0.05, n=40/arm
powMCT(contMat, alpha=0.05, altModels=mod1, n=40, sigma=0.34)
#       emax
#0.7067603
```

A sample size of $n = 40$ per arm provides $\approx 71\%$ power to detect a significant dose–response signal under the first $E_{\max}$ model from Table 13.1 in the candidate set.

Because MCP-Mod allows for multiple candidate models, the performance of the method in detecting a dose–response signal is better characterized by a vector of power values $\boldsymbol{\pi}(n) = (\pi_1(n), \dots, \pi_M(n))'$, where $\pi_m(n)$ is the power assuming that $\boldsymbol{\mu}_m$ is the true mean vector. For the purpose of deriving the sample size, $\boldsymbol{\pi}(n)$ needs to be mapped to a single overall measure of power using some summary function $g: [0, 1]^M \mapsto [0, 1]$ that is monotonically increasing in each of its arguments. A conservative choice for g would be the minimum (worst-case scenario under candidate models). Alternative choices could be a weighted average or a given quantile (e.g., median) of the individual power values.

We again use the COPD example and the `DoseFinding` package to illustrate the calculation of $\boldsymbol{\pi}(n)$ and the use of alternative summary functions.

```
## all candidate models
pw <- powMCT(contMat, alpha=0.05, altModels=mods, n=40, sigma=0.34)
pw
##   emax1     emax2   sigEmax quadratic
0.7068096 0.6791897 0.7714815 0.6040190

## different choices of summary function
c(min(pw), mean(pw), median(pw))
## [1] 0.6043546 0.6909600 0.6937901
```

We now consider the problem of determining the necessary sample size per dose n^* to ensure a prespecified summary power π^* for detecting a dose–response signal with MCP-Mod, under the assumed set of candidate models. That is, we want to find the smallest integer n^* such that $g[\boldsymbol{\pi}(n^*)] \geq \pi^*$.

```
## power values for different n, with min and mean summary functions
powSeq <- powN(upperN=100, lowerN=20, step=5, contMat=contMat,
               altModels=mods, sigma=0.34, alpha=0.05,
               alRatio=rep(1, 5), sumFct=c("min", "mean"))
powSeq
##       emax1 emax2 sigEmax quadratic   min  mean
## 20    0.451 0.434   0.506     0.379 0.379 0.443
## 25    0.526 0.506   0.587     0.442 0.442 0.516
.  .  .
## 65    0.881 0.855   0.925     0.789 0.789 0.862
## 70    0.902 0.878   0.941     0.816 0.816 0.884
.  .  .
## 90    0.955 0.939   0.977     0.893 0.893 0.941
## 95    0.964 0.949   0.983     0.908 0.908 0.951
```

```
## 100    0.970 0.957    0.986      0.920 0.920 0.959
```

```
## graphical display of the power curves
## plot(powSeq, lwd=2, ylab="Power")
```

From the output, more than 90 subjects per arm would be needed to ensure a minimum power of at least 90%.

Because g increases monotonically with n and as $n \to \infty$, $g[\pi(n)] \to 1$, there exists a unique minimum sample size n^* satisfying the power π^* condition. The sample size n^* can then be found using iterative root-finding algorithms, such as the one implemented in the `sampSizeMCT` function in `DoseFinding`, illustrated below for the COPD example (see Ref. [10] for details on the algorithm).

```
## sample size - min summary function
sampSizeMCT(upperN=100, lowerN=90, contMat=contMat, altModels=mods,
            sigma=0.34, alRatio=rep(1,5), power=0.9, alpha=0.05,
            sumFct=min)
## Total sample size: 465
## Sample size per arm: 93 93 93 93 93
## targFunc: 0.902
```

A sample size $n^* = 93$ per arm would be needed to ensure at least 90% power under any of the models in the candidate set. From the output above, it is clear that the quadratic model is associated with the lowest power values among the candidate models and, thus, is driving the sample size. If the quadratic model is deemed less important, the mean summary function could be used for the calculation of the sample size.

```
## mean sumary function
sampSizeMCT(upperN=100, lowerN=80, contMat=contMat, altModels=mods,
            sigma=0.34, alRatio=rep(1,5), power=0.9, alpha=0.05,
            sumFct=mean)
## Total sample size: 375
## Sample size per arm: 75 75 75 75 75
## targFunc: 0.9016
```

The resulting n^* of 75 subjects is smaller than that for the min summary function.

While the basic procedure for sample size calculation described here was based on the MCP part of MCP-Mod, the sample size could be calculated in a similar way also for other trend tests, i.e., by the specification of a candidate set of true models, defining the mean and every dose level and iterating the sample size until the smallest sample size with an adequate summary power value is achieved.

13.3.2 Estimation of dose–response and doses of interest

This section describes sample size calculation approaches motivated by the second question of interest in Phase II studies: estimation of the dose–response curve and doses of interest. As discussed in Chapter 11, this is of major importance for dose selection for Phase III. It is, however, more difficult to quantify this into one single performance metric. Consequently, different metrics will be discussed in this section. The resulting sample size methods fall into two categories related to (i) the estimation of a dose of interest, such as the target dose (TD) or the $\widetilde{ED}_p$ (defined in Chapter 11 in detail), and (ii) the estimation of the dose–response curve.

Contrary to the approach in Section 13.2, we will primarily focus on simulation methods to calculate sample sizes. In our experience, the performance of asymptotic approximations is rather unpredictable to evaluate performance metrics accurately (i.e., when not merely comparing different designs). In some situations, asymptotic approximations perform well, while in other situations, the performance is not adequate and often it is unclear which one applies without running a simulation.

For simplicity, we will initially evaluate the performance metrics by simulating from a single model and only fitting the corresponding dose–response model. Later, we will illustrate the recommended approach, where simulations are performed under multiple true candidate dose–response models, and in each case all candidate models are fitted and model selection is performed on each simulated data set. Similar to Section 13.3.1, one could then select the sample size so that a certain summary performance metric value is achieved under all model scenarios.

13.3.2.1   Estimation of doses of interest

We start with sample size methods focusing on dose estimation. One approach is to calculate the sample size needed to achieve a predetermined precision [e.g., length of confidence interval (C.I.)] for the estimated dose. To make the discussion more concrete, suppose that we want to find the smallest n such that the expected length of the 90% C.I. for the TD is less than or equal to some desired precision. Here, the TD is the smallest dose leading to a target improvement of Δ over placebo. In the COPD example, that value is set to 0.12 L. The expected length of the C.I. for an estimated dose of interest can be obtained using either asymptotic methods (see Ref. [8] for asymptotic variance formulas for target dose estimates) or simulation methods (e.g., bootstrapping for each of the simulated data sets to obtain the C.I. length and calculating the average over all simulated data-sets). Both an asymptotic and a simulation approach are implemented in the `planMod` function in `DoseFinding`. For simulation, however, not a bootstrap approach is taken. Here, the expected length of a $(1 - \alpha) \times 100\%$ C.I. is calculated as the difference between the $(1 - \alpha/2) \times 100\%$ and $\alpha/2 \times 100\%$ quantiles of the simulated TD distribution. This is computationally cheaper than using nested bootstrap simulations in each simulation run and can be expected to give similar answers.

It is clear from Figure 13.1 that the TD varies with the assumed dose–response model. Table 13.2 gives the exact TD corresponding to a target effect of 0.12 L for the candidates models in the COPD example.

The precision of the TD estimate will vary with the assumed dose–response curve and so will the sample size needed to achieve a predetermined precision. Consider the sigmoid

TABLE 13.2

True TD for $\Delta = 0.12$ and true $\widetilde{ED}_p$ for different selections of p for the candidate models in the COPD example.

Model	$E_{\max}(ED_{50} = 2.6)$	$E_{\max}(ED_{50} = 12.5)$	Sigmoid $E_{\max}$	Quadratic
TD (mg)	9.2	30.8	44.4	35.6
$\widetilde{ED}_{25}$ (mg)	0.8	3.6	22.2	8.6
$\widetilde{ED}_{50}$ (mg)	2.5	10.0	30.2	18.9
$\widetilde{ED}_{75}$ (mg)	7.1	25.0	41.0	32.2
$\widetilde{ED}_{90}$ (mg)	18.6	50.0	38.3	44.1
$\widetilde{ED}_{99}$ (mg)	71.5	91.7	86.6	58.0

$E_{\max}$ model in the candidate set from the COPD example for illustration. Initially, we evaluate, via simulations, the expected length of the 90% C.I. for the TD using $n = 93$ per arm, the sample size calculated in Section 13.3.1 to ensure at least 90% power under any of the candidate models

```
## doses and std. dev
doses <- c(0,12.5,25,50,100)
sig <- 0.34

## sigmoid Emax model
mod3 <- Mods(sigEmax=c(30.5, 3.5), placEff=0, maxEff=0.15,
          doses=c(0,12.5,25,50,100))
## length of 90% CI for TD, sigemax model
pObj3 <- planMod("sigEmax", mod3, n=93, sig, doses=doses,
          simulation=T, nSim=5000)
summary(pObj3, Delta=0.12)
##          Eff-vs-ANOVA  cRMSE lengthTDCI P(no TD) lengthEDCI
## sigEmax          1.58 0.0396       58.6    0.152         NA
```

The quantity of interest in the summary of the `planMod` object is `lengthTDCI`, the expected length of the 90% C.I. for TD (the default confidence level is 90%). Its value, 58.6 mg, is larger than the TD itself (44.4 mg in Table 13.2). Clearly, $n = 93$ does not provide sufficient precision for TD estimation, in this case. Another output of interest is `P(no TD)`, which gives the fraction of simulations, where no TD could be estimated (there is no dose that reaches an effect of 0.12 L). The complete output of the `planMod` function is explained on the help page for the function in R.

Consider now the second of the $E_{\max}$ models in the candidate set from Table 13.1.

```
## Emax model with ED50=12.5
mod2 <- Mods(emax=12.5, placEff=0, maxEff=0.15,
          doses=c(0,12.5,25,50,100))
## length of 90% CI for TD, sigemax model
pObj2 <- planMod(``emax'', mod2, n=93, sig, doses=doses,
          simulation=T, nSim=5000)
summary(pObj2, Delta=0.12)
##       Eff-vs-ANOVA  cRMSE lengthTDCI P(no TD) lengthEDCI
## emax          1.46 0.0411        164    0.139         NA
```

The expected length of the 90% C.I. for the TD is now nearly three times as large as under the sigmoid $E_{\max}$ model, for a smaller true TD of 30.8 mg. The sample size of $n = 93$ is also inadequate in this case. The better precision of the TD estimate under the sigmoid $E_{\max}$ model, compared to the second $E_{\max}$ model, is related to the steepness of the dose–response curve close to the TD (see Figure 13.1). The steeper the curve in the area around the true TD, the more precise the TD estimate (but also the higher the impact of misspecifying the TD on the average effect of the drug).

One can proceed to calculate the sample size needed to obtain a prespecified precision for the TD estimate under a given dose–response curve through repeated calls to `planMod`, varying the value of `n` in the call. For example, setting the desired precision for the TD in the COPD example to 20 mg will lead to about $n = 1650$ (sigmoid $E_{\max}$) or $n = 3800$ ($E_{\max}$) per arm. Both sample sizes would not be feasible for a Phase II study in practice, so one should consider relaxing the required precision. For example, if a precision of 30 mg were to be used, the required sample sizes for the sigmoid $E_{\max}$ and the second $E_{\max}$ models would be, respectively, $n = 700$ and 1800 per arm, still too high for most practical cases.

An alternative to utilizing the C.I. length for the TD estimate for sample size calculation is to consider the probability of achieving a response for an $\widehat{ED}_p$ estimate that is within a prespecified acceptable range. If the dose of interest is the $\widehat{ED}_{90}$, one could require that, with, say, 80% probability that the actual placebo-corrected response associated with the estimated dose will be within true 75% and 99% of the maximum response attainable within the dose range used in the Phase II study. That is, it will be within the interval $[\widetilde{ED}_{75}, \widetilde{ED}_{99}]$, where $\widetilde{ED}_{75}$ and $\widetilde{ED}_{99}$ denote the true values of the underlying dose–response curve with 80% probability. Note that, when focusing on efficacy, the lower bound of the response interval is of greater importance, but the upper bound is often relevant when safety is brought into consideration. Again, the `planMod` function can be used to explore the sample size needed to achieve a desired probability for the prespecified target response interval. The COPD example is used for illustration, with Table 13.2 showing the true $\widetilde{ED}_p$ values corresponding to the candidate models.

Under the sigmoid $E_{\max}$ candidate model, assuming the power calculation-based sample size of $n = 93$ per arm, we obtain the following.

```
## Pr(estimated ED_90 between true ED_75 and ED_99)
## sigmoid Emax, n=93/arm
planMod("sigEmax", mod3, n=93, sigma=sig, doses=doses, simulation=T,
        p=0.9, pLB=0.75, pUB=0.99, nSim=5000)
## Fitted Model: sigEmax
##
## Asymptotic Approximations
##          dRMSE Pow(maxDose) P(EDp)
## sigEmax 0.0414       0.877  0.447
##
## Simulation Results (nSim = 5000)
##          dRMSE Pow(maxDose) P(EDp)
## sigEmax  0.039       0.964  0.577
```

The quantity of interest in the output is `P(EDp)`, which gives the probability that the estimated $\widetilde{ED}_p$ is within the true $\widetilde{ED}_{pLB}$ and $\widetilde{ED}_{pUB}$ – in this example, the estimated $\widetilde{ED}_{90}$ being between the true $\widetilde{ED}_{75}$ and $\widetilde{ED}_{99}$. The function calculates those estimated probabilities using both asymptotic results and simulations. From the results above, it is clear that with a sample size of $n = 93$ per arm, the probability that the estimated $\widetilde{ED}_{90}$ gives a response between 75% and 99% of the true maximum effect is rather low. For comparison, consider the second $E_{\max}$ model in the candidate set, with the same sample size of 93 subjects per arm.

```
## Pr(estimated ED_90 between true ED_75 and ED_99)
## second Emax, n=93/arm
planMod(emax", mod2, n=93, sigma=sig, doses=doses, simulation=T,
        p=0.9, pLB=0.75, pUB=0.99, nSim=5000)
## Fitted Model: emax
##
## Asymptotic Approximations
##        dRMSE Pow(maxDose) P(EDp)
## emax  0.0431       0.915  0.765
##
## Simulation Results (nSim = 5000)
```

```
##           dRMSE Pow(maxDose) P(EDp)
## emax      0.041       0.936  0.796
```

The response coverage probabilities under the second $E_{\max}$ model are larger than those under the sigmoid $E_{\max}$ model. One reason for this might be the steeper slope of the dose–response curve around the $\widetilde{ED}_{90}$ under the sigmoid $E_{\max}$ model, which leads to a relatively narrow interval $[\widetilde{ED}_{75}, \widetilde{ED}_{99}]$. For the second $E_{\max}$ model, a wider interval results, see also Table 13.2 and Figure 13.4.

It is interesting that the steepness of the dose–response curve around the value of the dose of interest (TD or $\widetilde{ED}_p$) has different consequences depending on the performance metric considered for the sample size calculation: the steeper the curve, the smaller the required sample size if the focus is on the precision of the estimated TD and the other way around, if the focus is on the probability that the estimated $\widetilde{ED}_{90}$ has an effect between 75% and 99% of the maximum effect.

The sample size required to ensure a 90% probability that the estimated $\widetilde{ED}_{90}$ will be within $\widetilde{ED}_{75}$ and $\widetilde{ED}_{99}$ would be around $n = 1300$ per group under the sigmoid $E_{\max}$ model and $n = 250$ per group under the second $E_{\max}$ model. The respective sample sizes to ensure 80% response coverage probability would be $n = 650$ and 100 per arm. These results illustrate the possible impact of the assumed dose–response curve on design considerations.

13.3.2.2 Estimation of the dose–response curve

We now discuss sample size calculation approaches focusing on the estimation of the dose–response curve as a whole, instead of a particular dose of interest. The first method is a variation of the response coverage probability approach just presented. Instead of focusing on a dose of interest for possible utilization in Phase III, we consider instead a dose in the central region of the dose–response curve, namely the $\widetilde{ED}_{50}$. If that quantity can be properly estimated, then it is likely that the full dose–response curve will be well characterized. To make it more concrete, we are interested in ensuring adequate probability, say 90%, that the estimated $\widetilde{ED}_{50}$ will be within the interval $[\widetilde{ED}_{25}, \widetilde{ED}_{75}]$ (see Table 13.2 for the true values

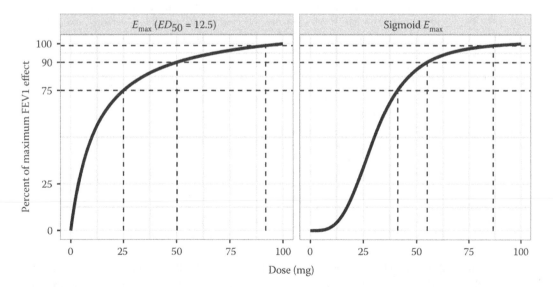

FIGURE 13.4
$\widetilde{ED}_{75}$, $\widetilde{ED}_{90}$, and $\widetilde{ED}_{99}$ for the second $E_{\max}$ model and the sigmoid $E_{\max}$ model.

TABLE 13.3

Sample sizes required to ensure response coverage probabilities for estimated $\widetilde{ED}_{50}$ under candidate models in COPD example.

Probability (%)	$E_{\max}$ ($ED_{50} = 2.6$)	$E_{\max}$ ($ED_{50} = 12.5$)	Sigmoid $E_{\max}$	Quadratic
80	770	180	200	10
90	1580	300	350	45

underlying the candidate models). Table 13.3 gives the sample sizes (per group) required to ensure 80% and 90% response coverage probabilities for the estimated $\widetilde{ED}_{50}$ under the candidate models in the COPD example. The wide variation observed in the sample sizes in Table 13.3 further illustrates the impact of the assumed dose–response curve and the need for combining information across candidate models. In this particular example, a sample size of $n = 200$ per arm provides reasonable $\widetilde{ED}_{50}$ response coverage probability for all but the first $E_{\max}$ model and is within the feasible range of trial sizes for this indication. Note that this calculation assumed that only the true dose–response model is fitted and used in each simulation scenario.

The final sample size calculation approach considered here focuses on the overall estimation error for the (placebo-corrected) dose–response curve itself. More specifically, we consider the root mean square error (RMSE) averaged over a fine grid of values covering the examined dose range in the study. The goal is to find the minimum sample size needed to provide an average RMSE less than or equal to a desired precision. One can set the desired precision for the average RMSE as a percentage of the target effect, say, 20% of $0.12\,L$, giving $0.024\,L$. The `planMod` function, together with its `summary` method, can be used to derive the appropriate n to meet the average RMSE precision requirement. We use a variation of the call to `planMod` considering a set of candidate model families for the first argument and different candidate dose–response curves for the second argument, instead of a single model family and a single dose response curve, as considered in the previous examples of this section. This causes all models to be fitted to the data. The model with the best Akaike information criterion (AIC) is selected for estimation for each simulated data set. This is similar to the MCP-Mod approach (with AIC model selection), except that the MCP step testing for the presence of a dose–response signal is omitted.

```
## sample size to ensure average RMSE max value of 0.024
prAll <- planMod(c("emax", "sigEmax", "quadratic"), mods, n=350,
                 sig, doses=doses, asyApprox=F, simulation=T,
                 nSim=5000)
summary(prAll)
##          Eff-vs-ANOVA  cRMSE lengthTDCI P(no TD) lengthEDCI
## emax1            1.27 0.0239         NA       NA         NA
## emax2            1.16 0.0229         NA       NA         NA
## sigEmax          1.09 0.0241         NA       NA         NA
## quadratic        1.36 0.0227         NA       NA         NA

plot(prAll)
```

The relevant column in the output is `cRMSE`, the average RMSE calculated over a grid of 101 equally spaced points in the dose range. The sample size of $n = 350$ meets the precision criterion for the average RMSE under all four candidate models considered. The estimation precision is graphically illustrated in Figure 13.5.

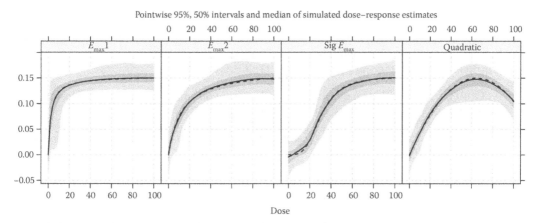

FIGURE 13.5
Fitted dose–response curves with condence bands in COPD example, with a sample size of $n = 350$ per arm.

Note that when an approach like MCP-Mod is used, the model selection should be simulated as well, as it is part of the procedure. Although this was only examined on the cRMSE metric in this chapter, it should be taken into account for any other performance metric for sample size calculation. Still, similar to the case for power calculations, different sample sizes will be associated with the different true candidate models and a summary function will be needed to combine the individual n's into a single sample size recommendation. A conservative, but often not feasible, approach is to take the maximum sample size. Alternatives would be the median or some weighted mean of the individual values.

In conclusion, sample size calculation approaches based on estimation of doses of interest or dose–response curves tend to produce considerably larger sample sizes than methods focusing on detection of a dose–response signal. In practice, to keep the size of the study feasible, one needs to find a compromise between dose–response signal detection and estimation precision as the criteria for sample size determination. Irrespective, it is important to properly evaluate the operating characteristics of a given design (including sample size) to understand its strengths and limitations.

References

1. B. Bornkamp, J. Pinheiro, and F. Bretz. *Dose Finding: Planning and Analyzing Dose Finding Experiments*. R Package Version 0.9-13, 2016.

2. ADDPLAN, Inc, an Aptiv Solutions Company. *ADDPLAN DF Version 3.1 Methodology Overview*, 2014.

3. A. Mullard. Regulators and industry tackle dose-finding issues. *Nature Reviews Drug Discovery*, 14:371–372, 2015.

4. European Medicines Agency. Report from dose finding workshop, 2015. http://www.ema.europa.eu/docs/en_GB/document_library/Report/2015/04/WC500185864.pdf.

5. B. Bornkamp, F. Bretz, A. Dmitrienko, G. Enas, B. Gaydos, C.-H. Hsu, F. König, M. Krams, Q. Liu, B. Neuenschwander, T. Parke, J. C. Pinheiro, A. Roy, R. Sax, and F. Shen. Innovative approaches for designing and analyzing adaptive dose-ranging trials. *Journal of Biopharmaceutical Statistics*, 17:965–995, 2007.

6. A. C. Atkinson, A. N. Donev, and R. D. Tobias. *Optimum Experimental Design, with SAS*. Oxford University Press, Oxford, UK, 2007.

7. V. V. Fedorov and S. L. Leonov. *Optimal Design for Nonlinear Response Models*. Chapman and Hall, Boca Raton, 2014.

8. H. Dette, F. Bretz, A. Pepelyshev, and J. C. Pinheiro. Optimal designs for dose finding studies. *Journal of the American Statisical Association*, 103:1225–1237, 2008.

9. F. Bretz, H. Dette, and J. Pinheiro. Practical considerations for optimal designs in clinical dose finding studies. *Statistics in Medicine*, 29:731–742, 2010.

10. J. C. Pinheiro, B. Bornkamp, and F. Bretz. Design and analysis of dose finding studies combining multiple comparisons and modeling procedures. *Journal of Biopharmaceutical Statistics*, 16:639–656, 2006.

11. S. Kotz and S. Nadarajah. *Multivariate t Distributions and Their Applications*. Cambridge University Press, Cambridge, 2004.

12. A. Genz and F. Bretz. Methods for the computation of multivariate t-probabilities. *Journal of Computational and Graphical Statistics*, 11:950–971, 2002.

13. A. Genz, F. Bretz, and T. Hothorn. *mvtnorm: Multivariate Normal and Distributions*, R package, 2008.

14

Two-Stage Designs in Dose Finding

Tobias Mielke

ICON Clinical Research

Vladimir Dragalin

Janssen Research & Development

CONTENTS

14.1 Introduction

Challenges in dose-finding studies were discussed in the previous chapters on MCP-Mod methodology and design of Phase II dose-finding studies. Problems related to design inefficiency in conventional Phase II studies were also examined in the first chapter with suggestions for more efficient dose allocations. However, the optimal dose allocation depends on the unknown dose–response relationship. Considering the dose allocation based on a guess of the true dose–response model may result in an inefficient design. Adaptive designs make use of accumulating information to safeguard against design misspecifications. The purpose of this chapter is to introduce and discuss adaptive two-stage dose-finding designs.

Bayesian and maximin optimality criteria help to determine robust study designs in case of uncertainties in the design stage (e.g., [1]). Compound optimal designs may be used to address multiple study objectives simultaneously (e.g., estimation of the entire dose–response model or of the target dose). In combination with the MCP-Mod approach, compound optimality criteria are used to address model uncertainty (e.g., [2]). Selected candidate models in MCP-Mod have an underlying motivation and might be considered for the determination of an efficient study design.

Although these designs will be efficient for a wide range of possible dose–response shapes, they may not be optimal for the true underlying model and not for all objectives of a dose-finding study. Taking an interim look at the data and adjusting the next-stage allocation based on observed responses may overcome these drawbacks. Different adaptive dose-finding designs were compared and contrasted by the PhRMA Working Group on Adaptive Designs [3, 4]. Mercier et al. [5] describe a model-based two-stage design with an application in a multiple sclerosis study reported by Selmaj et al. [6]. Different adaptive allocation strategies were compared to a fixed design with the result that response-adaptive allocations may reduce the risk of over- or underestimation of the target dose.

Objectives of Phase II dose-finding studies include the proof of drug-related effects, estimation of the dose–response, and the selection of doses for confirmatory testing. The benefit of adaptations in reaching these objectives depends greatly on the considered study design. Two-stage designs can be developed to address these objectives sequentially, e.g., including a proof of concept (PoC) objective within a dose-finding study. First-stage designs are frequently considered to partly answer the question of the existence of a drug-related effect. The designs seamlessly transition from the PoC stage into a dose-finding stage. Alternatively, the first-stage design might target the description of the dose–response relation and transition to an expansion phase enriching information on the most promising doses, see, e.g., adaptive Dc-optimal designs in [7].

Once the objectives of the study and potential adaptation rules are determined, the optimal timing for the adaptation needs to be evaluated. Considerations on the optimal timing in adaptive two-stage dose-finding designs are given in [8]. Early interim analyses are beneficial, as more patients will be allocated according to the updated design. However, due to the limited information in the interim analysis, the probability of suboptimal adaptations is increasing with decreasing stage one information. Late adaptations are better informed but will limit the benefit of the design, as only a few patients will be randomized according to the new rules.

Quinlan et al. [9] summarize operational challenges in the implementation of adaptive study designs. An appropriate technical infrastructure needs to support the implementation of the proposed study design changes. The relation between recruitment speed and time to endpoint will frequently limit the feasibility of adaptive approaches and should be studied up front. Longitudinal models ([10]) and surrogate endpoints not only mitigate this problem, but they may also introduce additional uncertainties in the interim decision.

This chapter is structured as follows. In this section, the statistical dose–response model will be introduced, and the Fisher information for a two-stage design will be defined. Six different two-stage designs will be introduced using the COPD study as an illustration. These six two-stage designs will illustrate the proposed adaptation rules in the following sections. Stopping rules at the end of the first stage and options for model selection for the second stage will be discussed in Section 14.2. Response-adaptive allocation rules for the second stage will be discussed in Section 14.3. The operating characteristics of the proposed two-stage designs are evaluated in Section 14.4 in a simulation study under three dose–response scenarios. The timing of interim analyses will briefly be examined in Section 14.5, before the chapter closes with a short discussion of the results and recommendations for the application of two-stage designs.

14.1.1 Statistical model and information matrix

In this chapter, the statistical model for the average response of n_{ij} subjects in stage i on the jth dose group d_j is considered to be normally distributed:

$$\overline{Y}_{ij} = \mu(d_j, \theta) + \epsilon_{ij} \sim N\left(\mu(d_j, \theta), \frac{1}{n_{ij}}\sigma^2\right), \quad i = 1, 2, \ j = 1, ..., k. \tag{14.1}$$

The mean response function is given by $\mu(d, \theta)$ and follows the structure described by Bornkamp et al. [11]:

$$\mu(d, \theta) = \theta_0 + \theta_1 \mu^0(d, \theta^*) = \left(1, \mu^0(d, \theta^*)\right)\theta_L,$$

where $\theta_L = (\theta_0, \theta_1)^\top$ denotes the linear model parameters and $\mu^0(d, \theta^*)$ is the standardized model. Multiple dose–response relationships will be considered throughout the chapter. The index g denotes the index of the considered models and related parameters $\mu_g(d; \theta_g)$, $g = 1, ..., m$.

The allocation proportions for the first stage of the study are fixed and given by $\mathbf{w}_1 = (w_{11}, ..., w_{1k})$. The first-stage Fisher information for the dose–response model μ_g with sample size N_1 and allocation $\mathbf{w}_1$ is defined by

$$\frac{N_1}{\sigma^2} M_{g;\theta_g}(w_1) := \frac{N_1}{\sigma^2} \sum_{j=1}^{k} w_{1j} \frac{\partial \mu_g(d_j, \theta)}{\partial \theta} \frac{\partial \mu_g(d_j, \theta)}{\partial \theta^\top}.$$

Given the second-stage allocation $\mathbf{w}_2 = (w_{21}, ..., w_{2k})$ and total sample size N, the total information is given by

$$\frac{N}{\sigma^2} M_{g;\theta_g}(\mathbf{w}) = \frac{N_1}{\sigma^2} M_{g;\theta_g}(w_1) + \frac{N - N_1}{\sigma^2} M_{g;\theta_g}(w_2), \tag{14.2}$$

where

$$w = (w_1, ..., w_k) = \frac{N_1}{N}(w_{11}, ..., w_{1k}) + \frac{N - N_1}{N}(w_{21}, ..., w_{2k}).$$

Note that the second-stage design w_2 depends on the first-stage observations. The exact Fisher information would need to take the uncertainty on the second-stage decision into account. Fedorov et al. [12] motivate the use of expression (14.2) for the interim design optimization based on consistency results for the maximum likelihood estimator. Dette et al. [8] use a more refined second-order Taylor approximation to the variance of the parameter estimator to examine the efficiency of two-stage designs.

Stage 1 and 2 data will be pooled for the final analysis:

$$\overline{y}_j = \frac{\overline{y}_{1j} n_{1j} + \overline{y}_{2j} n_{2j}}{n_{1j} + n_{2j}}, \quad j = 1, ..., k.$$

The false-positive rate of the adaptive model-based contrast test can be controlled using p-value combination methods. Comprehensive treatment of the family-wise error rate control in adaptive multi-armed trials is given in [13, 14].

14.1.2 COPD example revisited

The COPD study from the previous chapter will serve as an illustrative example. An adaptive design may be feasible in this situation given the short observation period of 7 days.

TABLE 14.1
Candidate dose–response models for the COPD study.

	Function	Standardized Model
M1:	$E_{\max}1$	$d/(5+d)$
M2:	$E_{\max}2$	$d/(15+d)$
M3:	Sigmoid $E_{\max}$	$d^3/(50+d^3)$
M4:	Quadratic	$d - d^2/160$
M5:	Exponential	$\exp(d/20) - 1$

The treatment effect assumptions (measured in liters as FEV1—forced expiratory volume within 1 s) are unchanged:

$$\mu_g(0, \theta_g) = 0.00, \quad \mu_g(d_g^*, \theta_g) = 0.15, \quad g = 1, ..., m \text{ and } \sigma = 0.34,$$

where d_g^* is the dose with maximum effect in the examined dose range for model g. The set of candidate models in Table 14.1 differs from the preceding chapter and covers the full response range. As another slight deviation from the previous settings, we consider that any multiple of the minimum dose (12.5 mg) up to 100 mg may be administered; therefore, the available doses are $\{0, 12.5, 25, 37.5, 50, 62.5, 75, 87.5, 100\}$. Basic concepts of experimental design theory were introduced in the preceding chapter on designing dose-finding studies. The allocation of patients according to a D-optimal design will also lead to an optimized variance around the estimated dose–response curve for standard statistical models and might hence be reasonable for design optimization [15]. The compound D-optimal design, taking all of the five considered candidate shapes from Table 14.1 into account, can be calculated using ADDPLAN DF [16] or the R package DoseFinding [17] and results in

$$w_{\text{COD}}^* = \begin{pmatrix} 0 & 12.5 & 25 & 37.5 & 50 & 62.5 & 75 & 87.5 & 100 \\ 0.26 & 0.18 & 0.00 & 0.10 & 0.00 & 0.08 & 0.12 & 0.00 & 0.26 \end{pmatrix}.$$

This chapter shall provide a basic understanding of the potential flexibility of adaptive dose-finding designs. Every considered study design will target in the following particular objectives. None of these designs may generally be stated as being the best design. The impact of different initial study designs and adaptation rules on the accrued information will be examined throughout the chapter using the following six study designs:

$\mathbf{D}_0$: The standard dose-finding design with fixed equal allocation to three active doses (25, 50, and 100 mg) and placebo serves as a benchmark.

$\mathbf{D}_1$: The top-down design starts with a balanced allocation to placebo and the maximum dose in the first stage ($\mathbf{D}_{11}$). The second-stage design is given by a balanced allocation to placebo and lower doses (12.5, 25, and 50 mg). This design is of particular interest if a positive-response signal is required before investing into a larger Phase II study with additional doses.

$\mathbf{D}_2$: A balanced first-stage allocation to all available doses ($\mathbf{D}_{12}$) with a following second-stage compound optimal design will address the question whether covering all doses adds any value in dose finding.

$\mathbf{D}_3$: The study starts with the standard dose-finding design $\mathbf{D}_0$. A rule-based adaptation (a detailed definition will be given in Section 14.3.2) will allocate the second-stage patients according to a set of candidate designs matching a range of predefined response patterns.

D_4: Design $\mathbf{D}_4$ will start with the compound D-optimal allocation w^*_{COD}. The weights for the five candidate models and their parameter estimates will be updated at the interim analysis. The second-stage patients will be allocated according to the updated compound D-optimal design.

D_5: Design $\mathbf{D}_5$ will start with the allocation w^*_{COD}. After the interim analysis, patients will be allocated according to the most efficient design out of a set of the predefined candidate designs.

The designs were selected mainly out of academic interest. Using these designs, the introduced adaptation rules will be displayed, and potential benefits and limitations of different approaches will be highlighted. The study designs will be evaluated based on three different underlying dose–response scenarios for (14.1):

$$E_{\max} \ \eta_1(d) = e_{\max} \frac{d}{d + 10},$$
$$\text{Sigmoid } E_{\max} \ \eta_2(d) = e_{\max} \frac{d^4}{d^4 + 35^4},$$
$$\text{Exponential } \eta_3(d) = e_{\max} \left(\exp\left\{ \frac{d}{15} \right\} - 1 \right),$$

with $\sigma = 0.34$. Adaptation options will be evaluated for different effect sizes $e_{\max}$ such that this parameter is kept unspecified in given scenario definition. The $E_{\max}$ scenario has the ED_{50} at 10% of the considered dose range, while the exponential scenario at 90%. The candidate models for the MCP-Mod approach in Table 14.1 do not meet any of these scenarios perfectly. The D-efficiency serves as a measure on the loss of information with suboptimal designs. The standard design $\mathbf{D}_0$ has a D-efficiency of 97% in the moderate scenario η_2. This means that the optimal design for this scenario requires 97% of the patients as compared to the design $\mathbf{D}_0$ to reach the same information. The D-efficiency of design $\mathbf{D}_0$ is small for the extreme scenarios η_1 (69%) and η_3 (18%). The efficiency of the compound optimum design w^*_{COD} is given by 86% (η_1), 57% (η_2), and 55% (η_3). Hence, there is still room for improvement in the last two cases using adaptive designs.

14.2 First-Stage Design

The two main objectives of the first stage are to establish the PoC and to determine the optimal dose allocation of the new subjects in the second stage. The former can be achieved by considering stopping for futility rules in case the data in the first stage do not show signs of treatment effect at any dose. We consider two such stopping rules in the next subsections. Dose allocation in the second stage depends on the interim modeling. The quality of interim modeling and model selection depending on the considered first-stage study design will be examined in the second part of this section.

14.2.1 Test for existence of any drug-related effects

The controlled false-positive probability in statistical tests makes these also interesting as quantitative decision criteria for development continuation. The simplest futility rule in multi-armed studies can be developed using a significance test for multiple hypotheses. The study is stopped for futility if none of the hypothesis H_{0i}: $\mu_i \leq \mu_1, i = 2, ..., k$ can be rejected at a multiplicity corrected level α_0. The notation μ_i describes here for simplicity the mean at dose group d_i. The critical value $\mathbf{c}_{1-\alpha_0}$ is calculated using the multivariate normal distribution with an appropriate correlation matrix. Rejection of $H_0 = \bigcap_{i=2}^{k} H_{0i}$ using pairwise comparisons implies that at least one dose is superior to placebo at level α_0. However, the multiplicity correction increases the required sample size of the first stage when patients are allocated to many doses, e.g., when using designs as $\mathbf{D}_{12}$. Hierarchical tests or trend tests, as in the MCP-Mod method, reduce the multiplicity penalty, but these will lead to a different interpretation of the test results. Futility stopping based on testing against a flat dose–response will control the probability to continue the study at the level α_0 in case there is no effect. The probability to continue development, in case there is a true benefit, is not controlled such that the first stage of the study requires an appropriate sample size to ensure continuation of promising developments with a high probability.

14.2.2 Testing against existence of target effects

The test for existence of any drug-related effects fixes the false continuation probability at level α_0. One may alternatively wish to fix the probability of false early study termination at level α_0. Consider a test for the null hypothesis:

$$H_0 : \{\mu_2 \geq \mu_1 + \mathrm{TV}\} \cup \{\mu_3 \geq \mu_1 + \mathrm{TV}\} \cup \cdots \cup \{\mu_k \geq \mu_1 + \mathrm{TV}\},$$

where TV is the target value of the commercially viable treatment effect. Rejection of H_0 implies that the effect at all doses is below the TV. The study is stopped for futility if H_0 can be rejected at some level α_0, see Lalonde et al. [18] for a similar approach in their dual go/no go framework. A multiplicity adjustment is not required for intersection–union tests: H_0 is rejected at level α_0 if all one-sided tests are rejected at local level α_0, see Berger and Hsu [19]. The probability to stop development in case of a true underlying effect TV is below α_0 in this framework, such that the study will continue to full enrollment with probability greater than $1 - \alpha_0$.

Model-based estimators may decrease the variance of the treatment effect estimator, increasing the power under the alternative. This translates into an increased probability of futility stopping in case the drug does not reach the TV. Consider the MCP-Mod approach with m-candidate models with the guesstimates θ^*. Using the design matrices

$$F_{g;\theta^*} := \begin{pmatrix} 1 & \mu_g^0(d_1, \theta^*) \\ \cdots & \cdots \\ 1 & \mu_g^0(d_k, \theta^*) \end{pmatrix}, \quad g = 1, \ldots, m, \tag{14.3}$$

and the weight matrix $W = \mathrm{diag}(w_{11}, \ldots, w_{k1})$, the least squares estimator for the linear parameter $\theta_{L,g}$ is given by

$$\widehat{\theta}_{L,g} := \left(F_{g;\theta^*}^\top W F_{g;\theta^*} \right)^{-1} F_{g;\theta^*}^\top W \overline{Y}_1.$$

Under model g, this estimator follows a normal distribution with

$$E(\widehat{\theta}_{L,g}) = \left(F_{g;\theta^*}^\top W F_{g;\theta^*} \right)^{-1} F_{g;\theta^*}^\top W \mu_g(d, \theta_g),$$

$$Cov(\widehat{\theta}_{L,g}) = \frac{\sigma^2}{N_1} \left(F_{g;\theta^*}^\top W F_{g;\theta^*} \right)^{-1}.$$

Let d_g^* denote the dose with maximum response in the examined dose range for the candidate model g. The maximum treatment effect for model g is then estimated as follows:

$$\widehat{\Delta} := c_g^\top \overline{Y}_1 := \left(0, \mu_g^0(d_g^*, \theta^*) - \mu_g^0(0, \theta^*) \right) \widehat{\theta}_{L,g}.$$

Stopping for futility should be recommended if

$$\min_{g=1,\ldots,m} \sqrt{N_1} \frac{TV - c_g^\top \overline{Y}_1}{\sqrt{\sigma^2 c_g^\top W^{-1} c_g}} > z_{1-\alpha_0}.$$

The model-based maximum effects are significantly below the TV in this situation. Modelling assumptions will introduce bias such that the false-termination risk is generally not controlled using this approach.

Example 14.1: Futility Stopping

Let the interim analysis in the COPD study be conducted after $N_1 = 150$ patients, and consider the E_{max} (η_1) and exponential (η_3) scenarios described in the introductory section. The significance level $\alpha_0 = 25\%$ is considered for the futility stop. Figure 14.1 displays the dependence of the first-stage power on the maximum effect. The power of the test for the existence of any drug-related effects is given on the left-hand side. The significance level α_0 controls here the probability to continue development in case there is no drug-related effect. The right-hand side displays the test for a targeted difference of 0.1 L. The probability to stop the study at a true effect of 0.1 L is at most α_0 due to the intersection–union test. The probability of development continuation is hence at least $1 - \alpha_0$ for this futility rule. The black lines in Figure 14.1 represent pairwise comparison procedures. The gray lines display the power for model-based tests using candidate models as described in Table 14.1. The most powerful design for futility stopping is given in all settings with $\mathbf{D}_{11}$, which is represented by

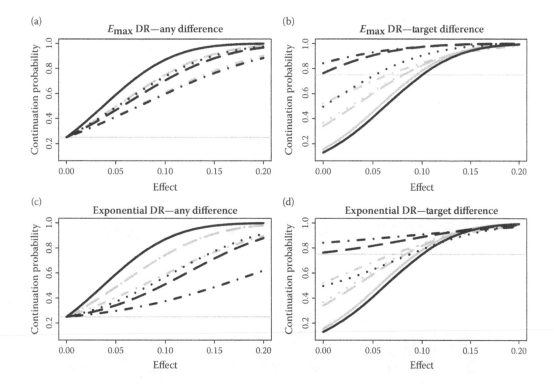

FIGURE 14.1
Continue if there is any difference (a and c) vs. stop if the difference at all doses is below the TV (b and d). Black lines: pairwise comparisons, gray lines: model-based test. First-stage designs: $\mathbf{D}_{11}$ (solid), $\mathbf{D}_{12}$ (dot-dash), $\mathbf{D}_0$ (dotted), and w^*_{COD} (dashed). Constant line: α_0.

the solid lines. For the test on any difference, continuation is proposed in working scenarios with maximum probability. For the test on the target difference, the probability of study termination in case of a true effect size below the TV is at maximum with the design $\mathbf{D}_{11}$. An equal allocation to all doses $\mathbf{D}_{12}$ (dot-dash) is the worst design for discrimination of promising and futile developments. The power for the compound optimal design w^*_{COD} (dashed) and the standard dose-finding design $\mathbf{D}_0$ (dotted) are very similar to each other for model-based approaches. The design w^*_{COD} loses power for pairwise comparisons when testing for the target effect. Wide confidence intervals for doses with few observations lead to a low number of stopped studies in these settings. The model-based test improves the stop probability for low-effect scenarios to the range of the design $\mathbf{D}_0$. The use of model-based techniques improves futility testing in both considered test settings.

14.2.3   Model selection

Particular interest in the interim analysis lies in the discrimination between different considered dose–response models. Model selection criteria offered in the MCP-Mod approach include the model-based trend test and the Akaike information criterion (AIC). As the size of the model-based trend test generally allows no direct conclusions on the appropriateness of the relating candidate models, one might alternatively consider to target the selection based on the squared deviation from the candidate models:

$$
\begin{aligned}
L_g(\overline{y}_1) &= \left(\overline{y}_1 - F_{g;\theta^*}\widehat{\theta}_{L,g}\right)^\top W \left(\overline{y}_1 - F_{g;\theta^*}\widehat{\theta}_{L,g}\right) \quad\quad\quad (14.4)\\
&= \overline{y}_1^\top W \left(W^{-1} - F_{g;\theta^*}(F_{g;\theta^*}^\top W F_{g;\theta^*})^{-1} F_{g;\theta^*}^\top\right) W \overline{y}_1, \quad g = 1, ..., m.
\end{aligned}
$$

One would typically select the model g that is closest to the data and provides hence the minimum value of $L_g(\overline{y}_1)$. Only the linear parameters $\theta_{L,g}$ will be estimated for this selection method such that there is no penalty on the number of model parameters as compared to the AIC.

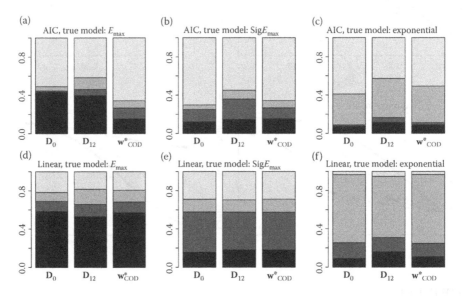

FIGURE 14.2
Interim modeling: model selection probability using the AIC (a–c) vs. L_g (d–f). Selected model from dark to bright: E_{max}, sigmoid E_{max}, exponential and quadratic.

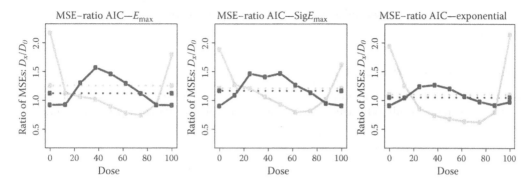

FIGURE 14.3
Estimation MSE of mean response for different doses of adaptive designs vs. fixed design.
Bright: $\mathbf{D}_{12}$ vs $\mathbf{D}_0$, dark: w^*_{COD} vs $\mathbf{D}_0$, and dotted: average MSE.

We consider in the following the three scenarios described in the introductory section for an interim analysis after 150 patients. Figure 14.2 displays the model selection probability given the true underlying E_{max}, sigmoid E_{max} and exponential scenarios with 0.15 L maximum difference in effect. The columns display the selection probability given the different designs and response scenarios. Properties of the AIC criterion are given in the upper three plots, whereas the lower plots summarize the selection using the linear criterion described above. The PoC design $\mathbf{D}_{11}$ was not studied in this example as it neither allows model discrimination nor modeling.

The quadratic model is selected frequently with the use of the AIC criterion. This model allows fitting both convex and concave shapes reasonably well. The designs $\mathbf{D}_{12}$ and w^*_{COD} reduce the selection probability of the quadratic model for the true underlying exponential model. However, generally the quadratic model is selected too often, leading to bias in the prediction. Observations at higher-dose groups support the discrimination between the quadratic, E_{max} and exponential shapes for the designs D_{12} and w^*_{COD}. Predefined candidate models for the model selection remove the penalty on the sigmoid E_{max} model. In case the true curve is close to the candidates, these predefined candidates may improve the probability to select the right model. Note, that it is recommended to take all models forward to the final analysis and to use the interim model selection only for design improvements.

Given the model selection procedure, the response may be predicted on the full dose range using the fitted models. The balanced allocation $\mathbf{D}_0$ provides the lowest average mean squared error (MSE) in the studied example for all considered dose–response scenarios (see Figure 14.3). The compound D-optimal design w^*_{COD} is best in estimating the response at placebo and the maximum dose. The MSE in the middle of the dose range is at a minimum with the use of the balanced allocation to all doses $\mathbf{D}_{12}$ in the studied example. Overall, the standard dose-finding design $\mathbf{D}_0$ and the optimal-design theory design w^*_{COD} provide a reasonable balance between modeling and effect estimation for the first stage in the considered example.

14.3 Second-Stage Design

The second-stage design takes the updated knowledge of the underlying dose–response relation into account. Shortcomings of first-stage designs may be reduced with appropriate adaptation rules for the second stage. Different adaptation rules will be presented in this section.

14.3.1   Optimal-design theory

Let the first-stage allocation proportion w_1 allow for any considered dose–response model μ_g the maximum likelihood estimation for the full parameter vector θ_g, $g = 1, ..., m$:

$$L_g(\theta_g; \overline{y}_1) = \sum_{j=1}^{k} w_{1j}(\overline{y}_{1j} - \mu_g(d_j, \theta_g))^2 \to \min_{\theta_g}.$$

$\widehat{\theta}_g$ describes the resulting parameter estimator for the response model μ_g of dimension p_g. Model weights may be calculated following the MCP-Mod approach, see Bornkamp et al. [20]:

$$\nu_{1;g} := \frac{\nu_g \times \exp(-0.5 \times (L_g(\widehat{\theta}_g; \overline{y}_1) + 2p_g))}{\sum\limits_{j=1}^{m} \nu_j \times \exp(-0.5 \times (L_j(\widehat{\theta}_j; \overline{y}_1) + 2p_g))},$$

where ν_g describes a weighting factor on the related model type that is defined prior to running the study. The compound optimality criterion Φ (e.g., D-optimality) is updated using the interim information on the model weights $\nu_{1;g}$ and parameter estimates $\widehat{\theta}_g$, as described in Bornkamp et al. [11]:

$$\Phi(w) := \sum_{g=1}^{m} \nu_{1;g} \Phi_{\mu_g;\widehat{\theta}_g}(w) = \sum_{g=1}^{m} \nu_{1;g} \Phi_{\mu_g;\widehat{\theta}_g}\left(\frac{N_1}{N} w_1 + \frac{N - N_1}{N} w_2\right).$$

Alternatively, the best fitting model might be selected for the design optimization. Selection of the best model for the design would not affect the candidate model set for the final MCP-Mod analysis in stage 2. Only the allocation weights would be optimized.

14.3.1.1   Adaptive optimal design

Standard design optimization for the total allocation w^* provides the second-stage design. The first-stage allocation enters the optimization for the total allocation as a lower bound:

$$\underline{w}_j = \frac{N_1}{N} w_{1j}, \quad j = 1, ..., k.$$

The optimized total allocation w^* hence takes already randomized first-stage patients into account. The optimal second-stage allocation is in a second step deduced from the total allocation:

$$w_{2j}^* = \frac{N w_j^* - N_1 w_{1j}}{N - N_1}, \quad j = 1, ..., k. \tag{14.5}$$

Second-stage designs not necessarily need to take the first-stage allocation into account. Locally optimal designs, given the interim parameter estimates, might also be considered as second-stage designs (e.g., [8]). Locally optimal designs may lead to a loss of efficiency for the preplanned total sample size N as compared to optimal second-stage designs w_2^*. However, in case enrollment is extended beyond the preplanned size N, these locally optimal designs may be superior to the optimal second-stage designs.

Example 14.2: Adaptive Optimal Design
Consider that 150 patients were allocated according to the design w_{COD}^* and that the following change from baseline was observed at the examined doses:

Dose	0	12.5	25	37.5	50	62.5	75	87.5	100
Response	0.03	0.02	—	0.04	—	0.07	0.16	—	0.17
Allocation	39	27	0	15	0	12	18	0	39

The pooled standard deviation is given by $0.34\,\mathrm{L}$. To reduce the selection probability of the quadratic model, we consider that model weights were chosen prior to the study as $\nu_1 = 10\%$ for the quadratic model and $\nu_j = 30\%$ for each other considered model type $j = 2, 3, 4$. Fitting candidate models to the data provides interim parameter estimates and model weights for the quadratic (14.2%), $E_{\max}$ (26.2%), exponential (40.6%), and sigmoid $E_{\max}$ (19.0%) models. The fitted curves are displayed in Figure 14.4. The updated compound D-optimal allocation proportions for a total of $N = 300$ subjects are given as follows:

$$w^* = \begin{pmatrix} 0 & 12.5 & 25 & 37.5 & 50 & 62.5 & 75 & 87.5 & 100 \\ 0.26 & 0.09 & 0.00 & 0.05 & 0.00 & 0.18 & 0.13 & 0.00 & 0.29 \end{pmatrix}.$$

Given formula (14.5), second-stage patients should be allocated according to

$$w_2^* = \begin{pmatrix} 0 & 12.5 & 25 & 37.5 & 50 & 62.5 & 75 & 87.5 & 100 \\ 0.26 & 0.00 & 0.00 & 0.00 & 0.00 & 0.27 & 0.13 & 0.00 & 0.32 \end{pmatrix}.$$

The compound optimal design for the second stage concentrates allocation on the doses with the highest increase in response, reducing the maximum uncertainty.

The second plot in Figure 14.4 compares the efficiency of locally optimal designs as a function of the total sample size. The dark dotted curve displays the efficiency of the locally compound optimal design (w^*) compared to the optimal second-stage design (w_2^*). The efficiency is high and tends to 1 as the total sample size increases. Locally optimal designs for selected dose–response models show loss in efficiency with increasing sample size. Locally optimal designs for the $E_{\max}$ model would place patients to low doses, to increase learning on the increasing part for this model. This leads to an allocation to the flat part of the observed dose–response curve in the given example. Note that the continuation with

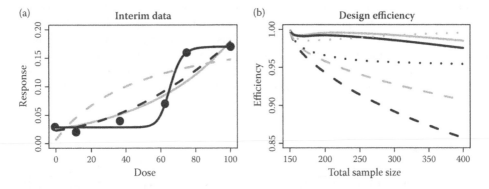

FIGURE 14.4
(a) Interim data with fitted models. (b) Design efficiency depending on total sample size. Black: SigEmax (solid) and quadratic (dashed), gray: exponential (solid) and $E_{\max}$ (dashed), and dotted: fixed (black) and locally optimal design (gray).

the fixed compound optimal starting design (w^*_{COD}, dark dotted line) is efficient for all considered sample sizes.

14.3.1.2   Optimal candidate designs

D-optimal allocation proportions are usually not applied in practice. Design theory may still support the interim decision by selecting an efficient design out of a set of predefined candidate designs. The candidate design with the minimum value of the interim optimality criterion $\Phi(w)$ is then selected for the allocation of the second-stage patients.

The selection of the most efficient design will depend on the interim model weights and parameter estimates. The model selection properties presented in the previous section underline the uncertainty in the definition of the interim optimality criterion. Instead of constructing separate candidate designs for each MCP-Mod shape, efficient designs for a combination of shapes might safeguard against design misidentifications.

Example 14.3: Optimal Candidate Designs

The considered design D_5 starts with an allocation according to w^*_{COD}. Table 14.2 displays a set of candidate designs for the second-stage allocation. Each of the candidate allocations targets a candidate response model with focused allocation to the increasing part of the underlying dose–response curve. The E_{max} design w_{M1} will allocate more patients to low doses. The design for the sigmoid E_{max} increases the learning on the medium dose range, whereas the exponential design targets the high doses. A high interim weight for the quadratic model may indicate weak interim information on the underlying dose–response relation. The proposed design w_{M4} screens the full dose range to improve the insight into the dose–response relation. The last column in Table 14.2 displays the efficiency of the candidate designs for the adaptive compound optimality criterion given the interim data from Example 14.2. Design w_{M4} would be selected for the adaptation as it leads to an efficiency of 94%.

14.3.2   Rule-based designs

General rules for the second-stage allocation that are not based on optimal-design theory may be considered for the determination of the second-stage allocation. A particular example is the best intention design that targets the allocation of patients in the second stage to the most promising dose levels. This idea is similar to the use of expansion cohorts in Phase I dose finding. The increased allocation to the promising doses shall improve information on these dose levels prior to confirmatory study initiation. This approach may be suboptimal for dose–response modeling. Second-stage designs targeting the full dose–response model instead will also provide good information on the effect at the most promising doses as the model will forward information to the doses. Given the first-stage data, one might wish to define certain design decisions based on observed response patterns to improve dose–response modeling.

TABLE 14.2

Candidate designs for $\mathbf{D}_5$ and efficiency given the data from Example 14.2.

Models	0	12.5	25	37.5	50	62.5	75	87.5	100	eff$_{COD}$ (%)
w_{M1}	0.20	0.40	0.10	—	0.10	—	—	—	0.20	85
w_{M3}	0.20	—	—	0.20	0.20	0.20	—	—	0.20	93
w_{M4}	0.20	—	0.20	—	0.20	—	0.20	—	0.20	94
w_{M5}	0.20	—	—	—	0.20	—	0.20	0.20	0.20	92

14.3.2.1 Scenario-based adaptive designs

Suppose that interim data on all active doses provide the same responses above placebo. Given such a response pattern in an interim analysis, examination of additional lower-dose groups would be of interest, to determine the increasing part of the dose–response curve. Mercier et al. [5] describe an approach to handle predefined reactions on observed patterns in a study on multiple sclerosis. The proposed approach defines candidate designs for different response patterns. In the interim analysis, the allocation rule selects the candidate pattern with maximum correlation to the observations and allocates patients accordingly.

Alternatively, one might target the distance of candidate models from the observed data. Candidate models as in MCP-Mod support the definition of response patterns, second-stage designs, and design selection rules. Note, however, that design and analysis models may be distinct. Models used for the definition of rule-based adaptation scenarios do not need to be in the candidate set for MCP-Mod and vice versa. The allocation rule for the design model with minimum squared deviation $L_g(\overline{y}_1)$ (as defined in Equation 14.4) from the observed data will typically be selected for the second stage. The definition of allocation rules for the considered models follows similar considerations as optimal candidate designs. Mercier et al. [5] try to fill the gaps in the dose–response curve by allocating the second-stage patients to doses that will help to describe the increasing part of the dose–response curve or the beginning of the plateau better. In contrast to optimal candidate designs, the selected second-stage design will not directly take efficiency considerations into account. Resulting designs may be inefficient, if not appropriately preplanned.

Example 14.4: Scenario-Based Adaptive Designs

Design $\mathbf{D}_3$ starts with the standard dose-finding allocation $\mathbf{D}_0$. After the interim analysis, patients will get randomized according to one selected candidate design. We consider the candidate designs as described in Table 14.2 and the first-stage data given in Example 14.2. The squared distances $L_g(\overline{y}_1)$ are given in the example by 3.36 and 2.40 for the two $E_{\max}$ models, 0.52 for the Sigmoid $E_{\max}$ model, 1.81 for the quadratic model, and 1.19 for the exponential model such that the allocation w_{M3} for the sigmoid $E_{\max}$ model would be selected for the next stage.

14.4 Operating Characteristics of the Designs

The theory on the efficiency of adaptive design and analysis approaches depends on asymptotic considerations. These results might be of limited accuracy for the common sample size in dose-finding studies, given the nonlinear response models. Simulations are frequently used to evaluate the operating characteristics of adaptive study designs. A selection of operating characteristics of the examined study designs will be highlighted in the following subsections. The presented results help to identify limitations and benefits of some adaptive design options and may support the fine-tuning in the planning stage of a dose-finding study. Designs were evaluated for the three response scenarios defined in the introductory section. Effect scenarios covered no effect and $0.1\,\mathrm{L}$ maximum effect for the evaluation of stopping probabilities. The maximum effect scenario of $0.15\,\mathrm{L}$ is used to study the properties of the dose estimation and response prediction.

14.4.1 Futility stopping

Futility stopping results for the $E_{\max}$ model (η_1) are summarized in Figure 14.5. The dark-colored area indicates final study success, which is defined by a positive MCP-Mod test at

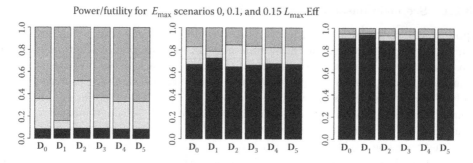

FIGURE 14.5
Dark: final success, bright: late failure, and medium: futility stop.

level 10%. The medium-colored area summarizes the percentage of studies stopped early for futility. A model-based futility stop for the targeted effect difference of $0.1\,L$ at $\alpha_0 = 25\%$ was used for the design evaluation. The area of the highest interest for the design comparison is the bright area, displaying the number of studies with failure after full study completion. Results for the sigmoid $E_{\max}$ (η_2) and exponential (η_3) scenario are very similar and will not be presented here. Design D_1 is most powerful in stopping nonworking medications early. This design is in addition most powerful in effective scenarios. The superior power of design $\mathbf{D}_1$ in establishing positive effects might be explained by the increased allocation to placebo, which increases the certainty on the response at low doses. Note that the targeted futility-stopping probability of $\alpha_0 = 25\%$ is met with design $\mathbf{D}_1$ in case of $0.1\,L$ effect change. All other designs are conservative, due to the intersection–union test. This carries forward to a decreased futility-stopping probability in the no-effect scenarios. The balanced allocation $\mathbf{D}_2$ is worst for futility stopping. The probability of failure after full study completion is given in this design with 42%. An allocation to many doses in the first design stage is hence not recommended in case there is high uncertainty on the efficacy of the compound.

14.4.2   Prediction

$E_{\max}$ curves may be fitted well using designs as $\mathbf{D}_0$. As long as the true ED_{50} in the $E_{\max}$ model is not too low, the design $\mathbf{D}_0$ will be appropriate for the modeling. The average MSE of the mean response estimation was examined over a grid of doses for the lower, middle, and upper thirds of the dose range in the three considered response scenarios. Table 14.3 displays the ratio of the average MSE for the adaptive design options and the fixed design. A value below 1 implies an improvement with the adaptive design and may be interpreted as the potential savings in sample size in comparison to the fixed design. The interesting dose range for the $E_{\max}$ scenario is given by the lower third, for the sigmoid $E_{\max}$ by the middle third and for the exponential scenario by the upper third. Any adaptation in the $E_{\max}$ scenario will potentially decrease the efficiency of the fixed design. Adaptations will improve the design $\mathbf{D}_0$ in case of a deviation from the expected efficacy onset, e.g., for a large ED_{50} as in the examined exponential model. The top-down design $\mathbf{D}_1$ is weak in the dose–response modeling across all examined scenarios. The increased allocation to placebo improves information on the low dose range, which is missing for the modeling of the dose–response in the medium and high dose range. The scenario-based design $\mathbf{D}_3$ provides a simple and efficient rule for the selection of updated allocations in the examined simulation scenarios.

TABLE 14.3

Ratio of estimation MSE of the mean response of adaptive designs vs. fixed design for the lower (L), middle (M), and upper (U) thirds of the examined dose range.

	E_{max}			Sigmoid E_{max}			Exponential		
	L	**M**	**U**	**L**	**M**	**U**	**L**	**M**	**U**
D_1	0.94	1.51	1.28	0.96	1.53	1.34	1.11	1.64	1.15
D_2	1.11	1.30	1.03	1.08	1.09	0.89	1.23	1.02	0.75
D_3	0.99	1.17	1.06	1.10	0.89	0.91	1.14	0.91	0.77
D_4	1.00	1.32	1.05	1.11	1.05	0.88	1.20	1.01	0.80
D_5	1.01	1.30	1.08	1.17	0.95	0.85	1.19	0.98	0.82

TABLE 14.4

Probability that the ED_p reaches the targeted effect range.

	E_{max}		Sigmoid E_{max}		Exponential	
	ED_{50}	ED_{90}	ED_{50}	ED_{90}	ED_{50}	ED_{90}
D_0	0.45	0.31	0.23	0.16	0.21	0.13
D_1	0.51	0.32	0.18	0.11	0.19	0.12
D_2	0.50	0.33	0.27	0.14	0.50	0.37
D_3	0.53	0.35	0.27	0.16	0.42	0.31
D_4	0.52	0.35	0.24	0.14	0.50	0.37
D_5	0.52	0.36	0.25	0.16	0.47	0.34

14.4.3 Dose estimation

The ED_{50} describes the location of the dose–response curve, whereas the ED_{90} defines the beginning of the plateau. The estimation of both doses was examined in the simulations. The probability that the estimated doses have indeed a relative effect close to the target effect was evaluated. The probability of relative effects between 25% and 75% was calculated for the estimated ED_{50}. For the ED_{90}, the range of relative effects between 85% and 95% was targeted. Table 14.4 summarizes the resulting estimation probabilities. The fixed design works relatively well in the E_{max} scenarios. An accurate estimation of the increasing part of the dose–response curve is, however, not possible for the exponential scenario. Adaptive designs improve the probability for the ED_{50} estimation in the range from 20% up to 50% for simple scenario-based adaptations. The same observation holds for the estimation of the ED_{90}.

14.4.4 Allocation

The allocation of patients to the increasing part of the response curve may be targeted to actually observe the response onset (e.g., to doses with 25–75% of the maximum effect). Observations at these doses will support the identification of the increasing part of the dose–response curve and support the dose selection for confirmatory studies. The considered fixed design D_0 misses the allocation of patients to these doses in all considered scenarios; see Table 14.5. The scenario-based adaptation (D_3) offers an intuitive way to increase allocation to these doses of interest. Designs based on optimal design theory target these doses already in the first stage of the study and will also continue allocation of second-stage patients to these doses.

TABLE 14.5

Percentage of patients in the interesting dose range.

	D_0	D_1	D_2	D_3	D_4	D_5
$E_{\max}$	0	12	13	12	16	18
Sigmoid $E_{\max}$	0	0	9	4	12	10
Exponential(%)	0	0	12	7	8	5

Adaptive design options add value in estimating the increasing part of the dose–response curve. Given the results on futility stopping, the first-stage allocation should not cover too many doses as this may limit the insight into the effect size in the interim analysis. In addition, a high number of doses will not improve modeling. It is recommended to start with a selection of doses and expand allocation to an updated set of doses after the interim analysis. On the other hand, not too few doses should be studied in the first stage. A first-stage design with only one dose and placebo might be powerful in determining the efficacy of the drug, but informed adaptations will not be possible. Complex study designs are not automatically better designs. Simple design adaptations following scenario-based allocation rules are easy to communicate to the teams and may provide significant improvements in Phase II dose finding.

14.5   Interim Timing

Interim timing defines the number of patients allocated to the first and second part of the two-stage design. Early interim analyses with small first-stage information lead to a higher uncertainty in adaptations, whereas late interim analyses decrease the number of patients allocated according to the updated design. Determination of the optimal interim timing depends on the candidate designs and on the variability of the endpoint. A bad study design is easily improved, whereas good study designs are better kept untouched.

Dette et al. [8] study the efficiency of two-stage designs depending on the interim timing using asymptotic considerations and analytical approximations to the interim uncertainty. Their idea of second-order Taylor approximations to the information matrix might also be extended to design criteria including model uncertainty, as in MCP-Mod designs. Fedorov et al. [12] examine properties of the study design depending on interim timing. Simulations may help to determine the most appropriate time for interim decision making. An example on the use of simulations for the specification of the interim timing is given in the following for the scenario-based design D_3. Simulations were programed covering interim timings after 10–90% of the total number of 300 patients. Figure 14.6 summarizes a selection of operating characteristics. It is obvious that the probability of selecting the correct working model in the interim analysis increases with increasing first-stage sample size. The increasing interim timing comes on the other hand with a decreased average number of patients on the interesting doses. Although the number of randomized patients to the interesting doses looks impressive for the $E_{\max}$ model (solid curve in Figure 14.6) with an interim analysis after 20% of the patients, the MSE is much worse as compared to the fixed design. The correct adaptation scenario gets selected in only 48% of the cases. With 18% probability, the study will continue with the allocation for the exponential model, which will add no value to the estimation of the $E_{\max}$ model.

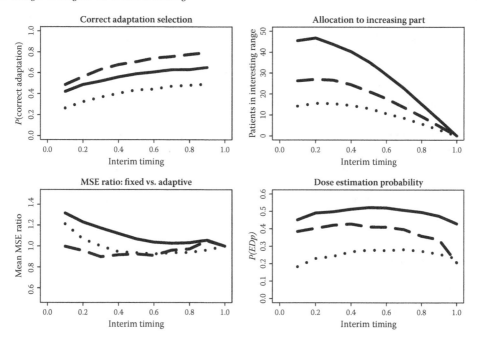

FIGURE 14.6
Design characteristics in dependence on interim timing. Solid: E_{max}, dotted: sigmoid E_{max}, dashed: exponential scenario.

The decreasing variability in the adaptation decision with increasing sample size leads to better model fits for the exponential and sigmoid E_{max} models. The lowest MSE is reached with an interim analysis after about 50% of the total study size. The accuracy of the ED_{50} estimation peaks at interim analyses after 40–60% of the patients for all considered models.

The resulting optimal proportion of first-stage patients is in the range of other published considerations on interim timing (e.g., [8, 21, 12]). Note, however, that this result will not hold for general two-stage designs in every study. The dependence of the design quality on interim timing should always be examined using a range of simulation scenarios addressing the uncertainty on the response model and effect sizes.

14.6 Discussion

Adaptive two-stage designs may increase efficiency in Phase II from several perspectives. Futility stopping and adaptive allocation rules were discussed within this chapter. Both adaptation rules help to combine the main objectives of Phase II within one study. Instead of running separate PoC and dose-finding studies, positive effects of the drug may be established, and the dose–response may be described within a single efficient study. The uncertainty on the dose–response, which might be present at the beginning of Phase II, is well addressed with potential allocation adaptations. The simulation study displayed that already simple rule-based adaptations may significantly enhance the identification of the interesting part of the dose–response curve. However, adaptive designs are not necessarily better than fixed designs. In the worst case, a good initial design might get spoiled by a suboptimal adaptation. Specially, the top-down design $\mathbf{D}_1$ is suboptimal for dose–response modeling, although this design is most powerful for futility stopping. Additional doses in the first stage of this design improve the modeling and may be used for allocation adaptations. Model-based effect estimators provide an efficient tool for futility stopping. The power of seamless PoC-dose-finding designs will hence not suffer heavily by additional doses if the dose–response model is utilized for effect estimation. Increasing the number of examined first-stage doses beyond four to five will decrease the efficiency of the PoC step, while not adding much value (if any) to the modeling. It is clear that the relation between benefit and risk of the considered adaptation rules should be well examined prior to initiating the study. Adaptation rules and simulations programs will need to be at hand during the interim analysis to review the considered rules, propose the most effective second-stage study design, and inform the relevant personal on the updated results and allocation in real time.

References

1. H. Dette, L. Haines, and L. Imhof. Maximin and Bayesian optimal designs for regression models. *Statistica Sinica*, 17:463–480, 2007.

2. H. Dette, F. Bretz, A. Pepelyshev, and J. Pinheiro. Optimal designs for dose-finding studies. *Journal of the American Statistical Association*, 103:1225–1237, 2008.

3. B. Bornkamp, F. Bretz, A. Dmitrienko, G. Enas, B. Gaydos, C. H. Hsu, F. Koenig, M. Krams, Q. Liu, B. Neuenschwander, et al. Innovative approaches for designing and analyzing adaptive dose-ranging trials (with discussion). *Statistics in Biopharmaceutical Research*, 17:965–995, 2010.

4. V. Dragalin, B. Bornkamp, F. Bretz, F. Miller, S. K. Padmanabhan, N. Patel, I. Perevozskaya, J. Pinheiro, and J. R. Smith. A simulation study to compare new adaptive dose-ranging designs. *Statistics in Biopharmaceutical Research*, 2:487–512, 2010.

5. F. Mercier, B. Bornkamp, D. Ohlssen, and E. Wallstroem. Characterization of dose–response for count data using a generalized MCP-Mod approach in an adaptive dose-ranging trial. *Pharmaceutical Statistics*, 14:359–367, 2015.

6. K. Selmaj, D. K. Li, H. P. Hartung, B. Hemmer, L. Kappos, M. S. Freedman, O. Stüve, P. Rieckmann, X. Montalban, T. Ziemssen, et al. Siponimod for patients with relapsing-remitting multiple sclerosis (BOLD): An adaptive dose-ranging, randomised, phase 2 study. *The Lancet Neurology*, 12:756–767, 2013.

7. S. K. Padmanabhan and V. Dragalin. Adaptive Dc-optimal designs for dose finding based on a continuous efficacy endpoint. *Biometrical Journal*, 52:836–852, 2010.

8. H. Dette, B. Bornkamp, and F. Bretz. On the efficiency of two-stage response-adaptive designs. *Statistics in Medicine*, 32:1646–1660, 2012.

9. J. Quinlan, B. Gaydos, J. Maca, and M. Krams. Barriers and opportunities for implementation of adaptive designs in pharmaceutical product development. *Clinical Trials*, 7:167–173, 2010.

10. V. Dragalin. Optimal design of experiments for delayed responses in clinical trials. In *mODa 10—Advances in Model-Oriented Design and Analysis*, D. Ucinski, A. C. Atkinson, M. Patan (eds), pp. 55–61. Springer, New York, 2013.

11. B. Bornkamp, F. Bretz, H. Dette, and J. Pinheiro. Response-adaptive dose-finding under model uncertainty. *Annals of Applied Statistics*, 5:1611–1631, 2011.

12. V. Fedorov, Y. Wu, and R. Zhang. Optimal dose-finding designs with correlated continuous and discrete responses. *Statistics in Medicine*, 31: 217–234, 2011.

13. F. Bretz, F. Koenig, W. Brannath, E. Glimm, and M. Posch. Adaptive designs for confirmatory clinical trials. *Statistics in Medicine*, 28:1181–1217, 2009.

14. ADDPLAN, Inc., An Aptiv Solutions Company. *ADDPLAN MC Version 6.1 User Manual*. Aptiv Solutions, Cologne, Germany, 2014.

15. J. Kiefer and J. Wolfowitz. The equivalence of two extremum problems. *Canadian Journal of Mathematics*, 12:363–366, 1960.

16. ADDPLAN, Inc., An Aptiv Solutions Company. *ADDPLAN DF—Adaptive Designs, Plans and Analysis—Dose Finding Module*. Aptiv Solutions, Cologne, Germany, 2014.

17. B. Bornkamp, J. Pinheiro, and F. Bretz. Dosefinding: Planning and analyzing dose finding experiments. *R Package Version 0.9–13*, 2015.

18. R. L. Lalonde, K. G. Kowalski, M. M. Hutmacher, W. Ewy, D. J. Nichols, P. A. Milligan, B. W. Corrigan, P. A. Lockwood, S. A. Marshall, L. J. Benincosa, et al. Model-based drug development. *Clinical Pharmacology and Therapeutics*, 82:21–32, 2007.

19. R. Berger and J. Hsu. Bioequivalence trials, intersection-union tests and equivalence confidence sets. *Statistical Science*, 11:283–319, 1996.

20. B. Bornkamp, J. Pinheiro, and F. Bretz. MCPMod: An R package for the design and analysis of dose-finding studies. *Journal of Statistical Software*, 29:1–23, 2010.

21. E. McCallum and B. Bornkamp. Accounting for parameter uncertainty in two-stage designs for phase II dose-response studies. In *Modern Adaptive Randomized Trials: Statistical and Practical Aspects*, pp. 427–450. CRC Press, Boca Raton, 2012.

15

Longitudinal Dose–Response Models

Heinz Schmidli and Markus R. Lange

Novartis Pharma AG

CONTENTS

In dose-finding clinical trials, patients are typically assessed several times during the course of the trial. Longitudinal dose–response models use data at all timepoints to describe the time-changing effect of a treatment regimen. These models are more efficient than dose–response models that focus on data at one specific timepoint. However, longitudinal dose–response models are also more complex and diverse than dose–response models. We describe here the most advanced longitudinal dose–response models, the so-called *dose–time–response models*. These have mainly been developed by pharmacologists and are closely related to pharmacokinetic/pharmacodynamic (PK/PD) models. We also discuss the value of dose–time–response models for the design of clinical trials, in particular for the choice of dosing regimens. Two applications illustrate dose–time–response models: an analysis of a dose-ranging phase II trial, and a joint analysis of three phase II/III trials. A discussion summarizes the main advantages and challenges of longitudinal dose–response modeling.

15.1   Introduction

In most dose-finding trials, patients are evaluated several times during the course of the trial. For example, in the dose-ranging study on the monoclonal antibody canakinumab, patients with gouty arthritis were assessed at baseline and at 2, 4, 8, 12, 16, 20, and 24 weeks after randomization to one of seven treatments [1]; see also Section 15.4.1. A common approach to analyze such trials is to choose a specific timepoint and then use a dose–response model to describe the effect of dose at this timepoint. However, this ignores valuable information collected at other timepoints and hence is not fully efficient. In this chapter, we describe longitudinal dose–response models that use data at all timepoints to describe the time-changing effect of a dosing regimen.

The choice of a longitudinal dose–response model depends both on the purpose of the model and on the degree of scientific understanding of the drug action. *Empirical models* may be sufficient if the main purpose is to descriptively fit the longitudinal data for the treatment regimens included in the dose-finding trial. Examples of empirical models are linear regression models with time and treatment regimen as categorical factors, or generalizations of the E_{max} model for longitudinal data [2, 3]. However, such models will often not allow reliable prediction of the effect for new treatment regimens, i.e., those not studied in the dose-finding trial. *Mechanistic models* are appropriate if the mechanism of drug action is sufficiently well understood, and prediction for new treatment regimens is important. Box and Draper [4] and Chapter 12 provide a detailed discussion of the roles of empirical and mechanistic models and note that the main advantage of mechanistic models is their ability to extrapolate and their parsimony. Mechanistic models typically used in drug development often include an empirical component, e.g., for describing the placebo effect; they are then often called semimechanistic.

The need for longitudinal dose–response models that allow us to predict the effect of a drug for untested treatment regimens is particularly evident for biologics. Biologics such as monoclonal antibodies have a long-lasting effect and hence are administered weekly to monthly. In dose-finding trials, just a few treatment regimens can be investigated, and the treatment regimen for phase III will often be different. The choice of the dosing regimen is then typically based on semimechanistic models. For example, in the development of the monoclonal antibody secukinumab for patients with psoriasis, the treatment regimen for phase III was different from the regimens studied in earlier phases and based on dose–response relationship data from four phase I–II studies [5].

We will focus in the following on longitudinal dose–response models that allow for extrapolation, namely *dose–time–response models*. These models are based on PK/PD models; however, they do not make use of drug concentration data. These semimechanistic models have been successfully used in various therapeutic areas after the initial proposal in the seminal paper by Levy [6].

In Section 15.2, we describe the most common dose–time–response models: the direct-response and the indirect-response models. Section 15.3 discusses the use of such models for the design of clinical trials. In Section 15.4, two applications illustrate clinical trial analysis with dose–time–response models. The chapter closes with a discussion of the main advantages and challenges of longitudinal dose–response modeling.

15.2   Dose–Time–Response Models

Dose–time–response models are based on PK/PD models [7]. However, in contrast to PK/PD models, dose–time–response models do not make use of pharmacokinetic (PK) data, such as drug concentration measurements in blood. They were first proposed by Levy [6], and have been further extended, in particular, by Verotta and Sheiner [8], Gabrielsson et al. [9], Jacqmin et al. [10], and Lange and Schmidli [11]. Various names have been used for dose–time–response models such as dose–response–time models, K-PD models, dose–response models with latent PK time profile, or composed models.

Initially, dose–time–response models were considered when PK measurements could not be taken or were not relevant, for example, in ophthalmology [12], asthma and COPD [13], or in pediatric studies [14]. However, dose–time–response models are also attractive in cases where PK data are available. Compared to PK/PD models, they are far simpler to use and faster to develop while still typically providing adequate predictions.

Dose–time–response models can be as diverse as the PK/PD models on which they are based. We will focus in the following on the simplest models and just consider endpoints which are normally distributed.

15.2.1 Drug concentration in the unobserved effect compartment

A drug administered to a subject is absorbed, distributed, metabolized, and excreted by the body. For mechanistic modeling of this process, the human body is considered to be divided into many compartments, such as gut, liver, kidney, brain, and so on. After a single dose of the drug is taken (e.g., as a tablet), the drug concentration in the different compartments will typically increase, reach a maximum, and then decrease. The compartment where the drug concentration is more directly related to the drug effect is called the *effect compartment*, first described by Segre [15]. The effect compartment may, for example, be interpreted as the brain for neuroscience drugs, the tumor for cancer drugs, or the skin for dermatology drugs, although this should not be taken too literally. The drug concentration in the effect compartment can typically not be measured in humans, and hence it is an unobserved latent variable [16].

Many drugs show the so-called linear pharmacokinetics. For these, the flow of the drug among the compartments can be described by a system of linear differential equations [17]. After taking a single oral dose D at time $t = 0$, the concentration $C(t)$ in the effect compartment is then a sum of exponential terms. In the simplest case, the concentration in the effect compartment is

$$C(t) = \frac{D\,\theta_1}{\theta_1 - \theta_2}\left(e^{-\theta_2 t} - e^{-\theta_1 t}\right), \tag{15.1}$$

with absorption rate θ_1 and elimination rate θ_2. As the drug concentration in the effect compartment is unobserved, it is only determined up to a scaling factor (the volume of distribution), which can be set to 1 [10].

For drugs with linear PKs, the drug concentration profile in the effect compartment for a dosing regimen of interest can easily be derived from the concentration profile of a single dose. For example, a doubling of the dose will result in a doubling of the concentration. And, for multiple doses, the single-dose concentration profiles can be superimposed, as illustrated in Figure 15.1.

The model for the unobserved drug concentration in the effect compartment contains unknown parameters. In the following, these will be indirectly estimated from response data by utilizing models that link the latent concentration in the effect compartment with the response. Two commonly used models are the *direct-response models* discussed in Section 15.2.2 and the *indirect-response models* discussed in Section 15.2.3.

15.2.2 Direct-response models

With *direct-response models*, the time-varying drug concentration in the unobserved effect compartment is directly linked to the observed drug effect, e.g., longitudinal measurements of a clinical efficacy endpoint. This relationship is quantified by a function $g(C)$ of the latent concentration C in the effect compartment. A common choice is the $E_{\max}$ model:

$$g(C(t)) = \theta_5 + \frac{\theta_4 C(t)}{\theta_3 + C(t)}, \tag{15.2}$$

where θ_5 is the expected placebo response (i.e., $C(t) = 0$), $\theta_5 + \theta_4$ is the maximal possible expected response (i.e., $C(t) \to \infty$), and θ_3 is the latent concentration for which the expected response is at half of the maximal possible effect.

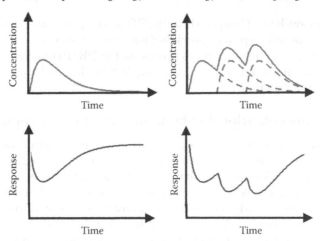

FIGURE 15.1
The upper two panels show typical time profiles of the concentration in the unobserved effect compartment for a single dose (left) and for multiple doses (right) of a drug. The time-changing concentration for multiple doses (three doses in this case) is obtained from the single-dose concentration profile (dashed lines) by superposition. The two lower panels show the corresponding longitudinal response profiles.

Suppose that longitudinal measurements of a continuous response y_{ij} are available, taken at time t_j, $j = 1, ..., J$, for patients $i = 1, ..., N$. For a patient i who receives a single drug dose D_i, the simplest model combines (15.1) and (15.2) to obtain

$$y_{ij} = \theta_5 + \frac{\theta_4 D_i(e^{-\theta_2 t_j} - e^{-\theta_1 t_j})}{\theta_3(1 - \theta_2/\theta_1) + D_i(e^{-\theta_2 t_j} - e^{-\theta_1 t_j})} + \epsilon_{ij}. \qquad (15.3)$$

Here, the residuals are assumed to be normally distributed, $\epsilon_i = (\epsilon_{i1}, ..., \epsilon_{iJ})^T \sim \mathcal{N}(0, \Sigma)$ i.i.d.

For multiple doses, the latent concentration in the effect compartment is obtained by superposition, as discussed in Section 15.2.1. Figure 15.1 shows typical time profiles for the response, based on a dose–time–response model such as (15.3).

The basic dose–time–response model can be extended in various ways, and these are discussed in more detail in Lange and Schmidli [11]. First, model (15.3) assumes a placebo effect that does not change with time; replacing θ_5 by a function of time, such as a linear trend, may be necessary in some applications. Second, the model parameters in (15.3) were assumed to be the same for all patients; using random-effects models and including baseline covariates may be more appropriate. Third, different residual error models may better describe the measurement errors.

15.2.3   Indirect-response models

Indirect-response models, also called *turnover models*, link the latent drug concentration in the effect compartment indirectly to the drug response. The basic models and various extensions are described by Gabrielsson et al. [9, 18]. With the same setting as in model (15.3), the simplest indirect-response model assumes that

$$y_{ij} = R_i(t_j) + \epsilon_{ij}, \qquad (15.4)$$

where the expected response profile $R_i(t)$ is defined through the differential equation

$$dR_i(t)/dt = \theta_6 g(C(t)) - \theta_7 R_i(t), \qquad (15.5)$$

with turnover parameters θ_6 and θ_7, and $\theta_5 = 1$. Here, as in (15.2), the $E_{\max}$ model is typically used as the function $g(C)$ of the concentration in the effect compartment. Depending on the parameters in the $E_{\max}$ model, the drug may either inhibit (decrease) or stimulate (increase) the production parameter θ_6.

Also useful is another differential equation model for the expected response profile

$$dR_i(t)/dt = \theta_6 - \theta_7 g(C(t))R_i(t). \tag{15.6}$$

Here, the drug may either inhibit (decrease) or stimulate (increase) the elimination parameter θ_7.

The choice among the different indirect-response models, as well as the direct-response models, described in Section 15.2.2 is ideally based on a good understanding of the mechanism of drug action. If this knowledge is limited, then an empirical selection of the model based on the observed longitudinal response data may be necessary.

15.2.4   Statistical inference and prediction

Longitudinal data from one or more clinical trials allow us to develop dose–time–response models, estimate model parameters, and predict outcomes. As dose–time–response models are nonlinear regression models, available general methods for inference and prediction can be used [19–22]. Both Bayesian and maximum likelihood (ML) approaches have been considered for fitting of dose–time–response models; see Lange and Schmidli [11] for a more detailed discussion.

Within a Bayesian framework, the posterior distribution of the model parameters is derived from the prior and the likelihood. If relevant historical information is available for some parameters of the dose–time–response model, the relevant information may be included as informative priors [11, 23]; this is particularly helpful for parameters that are not well identified by the data. Otherwise, weakly informative priors may be used [24]. For deriving the posterior distribution, Markov chain Monte Carlo (MCMC) methods are needed, and these generate a sample from the posterior distribution of the parameters [25]. Software programs that greatly facilitate this are WinBUGS [26], JAGS [27], Stan [28], NONMEM (Icon Development Solutions, Ellicott City, MD), and the SAS procedure MCMC (SAS Institute, Inc., Cary, NC). The direct-response models (Section 15.2.2) are typically easy to implement, whereas the indirect-response models (Section 15.2.3) are more challenging, as a numerical differential equation solver is needed such as used by RxODE [29].

ML methods provide point estimates for the model parameters with approximate confidence intervals. Although fitting dose–time–response models with ML is much faster than with Bayesian methods, the confidence intervals based on asymptotic theory may not be reliable, especially if some parameters are weakly identified by the data. The R package nlme [30], NONMEM (Icon Development Solutions, Ellicott City, MD), or the SAS procedure NLMIXED (SAS Institute, Inc., Cary, NC) may be used for ML estimation.

15.3   Clinical Trial Design Based on Dose–Time–Response Models

The outcomes of a clinical trial are influenced by two types of factors [31]: those that cannot be controlled and those that can. An example for the first type is the mechanism of drug action, comprised in the parameters θ of the dose–time–response model. Examples for the second type are design factors, such as the number of different doses or dosing regimens, the type of dosing regimens (e.g., once or twice daily), and the respective allocation of the patients to these dosing regimens. Another example is the selection of timepoints at which the patients should be observed. A particular choice of these design factors is called a design ξ.

Obviously, the design of a clinical trial has a big impact on the quality and interpretability of the final analysis. Hence, a study should be planned carefully. In current clinical practice, some of these design factors are often chosen in an *ad hoc* manner, relying on tradition, intuition, and experience. A more systematic and quantitative approach seems desirable as this may lead to more precise estimation of parameters of the dose–time–response model and to more informative clinical trials.

Clearly, there is not just one design that is best for every situation. As Sheiner [32] noted, clinical trials typically focus on either learning or confirming, and different designs are optimal in the two situations. For dose-finding trials, the learning aspect is more relevant. A good design should shed light on the functional relationship between dose and response, which directly translates to estimating the parameters of the dose–time–response model with high precision. The area in statistics that focuses on quantitative methods for the design of experiments (such as clinical trials) is called optimal design theory. Three main approaches are used for finding optimal design: *classical optimal designs, conservative Bayesian optimal designs*, and *Bayesian optimal designs*. We will briefly discuss these in connection with dose–time response models.

For *classical optimal design* approaches, it is supposed that the dose–time–response model is fitted by ML methods. The asymptotic variance–covariance matrix of the ML estimator of θ is the inverse of the Fisher information matrix (FIM) $F(\xi, \theta)$ under some mild regularity conditions [33]. Hence, a good design should yield a "large" FIM. A popular choice is to use the so-called D-optimal designs, which maximize the logarithm of the determinant $\log \det F(\xi, \theta)$ of that matrix. This increases the precision of the parameter estimator $\hat{\theta}$ as it is equivalent to minimizing the volume of the asymptotic confidence ellipsoid for $\hat{\theta}$. For nonlinear models, including dose–time–response models, the optimality of the designs depends on the true values of the parameters θ. A common approach to this problem is to work with a (hopefully) good guess $\tilde{\theta}$, which leads to a locally D-optimal design. This is critical, as using a bad guess can lead to very inefficient designs. For a detailed discussion of optimal designs for nonlinear models, we refer to Ref. [33]. Fang et al. [34] considered the models in Section 15.2.2 and provide locally D-optimal designs regarding the optimal choice of the observation times. In an attempt to make them more robust toward parameter misspecification, they consider adding one or more observation times to a locally D-optimal design. Dette et al. [35] also consider the optimal choice of observation times for dose–time–response models and provide a fully analytical solution to this problem. In order to decrease the dependency on the model parameters, they consider maximin optimal designs, which maximize the minimal efficiency of the estimates across a candidate set of parameter values. Lange and Schmidli [36] discuss locally D-optimal designs for dose–time–response models with respect to the choice of doses.

For *conservative Bayesian optimal design* methods, it is again supposed that the dose–time–response model is analyzed by ML. However, in order to obtain more robust designs, a prior distribution $p(\theta)$ is used instead of a best guess $\tilde{\theta}$ [37]. Hence, rather than just optimizing $\log \det F(\xi, \tilde{\theta})$, conservative Bayesian D-optimal designs optimize $\int \log \det F(\xi, \theta) p(\theta) d\theta$. Conservative Bayesian designs perform well on average over a set of parameters where the importance of different parameter values is described by the prior distribution. Lange and Schmidli [36] consider conservative Bayesian designs for the optimal selection of the dosing regimens, and they also discuss algorithms for the implementation.

For *Bayesian optimal design*, it is supposed that the clinical trial data are analyzed by Bayesian methods. To obtain a good design, the expected gain of information in the experiment is maximized, i.e., the expected difference between what we know after the experiment and what we already knew before [38]. This can be quantified by the expected Kullback-Leibler divergence between prior and posterior distributions of the model parameters, i.e., $\int \log \frac{p(\theta|y,\xi)}{p(\theta)} p(y,\theta|\xi) d\theta dy$. An advantage of this approach is the fact that it does not rely on any asymptotics. A disadvantage of Bayesian optimal designs is that computations can be very demanding. However, with increasing computer power and the possibility to parallelize calculations, Bayesian optimal designs have become feasible [39, 40].

15.4 Applications

In this section, we illustrate that parsimonious dose–time–response models are able to describe time-changing drug effects for various treatment regimens. We show this for two cases: first, for a dose-finding clinical trial, where both single and multiple doses of a drug were investigated; and second, for three phase II/III trials, which compared various very diverse drug regimens.

15.4.1 Dose-finding trial in patients with gout

We consider here the analysis of a dose-finding clinical trial for the monoclonal antibody canakinumab in patients with acute gouty arthritis, a painful inflammatory disease. The phase II trial lasted 24 weeks, and the participating patients were randomized to one of seven treatment groups [1]. More precisely, five groups received a single subcutaneous injection of canakinumab (25, 50, 100, 200, or 300 mg, respectively), and one group received multiple injections of canakinumab (50 mg at baseline and at week 4, and then 25 mg at weeks 8 and 12). The last group received an active comparator on a daily basis; we will ignore this treatment arm in the following. About 50 patients were randomized to each of the six canakinumab groups. An important endpoint in the study was the C-reactive protein (CRP) level, which can be considered as an indicator of the severity of the disease. Measurements of CRP were taken at baseline, week 2, week 4, and then every 4 weeks. For the analysis, the logarithm of CRP values was used.

For the Bayesian analysis, we fitted the model described in (15.3) to the data from the clinical trial; see Lange and Schmidli [11] for more details. Figure 15.2 shows that the simple dose–time–response model well describes the response after single or multiple doses of canakinumab.

15.4.2 Phase II/III trials in patients with urticaria

We discuss here the joint modeling of three randomized phase II/III trials that studied various treatment regimens for the monoclonal antibody omalizumab in patients with urticaria. Each trial lasted at least 28 weeks. Urticaria is a painful inflammatory disease which is more commonly referred to as hives.

In trial I [41], patients received placebo or six subcutaneous injections of omalizumab at weeks 0, 4, 8, 12, 16, and 20, with doses of either 75, 150, or 300 mg. Each of the four treatment groups consisted of about 80 patients. In trial II [42], patients received placebo or three subcutaneous injections of omalizumab at weeks 0, 4, and 12, again with doses of 75, 150, or 300 mg. About 80 patients were recruited in each of the four groups. Finally, trial III [43] only had two different treatment groups. The first group consisted of about 250 patients, and they received six subcutaneous injections of 300 mg omalizumab. The second group of 80 patients received placebo. An important clinical endpoint in all three studies

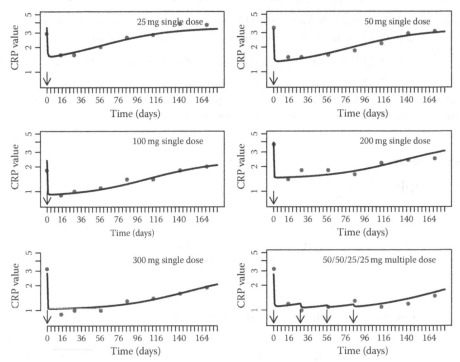

FIGURE 15.2
Bayesian dose–time–response modeling of a clinical trial in patients with gout. Each panel summarizes results for one treatment arm, where arrows indicate the drug injection times. Shown are mean CRP values (dots) and the median of the posterior distribution for the expected time profile (solid line).

was the itch severity score, which ranges from 0 to 21 and indicates how itchy (and thus how sick) a patient has been over the past week; it was measured each week.

For the analysis, we pooled the published summary data from all three trials [41–43], using the dose–time–response model (15.3), however, with a nonconstant placebo model, i.e., replacing θ_5 by $\theta_5 + \theta_6 \left(e^{-\theta_7 t} - 1\right) + \theta_8 t$. Figure 15.3 summarizes the results of a Bayesian analysis with vague priors. This illustrates that a simple dose–time–response model with a few parameters can well describe the main features of the drug effect for diverse treatment regimens.

15.5   Discussion

In a dose-finding clinical trial, numerous measurements on efficacy, safety, biomarkers, PKs, etc. are taken during the course of the trial. Integrating all these data into a joint model is not realistic. The desire to make use of relevant available data has to be balanced against the complexity of the models, the resources available, and the time needed.

Dose–response models at one timepoint are the simplest models. These models are well understood and also fast to fit and diagnose. They may be sufficient to answer key questions, especially if treatment effects do not much change with time, and no extrapolation for untested treatment regimens is needed.

Dose–time–response models can often provide more precise, reliable, and useful information than dose–response models, especially if the effect of a drug is time-changing or

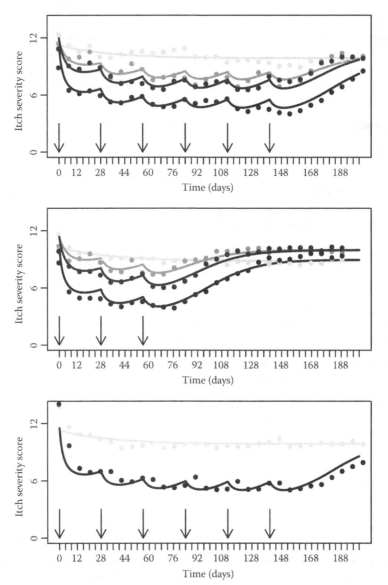

FIGURE 15.3
Joint Bayesian dose–time–response modeling of three clinical trials in patients with urticaria. Each panel summarizes results for one study, where the arrows indicate the drug injection times, and the brightness indicates the magnitude of the administered dose, ranging from placebo (light grey) to 300 mg (black). Shown are mean itch severity scores (dots) and the median of the posterior distribution for the expected time profiles (solid line).

if the variability in the data makes it difficult to discriminate between doses [11]. Dose–time–response models are also essential for biologic drugs such as monoclonal antibodies to understand and predict the time-changing effect of various regimens. Although dose–time–response models are more complex than dose–response models, model fitting and diagnosis do not need much more effort than for dose–response models.

PK/PD models allow us to also integrate drug concentration data. However, as drug concentrations can typically only be measured in the blood compartment, rather than in the more relevant latent effect compartment, a model to link the compartments is required. Building and evaluating such models are considerably more difficult and time-consuming, and PK/PD models are also more challenging to communicate. However, these models can provide a more detailed scientific understanding of the drug effect as they are able to describe the time-changing dose–exposure–response relationship.

References

1. N. Schlesinger, E. Mysler, H.-Y. Lin, M. De Meulemeester, J. Rovensky, U. Arulmani, A. Balfour, G. Krammer, P. Sallstig, and A. So. Canakinumab reduces the risk of acute gouty arthritis flares during initiation of allopurinol treatment: Results of a double-blind, randomised study. *Annals of the Rheumatic Diseases*, 70(7):1264–1271, 2011.

2. H. Tan, D. Gruben, J. French, and N. Thomas. A case study of model-based Bayesian dose response estimation. *Statistics in Medicine*, 30(21):2622–2633, 2011.

3. G. D. Schmith, R. Singh, R. Gomeni, O. Graff, A. G. Hamedani, J. S. Troughton, and S. M. Learned. Use of longitudinal dose–response modeling to support the efficacy and tolerability of alitretinoin in severe refractory chronic hand eczema (CHE). *CPT: Pharmacometrics & Systems Pharmacology*, 4(4):255–262, 2015.

4. G. E. P. Box and N. R. Draper. *Empirical Model-Building and Response Surfaces*. John Wiley & Sons, New York, 1987.

5. R. G. Langley, B. E. Elewski, M. Lebwohl, K. Reich, C. E. M. Griffiths, K. Papp, L. Puig, H. Nakagawa, L. Spelman, B. Sigurgeirsson, et al. Secukinumab in plaque psoriasis—Results of two phase 3 trials. *New England Journal of Medicine*, 371(4):326–338, 2014.

6. G. Levy. Kinetics of pharmacological effects. *Clinical Pharmacology & Therapeutics*, 7(3):362–363, 1966.

7. J. Gabrielsson and D. Weiner. *Pharmacokinetic and Pharmacodynamic Data Analysis: Concepts and Applications*, 3rd edn. CRC Press, Boca Raton, FL, 2001.

8. D. Verotta and L. B. Sheiner. Semiparametric analysis of non-steady-state pharmacodynamic data. *Journal of Pharmacokinetics and Biopharmaceutics*, 19(6):691–712, 1991.

9. J. Gabrielsson, W. J. Jusko, and L. Alari. Modeling of dose–response-time data: Four examples of estimating the turnover parameters and generating kinetic functions from response profiles. *Biopharmaceutics & Drug Disposition*, 21(2):41–52, 2000.

10. P. Jacqmin, E. Snoeck, E. A. van Schaick, R. Gieschke, P. Pillai, J.-L. Steimer, and P. Girard. Modelling response time profiles in the absence of drug concentrations: Definition and performance evaluation of the K-PD model. *Journal of Pharmacokinetics and Pharmacodynamics*, 34(1):57–85, 2007.

11. M. R. Lange and H. Schmidli. Analysis of clinical trials with biologics using dose–time–response models. *Statistics in Medicine*, 34(22):3017–3028, 2015.

12. F. G. Holz, J.-F. Korobelnik, P. Lanzetta, P. Mitchell, U. Schmidt-Erfurth, S. Wolf, S. Markabi, H. Schmidli, and A. Weichselberger. The effects of a flexible visual acuity-driven ranibizumab treatment regimen in age-related macular degeneration: Outcomes

of a drug and disease model. *Investigative Ophthalmology & Visual Science*, 51(1):405–412, 2010.

13. K. Wu, M. Looby, G. Pillai, G. Pinault, A. F. Drollman, and S. Pascoe. Population pharmacodynamic model of the longitudinal FEV1 response to an inhaled long-acting anti-muscarinic in COPD patients. *Journal of Pharmacokinetics and Pharmacodynamics*, 38(1):105–119, 2011.

14. M. Tod. Evaluation of drugs in pediatrics using K-PD models: Perspectives. *Fundamental & Clinical Pharmacology*, 22(6):589–594, 2008.

15. G. Segre. Kinetics of interaction between drugs and biological systems. *Farmaco-Edizione Scientifica*, 23(10):907–918, 1968.

16. T. Jacobs, R. Straetemans, G. Molenberghs, J. A. Bouwknecht, and L. Bijnens. A latent pharmacokinetic time profile to model dose-response survival data. *Journal of Biopharmaceutical Statistics*, 20(4):759–767, 2010.

17. M. Gibaldi and D. Perrier. *Pharmacokinetics*. CRC Press, Boca Raton, FL, 1982.

18. J. Gabrielsson and L. A. Peletier. Dose-response-time data analysis involving nonlinear dynamics, feedback and delay. *European Journal of Pharmaceutical Sciences*, 59:36–48, 2014.

19. D. M. Bates and D. G. Watts. *Nonlinear Regression: Iterative Estimation and Linear Approximations*. John Wiley & Sons, New York, 1988.

20. M. Davidian and D. M. Giltinan. *Nonlinear Models for Repeated Measurement Data*. CRC Press, Boca Raton, FL, 1995.

21. J. Pinheiro and D. Bates. *Mixed-Effects Models in S and S-PLUS*. Statistics and Computing. Springer, New York, 2000.

22. G. A. F. Seber and C. J. Wild. *Nonlinear Regression*. John Wiley & Sons, New York, 1989.

23. H. Schmidli, S. Gsteiger, S. Roychoudhury, A. O'Hagan, D. Spiegelhalter, and B. Neuenschwander. Robust meta-analytic-predictive priors in clinical trials with historical control information. *Biometrics*, 70(4):1023–1032, 2014.

24. B. Bornkamp. Functional uniform priors for nonlinear modeling. *Biometrics*, 68(3):893–901, 2012.

25. A. Gelman, J. B. Carlin, H. S. Stern, D. B. Dunson, A. Vehtari, and D. B. Rubin. *Bayesian Data Analysis*. Chapman & Hall, New York, 2014.

26. D. Lunn, C. Jackson, N. Best, A. Thomas, and D. Spiegelhalter. *The BUGS Book: A Practical Introduction to Bayesian Analysis*. Chapman & Hall/CRC Texts in Statistical Science. CRC Press, Baco Raton, FL, 2012.

27. M. Plummer. JAGS: A program for analysis of Bayesian graphical models using Gibbs sampling. In *Proceedings of the 3rd International Workshop on Distributed Statistical Computing*, Vol. 124, p. 125. Technical University Vienna, Austria, 2003.

28. A. Gelman, D. Lee, and J. Guo. Stan: A probabilistic programming language for Bayesian inference and optimization. *Journal of Educational and Behavioral Statistics*, 40(5):530–543, 2015.

29. W. Wang, K. M. Hallow, and D. A. James. A tutorial on RxODE: Simulating differential equation pharmacometric models in R. *CPT: Pharmacometrics & Systems Pharmacology*, 2015.

30. J. Pinheiro, D. Bates, S. DebRoy, D. Sarkar, and R Core Team. *nlme: Linear and Nonlinear Mixed Effects Models*, R Package Version 3.1-123, 2016.

31. S. D. Silvey. *Optimal Design*. Chapman & Hall, New York, 1980.

32. L. B. Sheiner. Learning versus confirming in clinical drug development. *Clinical Pharmacology & Therapeutics*, 61(3):275–291, 1997.

33. V. V. Fedorov and S. L. Leonov. *Optimal Design for Nonlinear Response Models*. CRC Press, Boca Raton, FL, 2013.

34. X. Fang and A. S. Hedayat. Locally D-optimal designs based on a class of composed models resulted from blending $E_{\max}$ and one-compartment models. *The Annals of Statistics*, 36(1):428–444, 2008.

35. H. Dette, A. Pepelyshev, and W. K. Wong. Optimal designs for composed models in pharmacokinetic–pharmacodynamic experiments. *Journal of Pharmacokinetics and Pharmacodynamics*, 39(3):295–311, 2012.

36. M. R. Lange and H. Schmidli. Optimal design of clinical trials with biologics using dose–time–response models. *Statistics in Medicine*, 33(30):5249–5264, 2014.

37. K. Chaloner and I. Verdinelli. Bayesian experimental design: A review. *Statistical Science*, 10(3):273–304, 1995.

38. D. V. Lindley. On a measure of the information provided by an experiment. *The Annals of Mathematical Statistics*, 26:986–1005, 1956.

39. E. G. Ryan, C. C. Drovandi, M. H. Thompson, and A. N. Pettitt. Towards Bayesian experimental design for nonlinear models that require a large number of sampling times. *Computational Statistics & Data Analysis*, 70:45–60, 2014.

40. E. G. Ryan, C. C. Drovandi, J. M. McGree, and A. N. Pettitt. A review of modern computational algorithms for bayesian optimal design. *International Statistical Review*, 84:128–154, 2015.

41. S. S. Saini, C. Bindslev-Jensen, M. Maurer, J.-J. Grob, E. B. Baskan, M. S. Bradley, J. Canvin, A. Rahmaoui, P. Georgiou, O. Alpan, et al. Efficacy and safety of omalizumab in patients with chronic idiopathic/spontaneous urticaria who remain symptomatic on H 1 antihistamines: A randomized, placebo-controlled study. *Journal of Investigative Dermatology*, 135(1):67–75, 2015.

42. M. Maurer, K. Rosén, H.-J. Hsieh, S. Saini, C. Grattan, A. Giménez-Arnau, S. Agarwal, R. Doyle, J. Canvin, A. Kaplan, et al. Omalizumab for the treatment of chronic idiopathic or spontaneous urticaria. *New England Journal of Medicine*, 368(10):924–935, 2013.

43. A. Kaplan, D. Ledford, M. Ashby, J. Canvin, J. L. Zazzali, E. Conner, J. Veith, N. Kamath, P. Staubach, T. Jakob, et al. Omalizumab in patients with symptomatic chronic idiopathic/spontaneous urticaria despite standard combination therapy. *Journal of Allergy and Clinical Immunology*, 132(1):101–109, 2013.

16

Multiple Test Strategies for Comparing Several Doses with a Control in Confirmatory Trials

Frank Bretz and Bjorn Bornkamp

Novartis Pharma AG

Franz König

Medical University of Vienna

CONTENTS

16.1 Introduction

The focus in the previous chapters has been on dose–response curve estimation in Phase II clinical trials. In this chapter, we focus on confirmatory clinical trials (Phase III trials), with emphasis on statistical testing rather than estimation.

When comparing several doses with a control, regulatory guidance mandates overall type I error rate control across all comparisons [1, 2]. That is, the maximum probability of rejecting any true null hypothesis is bounded by a pre-specified significance level α. If no adjustments are made to the testing strategy, the overall type I error rate will be inflated when more than one test is performed. As the number of tests increases, the inflation will be more pronounced.

In this chapter, we focus on the general concepts behind multiplicity in the context of confirmatory trials that compare several doses with a control. We introduce basic techniques to correct for multiplicity and describe their relative merits.

16.2   Methodology

16.2.1   Error rates

Consider the problem of comparing k active dose levels with placebo, resulting in k null hypotheses $H_1, \ldots, H_k$ that dose i is not better than placebo, $i = 1, \ldots, k$. Multiple test strategies aim at controlling the overall type I error rate for the entire set of hypotheses $\{H_1, \ldots, H_k\}$. A common error rate is the family-wise error rate (FWER), defined as the probability of rejecting at least one true null hypothesis [3]. Furthermore, the FWER is said to be controlled in the weak sense if FWER $\leq \alpha$ under the global null hypothesis $H = H_1 \cap \ldots \cap H_k$, that is, if all k null hypotheses are true. However, weak control is often not sufficient as it requires that none of the k doses be better than placebo. In practice, one is interested in controlling the FWER in the strong sense, that is, FWER $\leq \alpha$ under any configuration of true/false null hypotheses.

As an example, if a study compares $k = 4$ different doses with placebo, then a procedure controlling the FWER in the weak sense would only protect the type I error rate if the drug had no effect on any of the four doses. However, it would not protect the FWER if one or more doses had an effect. If the FWER were protected in the strong sense, then the probability of incorrectly concluding a dose had an effect would be less than α, no matter how many doses did or did not have an effect. All methods described in this chapter control the FWER in the strong sense.

16.2.2   Common multiple test procedures

Multiple test procedures can generally be divided into two categories: single-step tests and stepwise test procedures. Single-step procedures are characterized by the fact that the rejection or nonrejection of a null hypothesis does not take the decisions for any other hypothesis into account. Examples of single-step procedures include the tests by Bonferroni and Simes. In contrast, for stepwise procedures, the rejection or nonrejection of a null hypothesis may depend on the decision of other hypotheses. Examples of stepwise test procedures include the test procedures by Holm and Hochberg, which are stepwise extensions of the single-step procedures by Bonferroni and Simes, as we will see later. Stepwise test procedures are typically constructed using the closed test procedures described in Section 16.2.3. As seen later, they are more powerful in their construction than their respective single-step tests in the sense that any hypothesis rejected by the latter procedure will also be rejected by the former.

The aforementioned approaches have in common that they are based on the p-values derived from the marginal test statistics and are thus easy to perform and universally applicable with only minimal requirements. In contrast, the Dunnett test and its stepwise extensions fully exploit the correlation between the m pairwise dose–control comparisons. In the following, we introduce the common multiple test procedures mentioned above. All of the above procedures are implemented with the `multcomp` package in R [4]. Using the closed testing framework, we describe in addition the fixed-sequence test, which is often used in dose–response studies.

16.2.2.1   Bonferroni test and its stepwise extension by Holm

The simplest method for controlling the FWER is the Bonferroni test, which divides the significance level equally among all of the hypothesis tests. For example, if there are $k = 4$ tests to be performed at an overall level $\alpha = 0.05$, then each of the four tests would be conducted using the adjusted significance level $0.05/4 = 0.0125$. Although it is the simplest adjustment to make, it is also a very conservative adjustment, since it is applicable irrespective of the correlation between the test statistics.

The stepwise extension due to Holm [5] is more powerful than the single-step Bonferroni test as it allows the nonrejected hypotheses to be tested at a higher significance level once other hypotheses have already been rejected. Thus, once a hypothesis has been rejected, it is removed from the set of hypotheses to be tested, and the Bonferroni test is performed on the remaining tests. In the example above, if one hypothesis, say H_1, is rejected at the Bonferroni adjusted level of 0.0125, then the remaining three hypotheses, H_2, H_3, and H_4, could now be tested at level $0.05/3 = 0.0167$. In general, for hypotheses $H_{(1)}, H_{(2)}, \ldots, H_{(k)}$ associated with the ordered p-values $p_{(1)} \leq p_{(2)} \leq \cdots \leq p_{(k)}$, the Holm procedure is implemented as follows:

- If $p_{(1)} \leq \alpha/k$, then reject $H_{(1)}$ and continue, otherwise stop;

- If $p_{(2)} \leq \alpha/(k-1)$, then reject $H_{(2)}$ and continue, otherwise stop;

  ...

- If $p_{(k)} \leq \alpha$, then reject $H_{(k)}$.

Thus, the procedure keeps on testing further hypotheses at increased levels as long as a hypothesis in the sequence given by the ordered p-values cannot be rejected. All remaining null hypotheses have to be retained. Clearly, the Holm procedure is more powerful than the Bonferroni test as it uses the Bonferroni adjusted significance level α/k only at its first step.

16.2.2.2   Simes test and its stepwise extension by Hochberg

Simes [6] proposed a test for the global null hypothesis $H = H_1 \cap \ldots \cap H_k$, which is more powerful than the respective global test by Bonferroni. For the Simes test, let $p_{(1)} \leq \cdots \leq p_{(k)}$ denote again k individual p-values ordered by magnitude from smallest to largest. Then, the global null hypothesis H is rejected if $p_{(j)} \leq j\alpha/k$ for at least one $j \in \{1, \ldots, k\}$. Consider as an example the case $k = 2$, and let p_1 and p_2 denote the individual p-values for testing H_1 and H_2, respectively. Then, the Bonferroni test rejects $H = H_1 \cap H_2$ if $p_1 \leq \alpha/2$ or $p_2 \leq \alpha/2$. In contrast, the Simes test rejects H if $p_{(1)} \leq \alpha/2$ or $p_{(2)} \leq \alpha$. This illustrates that the Simes test is more powerful than the Bonferroni test as it uses larger adjusted significance levels. Note that FWER is only controlled when the test statistics satisfy a certain positive dependency, which, however, is the case in comparing several doses with a control; see, for example, Ref. [7] and the references therein.

Note that the Simes method tests only the global null hypothesis H without providing a conclusion about the individual null hypotheses $H_1, \ldots, H_k$. This can be achieved by using its stepwise extension described by Hochberg [8]. This procedure uses the same adjusted significance levels as the Holm procedure, but in a reverse order. To implement the Hochberg procedure, the following sequential procedure can be used:

- If $p_{(k)} \leq \alpha$, then reject $H_{(1)}, \ldots, H_{(k)}$ and stop, otherwise continue;

- If $p_{(k-1)} \leq \alpha/2$, then reject $H_{(1)}, \ldots, H_{(k-1)}$ and stop, otherwise continue;

  ...

- If $p_{(1)} \leq \alpha/k$, then reject $H_{(1)}$.

Consider as an example the case $k = 2$ and let $p_{(1)} \leq p_{(2)}$ denote the ordered individual p-values. Then, the Holm procedure rejects $H_{(1)}$ if $p_{(1)} \leq \alpha/2$ and rejects $H_{(2)}$ if $p_{(1)} \leq \alpha/2$

and $p_{(2)} \leq \alpha$. In contrast, the Hochberg procedure rejects $H_{(1)}$ if $p_{(1)} \leq \alpha/2$ and rejects $H_{(2)}$ if $p_{(2)} \leq \alpha$. This illustrates that the Hochberg procedure is more powerful than the Holm procedure. Note, however, that the Hochberg procedure shares the same limitation as the Simes test in that it controls the FWER only when the test statistics satisfy a certain positive dependency.

16.2.2.3   Dunnett test and its stepwise extension

If the correlation between the test statistics is known, as is typically the case when comparing several doses with a control, the single-step Dunnett test can be used [9]. The respective adjusted significance levels are slightly larger than those of the Bonferroni test as they exploit the correlation structure. Let

$$y_{ij} = \mu_i + \varepsilon_{ij} \tag{16.1}$$

denote the jth observation in treatment group i, $j = 1, \dots, n_i$, where n_i denotes the sample size of group i, μ_i the mean effect of treatment group $i = 0, \dots, k$, and $\varepsilon_{ij} \sim N(0, \sigma^2)$ the independent and identically distributed error terms. Note that $i = 0$ denotes the placebo group with which the k dose levels are compared. Let further

$$t_i = \frac{\bar{y}_i - \bar{y}_0}{s\sqrt{\frac{1}{n_i} + \frac{1}{n_0}}}$$

denote the t test for the null hypothesis H_i, $i = 1, \dots, k$, where $\bar{y}_i = \sum_{j=1}^{n_i} y_{ij}/n_i$ denotes the arithmetic mean of group $i = 0, \dots, k$ and $s^2 = \sum_{i=0}^{k} \sum_{j=1}^{n_i} (y_{ij} - \bar{y}_i)^2/\nu$ the pooled variance estimate with $\nu = \sum_{i=0}^{k} n_i - (k+1)$ degrees of freedom.

Each test statistic t_i is univariate t distributed. The vector of test statistics $(t_1, \dots, t_k)$ follows an m-variate t distribution with ν degrees of freedom and correlation matrix $R = (\rho_{ij})_{ij}$, where for $i \neq j$,

$$\rho_{ij} = \sqrt{\frac{n_i}{n_i + n_0}} \sqrt{\frac{n_j}{n_j + n_0}}, \quad i, j = 1, \dots, k.$$

In the balanced case, $n_0 = n_1 = \cdots = n_k$, and the correlations are constant, $\rho_{ij} = 0.5$ for all $i \neq j$. Multidimensional integration routines [10] can be used to calculate the adjusted significance levels.

The single-step Dunnett test described above can be improved by using a stepwise extension in a very similar way as the Holm procedure improves the Bonferroni test. Recall from Section 16.2.2.1 that the Holm procedure repeatedly applies the Bonferroni test. However, because the Bonferroni test does not account for the correlations between the test statistics, the Holm procedure can be improved as follows. Let $t_{(1)} \geq t_{(2)} \geq \cdots \geq t_{(k)}$ denote the ordered test statistics associated with the hypotheses $H_{(1)}, H_{(2)}, \dots, H_{(k)}$. The stepwise Dunnett procedure (subsequently called "step-down Dunnett") is implemented as follows:

- If $t_{(1)} \geq c_{k,1-\alpha}$, then reject $H_{(1)}$ and continue, otherwise stop;

- If $t_{(2)} \geq c_{k-1,1-\alpha}$, then reject $H_{(2)}$ and continue, otherwise stop;

  ...

- If $t_{(k)} \geq c_{1,1-\alpha}$, then reject $H_{(k)}$.

In the algorithm above, $c_{i,1-\alpha}$ denotes the $1 - \alpha$ quantile of the distribution of the maximum of i t-distributed random variables for $i = k, \dots, 1$, and is computed from the corresponding multivariate t distribution.

16.2.2.4   Fixed-sequence test

If the hypotheses are ordered *a priori*, based on their relative importance or expected treatment effect, they can be tested using a fixed-sequence test [11]. For example, if the k null hypotheses $H_1, \ldots, H_k$ denote the pairwise comparisons of the k active dose levels with placebo, it is reasonable to assume that the effect at the highest dose (indexed by k) is higher than for the next lower dose (indexed by $k - 1$), and so on. The fixed-sequence test then tests H_i at full level α as long as all previous hypotheses $H_k, \ldots, H_{i+1}$ are rejected and testing stops with the first nonsignificant result. Formally, it is implemented as follows:

- If $p_k \leq \alpha$, then reject H_k and continue, otherwise stop;

- If $p_{k-1} \leq \alpha$, then reject H_{k-1} and continue, otherwise stop;

    ...

- If $p_1 \leq \alpha$, then reject H_1.

The fixed-sequence approach has the advantage of being simple, and it controls the FWER in the strong sense. The approach is optimal when early tests in the sequence have the largest treatment effect and performs poorly when this assumption is violated [12]. Note that the hypotheses sequence has to be determined at the trial design stage, in contrast to the stepwise procedures by Holm, Hochberg, and Dunnett, which rely on data-driven ordering of the tests.

16.2.3   Closed test procedures

The closed test procedure [13] is a key principle for constructing multiple test procedures. In fact, all of the stepwise test procedures described above can be formally derived using a suitable closed test procedure. In a nutshell, it allows one to reject a single null hypothesis by looking at every possible intersection of that hypothesis with any other available hypotheses. If all intersection hypotheses can be rejected at level α, then the original elementary hypothesis can also be rejected at the same level α, with the FWER being maintained in the strong sense.

Consider as an example the case of testing three elementary null hypotheses H_1, H_2, and H_3 (Figure 16.1). According to the closed test procedure, we construct all intersection hypotheses $H_I = \bigcap_{i \in I} H_i$, $I \subseteq \{1, 2, 3\}$, $i = 1, 2, 3$. For every intersection hypothesis H_I, we

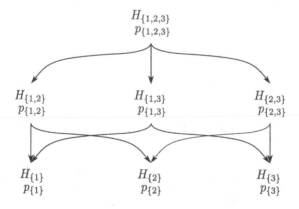

FIGURE 16.1

Closed testing principle for three elementary hypotheses H_1, H_2, and H_3.

obtain the corresponding p-value p_I using a suitable α-level test. An individual hypothesis is then rejected if all intersection hypotheses contained therein are rejected. For example, H_1 is rejected only if all intersection hypotheses $H_{\{1,2,3\}}, H_{\{1,2\}}$, and $H_{\{1,3\}}$ and the individual hypothesis $H_{\{1\}} = H_1$ itself are rejected by their α-level tests.

Note that the choice of how to test the intersection hypotheses is free. Consider the case of testing two hypotheses, H_1 and H_2, and assume that we use the Bonferroni test for $H = H_1 \cap H_2$. Then, we can reject H if $p_1 \leq \alpha/2$ or $p_2 \leq \alpha/2$. Assume that $p_1 \leq \alpha/2$. Then, $p_1 \leq \alpha$ as well, and we can immediately reject H_1. What remains is to test H_2, and we reject it if $p_2 \leq \alpha$. The analogous procedure applies if at the first step we reject H because $p_2 \leq \alpha/2$. In summary, this closed Bonferroni procedure rejects $H_{(1)}$ if the smaller p-value $p_{(1)} \leq \alpha/2$ and rejects $H_{(2)}$ if $p_{(1)} \leq \alpha/2$ and $p_{(2)} \leq \alpha$, which in turn is exactly the Holm procedure described in Section 16.2.2.1. Similarly it is shown that for $k = 2$, the Hochberg procedure is a closed Simes test (for $k > 2$, it is conservative and can be improved using the Hommel procedure [14]). The step-down Dunnett test is a closed version of the single-step Dunnett test (for any value of k), while the fixed-sequence test is a closed version of the weighted Bonferroni test.

16.2.4 Closed MCP-Mod

The standard MCP-Mod approach described in Chapter 12 only allows testing for a dose–response trend, but it does not make statements about the individual dose–control comparisons. In this section, we describe an extension of the MCP-Mod approach using the closed test procedure, which does allow such individual statements. We describe this closed MCP-Mod approach for a single, normally distributed endpoint following Section 12.1 in Chapter 12, although extensions to general general parametric models following Section 12.2 are possible.

Based on the closed test principle, for each intersection hypothesis, we need to define a suitable α-level test. We propose to use the MCP-Mod contrast test for testing every individual intersection hypothesis. Instead of using all doses, we use only those doses that are part of the intersection hypothesis. For testing every intersection hypothesis, we use the same set of predefined models, but recalculating optimal contrasts based on the set of doses. Of course, for the elementary hypotheses, all contrasts reduce to pairwise comparisons. The closed MCP-Mod procedure is defined then as follows:

1. Let $H_1, \dots, H_k$ denote the k hypotheses for the pairwise dose–control comparisons.

2. Construct all intersection hypotheses $H_I = \bigcap_{i \in I} H_i$, $I \subseteq \{1, \dots, k\}$.

3. Define a set $\mathcal{M}$ of prespecified candidate models to be used for testing every intersection hypothesis H_I.

4. Test every intersection hypothesis H_I using MCP-Mod contrast tests by recalculating anew the optimal contrasts for each H_I and model, based on the doses d_j, where $j \in J$, $J = 0 \cup I$, and d_0 denotes placebo.

5. Reject an elementary hypothesis H_i if all hypotheses H_I with $i \in I$ are rejected by their α-level test.

In other words, within each intersection hypothesis H_I, a multiple-contrast test is performed. The single-contrast test for detecting the mth model shape only uses data of doses d_j, $J \in 0 \cup I$. Thus, the modified test statistic $T_{m,I}$ is utilized that uses contrasts $c_{m,I} = (c_{m0,I}, c_{m1,I}, \dots, c_{mk,I})'$ with coefficients $c_{mi,I}, j \in \{J\}$, that are the optimal contrasts for testing model shape m using doses $j \in J$ and the control group $i = 0$ only. For any dose

$j \notin \{J\}$ being used in the calculation, the coefficient $c_{mj,I}$ is set to 0 in the vector. For testing the intersection hypothesis H_I, the final test statistic $T_{\max,I} = \max_m T_{m,I}$ is the maximum of all single-contrast tests for H_I. An intersection hypothesis H_I can hence be rejected if $T_{\max,I} \geq q_{1-\alpha,I}$, where $q_{1-\alpha,I}$ is the multiplicity-adjusted critical value from the multivariate t distribution.

Thus, the level α-test for the global null hypothesis $H_{1,...,k} = \bigcap_{i=1}^{k} H_i$ is given by the original contrast test from MCP-Mod. As mentioned earlier, for testing an elementary null hypothesis H_i, $i = 1, ..., k$, the contrast coefficients of all model shapes m reduce to a pairwise comparison between placebo and the corresponding active dose. Note that the used optimal contrasts are further constrained by requiring that the sign of the contrast coefficients of the active doses and placebo need to be different. For a more detailed description of this topic and of the closed MCP-Mod procedure itself, including a detailed investigation of type I error control, we refer to Ref. [15].

16.3   Simulations

In this section, we compare various multiple test procedures introduced in the previous sections by means of a simulation study.

16.3.1   Design of simulation trial

The simulation settings are motivated by a real confirmatory dose-finding trial, where the details have been modified for confidentiality reasons. We assume that there was a placebo arm and three active doses, $0.05, 0.4$, and 1, in the trial. The standard deviation was assumed as 1, and the sample size was 100 patients per group. Hypothesis testing is performed at a significance level of 2.5% one sided. Three different maximum values were of interest for power investigations: $0.3, 0.4$, and 0.5. In addition, the candidate model set for MCP-Mod was based on three $E_{\max}$ shapes, with $ED_{50} = 0.05, 0.3, 0.7$, and two sigmoid $E_{\max}$ shapes with $(ED_{50}, h) = (0.25, 3), (0.6, 1.5)$. The basic assumption of this model set is that the dose–response curve increases monotonically. In addition, all shapes assume that the steep part of the curve occurs in the low dose range. Figure 16.2 displays the standardized model shapes with a maximum effect of 1.

To investigate the power under misspecification of the model shape, we also investigated the power for a nonmonotonic shape, assuming a beta model with parameters $\delta_1 = 0.27, \delta_2 = 0.55$ and a scale parameter of 1.2 as well as an exponential model with $(\delta = 0.4)$. These were not included in the candidate model set for MCP-Mod. For details on the definition of these model functions, we refer to Chapter 11.

The `multcomp` and `DoseFinding` packages in R [16] were used to run the simulations. Each simulation scenario was repeated 10,000 times to ensure adequate precision in the determined power values.

16.3.2   Simulation results

In Figures 16.3, one can observe the simulation results under the model shapes used for MCP-Mod. One can see that the power to reject at least one (RAO) hypothesis is comparable for closed MCP-Mod and the fixed-sequence test. These two methods outperform step-down Dunnett, Hochberg, and Bonferroni. The latter three methods perform similarly, while Bonferroni is always the least powerful of these three multiplicity adjustments, as

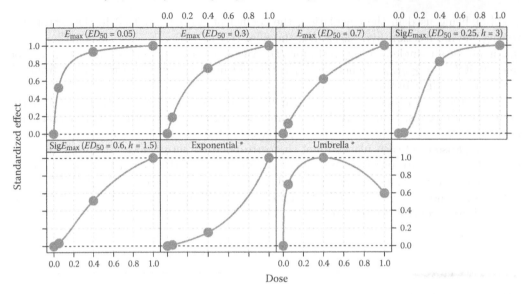

FIGURE 16.2

Dose–response model shapes used in the example.

Note that the shapes marked with an asterisk are not used in the candidate models for MCP-Mod.

the other two exploit the positive correlation between the test statistics. When observing the expected number of rejections divided by 3 (ENR/3), a similar overall picture emerges; closed MCP-Mod and fixed-sequence test again perform better than step-down Dunnett, Hochberg, and Bonferroni, and again Bonferroni performs slightly worse than step-down Dunnett and Hochberg. This is probably due to the fact that for the standard Bonferroni, for a hypothesis to be rejected, it needs to be rejected at level $\alpha/3$. Thus, one of the main advantages of stepwise (closed) methods compared to single-step methods is that more hypotheses can eventually be rejected. From the results for the individual dose–placebo comparisons, we can see that for the dose with the highest treatment effect, this is less relevant, but if low doses are still efficacious, the differences are more pronounced.

In Figure 16.4, one can observe the scenarios not included in the MCP-Mod candidate set. Here, the closed MCP-Mod procedure still has good power for the exponential shape, despite the fact that it was not included as one of the candidate shapes. For the non-monotonic shape, one can see that the methods that utilize information on monotonicity (the fixed-sequence test and closed MCP-Mod) perform worse than step-down Dunnett, Hochberg, and Bonferroni. The loss of power is larger for the fixed-sequence test than that for the closed MCP-Mod approach.

In summary, both the closed MCP-Mod and the fixed-sequence test perform well for the first set of model shapes. Among these two, closed MCP-Mod performs better in the second set of simulations. It appears that closed MCP-Mod is a bit more robust against misspecification of the model set than the fixed-sequence test, which is not robust against deviations from monotonicity. For example, contrast corresponding to the $E_{\max}$ ($ED_{50} =$ 0.05) shape will also have good power if the umbrella shape is true. For the fixed-sequence test, rejecting the high dose versus placebo comparison is a "fixed" gatekeeper, whereas for the closed MCP-Mod approach, one always tests linear combinations of the responses at all dose levels, which is probably why a misspecification of the contrasts to be used has less of an impact.

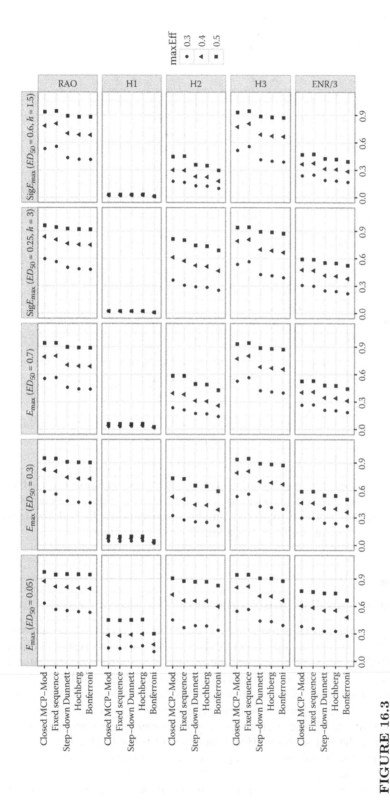

FIGURE 16.3
Simulation results for the scenarios. RAO: power to reject the corresponding dose–placebo comparison; ENR/3: expected number of rejections divided by 3. maxEff denotes the maximum effect in the dose range for all candidate shapes.

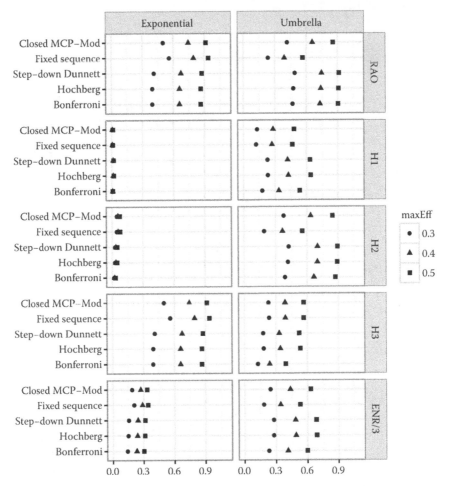

FIGURE 16.4
Simulation results for scenarios not included in the MCP-Mod candidate set of models. RAO: power to reject at least one hypothesis; H1–H3: power to reject the corresponding dose–placebo comparison; ENR/3: expected number of rejections divided by 3. maxEff denotes the maximum effect in the dose range for all candidate shapes.

16.4 Discussion and Recommendations

The topic of multiple comparisons is receiving increasing attention for the design and analysis of clinical trials in late-stage pharmaceutical drug development. Not accounting and adjusting for multiplicity could cause misleading results or inaccurate conclusions. In this chapter, several methods have been briefly introduced that could be used to address these concerns. The simplest methods of single-step methods, though conservative, are the most straightforward to implement. The closed test procedure is a powerful and flexible construction principle that allows the derivation of more powerful stepwise methods, either based on prespecifying the test sequence (fixed-sequence tests) or testing the hypotheses in a data-driven order (Holm, Hochberg, and step-down Dunnett tests). The closed MCP-Mod approach is an example of a recent application of the closed tests that uses optimal contrasts tests based on *a priori* information about plausible dose–response shapes available at the planning stage of a clinical trial. The simulation study in this chapter illustrates the performance of the several methods for a real study.

The methods described in this chapter are tailored to confirmatory trials that could potentially serve later as bases for regulatory decision making. The need to control strongly the FWER in this context is clear and mandated by regulatory guidelines. However, one should always be aware that multiplicity has a broad impact that raises challenging problems, which affect almost every decision throughout drug development. Good decision making and reproducibility need to account for multiplicity and might need different solutions at different drug development stages; this is even more true when it comes to the critical step of selecting the right dose of the right medicine for the right patients.

References

1. ICH. *ICH Topic E9: Notes for Guidance on Statistical Principles for Clinical Trials.* International Conference on Harmonization, London, UK, 1998.

2. EMEA. *CPMP: Points to Consider on Multiplicity Issues in Clinical Trials.* Committee for Medical Product for Human Use, London, UK, 2002.

3. Y. Hochberg and A. C. Tamhane. *Multiple Comparison Procedures.* John Wiley, New York, 1987.

4. F. Bretz, T. Hothorn, and P. Westfall. *Multiple Comparisons Using R.* CRC Press, Boca Raton, FL, 2010.

5. S. Holm. A simple sequentially rejective multiple test procedure. *Scandinavian Journal of Statistics*, 6:65–70, 1979.

6. R. J. Simes. An improved Bonferroni procedure for multiple tests of significance. *Biometrika*, 73:751–754, 1986.

7. K. Lu. Graphical approaches using a Bonferroni mixture of weighted Simes tests. *Statistics in Medicine*, 35(22):4041–4055, 2016.

8. Y. Hochberg. A sharper Bonferroni procedure for multiple significance testing. *Biometrika*, 75:800–802, 1988.

9. C. W. Dunnett. A multiple comparison procedure for comparing several treatments with a control. *Journal of the American Statistical Association*, 50(272):1096–1121, 1955.

10. A. Genz and F. Bretz. Methods for the computation of multivariate t-probabilities. *Journal of Computational and Graphical Statistics*, 11:950–971, 2002.

11. W. Maurer, L. A. Hothorn, and W. Lehmacher. Multiple comparisons in drug clinical trials and preclinical assays: A priori ordered hypotheses. *Biometrie in der Chemisch-Pharmazeutischen Industrie*, 6:3–18, 1995.

12. P. H. Westfall and A. Krishen. Optimally weighted, fixed sequence and gatekeeper multiple testing procedures. *Journal of Statistical Planning and Inference*, 99(1):25–40, 2001.

13. R. Marcus, E. Peritz, and K. R. Gabriel. On closed testing procedures with special reference to ordered analysis of variance. *Biometrika*, 63(3):655–660, 1976.

14. G. Hommel. A stagewise rejective multiple test procedure based on a modified Bonferroni test. *Biometrika*, 75:383–386, 1988.

15. F. König. Confirmatory testing for a beneficial treatment effect in dose-response studies using MCP-Mod and an adaptive interim analysis, July 9, 2015. Isaac Newton Institute, http://www.turing-gateway.cam.ac.uk/sites/default/files/asset/doc/1606/Franz %20Konig.pdf.

16. B. Bornkamp, J. Pinheiro, and F. Bretz. DoseFinding: Planning and analyzing dose finding experiments. *R Package Version 0.9–13*, 2016.

17

A Regulatory View on Dose-Finding Studies and on the Value of Dose–Exposure–Response Analysis

Sofia Friberg Hietala

Pharmetheus AB

Efthymios Manolis

European Medicines Agency

Flora Musuamba Tshinanu

University College London

CONTENTS

17.1   Background

The critical assessment of a marketing authorization application involves a comprehensive evaluation of product quality, nonclinical, and clinical data. The separate assessments come together in an evaluation of the benefit/risk (B/R) balance for the selected dose in the proposed indication and of the associated uncertainties. For a positive balance, the applicant needs to illustrate that the benefit of the treatment outweighs the risks. A negative balance may result not only from failure to demonstrate clinical efficacy and/or an acceptable safety profile but also from substantial uncertainty about positive or negative effects. An important part of the evaluation is the dosing rationale. The basis for dose selection should be addressed throughout the dossier; from the pharmaceutical development of an appropriate formulation, through *in vitro* drug action and preclinical toxicology coverage to supportive dose-finding and confirmatory clinical studies.

Current regulatory experience shows that the dose selection process and dose–exposure–response (D–E–R) characterization are often suboptimal [European Medicines Agency (EMA), 2015b]. Frequently, dose-finding studies comprise one or two active doses, and the primary analysis consists of pairwise comparisons against placebo, a design resulting in poor characterization of the D–E–R relationship. The competitive nature of drug development, where accelerated access to the market is a considerable incentive for sponsors, is one cited reason for the reduced standards in this stage. Yet, it appears that poor dose selection and poor understanding of D–E–R may lead to failed confirmatory trials, delays, or denials of regulatory approval, and necessitate changes in doses post approval (Sacks et al., 2014; Cross et al., 2002). Additional postmarketing commitments, further requirements for development in special populations, or withdrawal of marketing authorization may also result, all of which appear to reduce any initial gains from rushing through the dose-finding stage. It should be noted that beyond these (economical) considerations by the industry, the most harmful consequences of inadequate dose selection are related to public health: exposing patients to suboptimal doses with increased risks of experiencing adverse events and/or lack of efficacy.

A perceived lack of regulatory interest and scarce regulatory guidance in the area, particularly concerning the use of model-based approaches in drug development, are other contributing factors to poor dose-finding strategies according to the same report (EMA, 2015b). Although scientifically rigorous and optimal dose selection is not a formal requirement by either US or European Union law, there are regulatory guidelines addressing dose-finding strategies both in general terms and as therapy area-specific guidance. The overarching International Conference on Harmonisation (ICH) E4 guidance on Dose–Response Information to Support Drug Registration states that study designs should emphasize elucidation of the dose–response function, not individual pairwise comparisons. Similarly, the FDA guidelines (FDA, 2014) also state that being able to detect a statistically significant difference in pairwise comparisons between doses is not necessary if a statistically significant trend across doses can be established. This means that studying a trend across multiple dose levels is preferable to studying only one or two doses in the dose-finding study.

In this chapter, we will discuss some basic principles of D–E–R characterization and describe how regulatory assessors may use this information to assess the suitability of dose for Phase III, inform the dosing strategy as stated in the Summary of Product Characteristics (SmPC), in particular for special populations, and how this information is factored into B/R assessments and associated uncertainties discussions.

17.2 Cross-Sectional Dose–Response or Exposure–Response Analyses

D–E–R can be characterized using cross-sectional or longitudinal, model-based analyses. Both of these approaches have their merits and are complementary for the understanding and quantification of the D–E–R space.

A cross-sectional analysis of dose or exposure versus response is usually performed by nonlinear regression and represents a straightforward way to assess the therapeutic window of a medicinal product. The resulting D–E–R relationship can be easily communicated to regulators and used to support the choice of dosing for confirmatory trials. In addition, cross-sectional D–E–R relationships enable informed decisions from regulatory agencies on the choice of dose with an optimal B/R balance and on product labeling with respect to its use in special populations.

Provided that D–E–R analyses are adequate and well conducted, the decision on the dose to be labeled should be made on the totality of data and not necessarily restricted to Phase III doses tested. This is important when, for example, Phase III studies or postmarketing data identify safety concerns that need to be addressed by dose modifications. One recent regulatory decision that can be cited to this regard is that of the marketing authorization of lenvatinib in differentiated thyroid cancer, where a Postauthorization Safety Study (PASS) has been recommended by both the FDA and the EMA due to high rates of patients who needed dose reduction with the proposed starting dose. A refinement of the PK/PD model for drug efficacy for better characterization of the D–E–R was proposed as part of the commitments in the PASS (FDA, 2014).

The value of a D–E–R analysis will depend not only on the evaluated dose range but also on the timing of the analysis in relation to the time course of response, on design factors (such as the number of patients per dose level, covariate distribution, and dropout patterns), and on the relative impact and the covariance of predictors related to PK, disease progression, and PD. The predictive value of an E–R analysis performed on single dose-level data, i.e., where all variability in exposure is due to intrinsic variation in PK, may be limited by significant covariance between PK- and PD-associated predictors, as well as nonrandom dropout due to lack of efficacy or safety concerns. These limitations may be addressed by appropriate model diagnostics and mechanistic modeling (see Section 17.3). Nevertheless, the full characterization of D–E–R requires an evaluation of an adequate number and distribution of doses. Optimization of study design including dose range, number of patients per dose level, number of PK and PD measures, and sampling schedule is highly recommended in order to achieve adequate parameter precision. As recommended also in the FDA guidance on exposure–response, critical dose-finding studies should prospectively define hypotheses/objectives, include an appropriate control group, use randomization to ensure comparability of treatment groups and to minimize bias, and use acknowledged methods for assessing response variables.

The limitations of a cross-sectional D–E–R analysis lie in the convolution of diverse processes that contribute to the observed relationship and in the assumption of a time-invariant system. The approach should be used with caution in the evaluation of different dose regimens (e.g., immediate release versus slow release) where the relationship between exposure parameters (such as maximum concentration and total exposure) is likely to be significantly altered. Cross-sectional analyses are also sensitive to rate and severity of disease progression, which can impact the apparent magnitude of drug effects. In this case, the timing of the analysis should be optimized based on an understanding of the time course of drug effect and disease progression. Moreover, given that mechanistic thinking is not included, it is implicitly assumed that the distribution of relevant determinants of D–E–R in the data reflects that in the target population. This is not always true given the relatively small size of conventional dose-finding studies.

17.3 Longitudinal Exposure–Response Analysis

The analysis of D–E–R data and dose selection for confirmatory trials can be strengthened by longitudinal, model-based analysis. Longitudinal exposure–response analyses can enable a more efficient use of data than cross-sectional analyses. If there is a low signal-to-noise ratio, which would normally translate into large dose-finding studies, a longitudinal analysis is likely to allow for a smaller sample size. In addition, using individual observations rather than mean values for PK and PD increases the amount of data used in the analysis and allows for a description of both within- and between-subject variability (Karlsson et al., 2013). For slowly developing effects, such as the lowering of glycosylated hemoglobin (HbA1c) during treatment of diabetes, this approach may be informative with respect to dose separation, even with a relatively short study duration. The longitudinal analysis is also apt to time-variant systems and can inform optimal time for characterization of the D–E–R. However, the limitation described for cross-sectional analysis related to lack of mechanistic thinking will also apply when an empirical and data-driven approach is used for longitudinal exposure–response analysis. Model misspecification due to poor quality of data (e.g., protocol violation, poor patient compliance) or due to inappropriate study design will not always be ruled out.

17.4 Pharmacometrics and Model-Informed Drug Discovery and Development

Pharmacometrics as applied in Model-Informed Drug Discovery and Development (MID3) (Marshall et al., 2015) offers a "quantitative framework for prediction and extrapolation, centered on knowledge and inference generated from integrated models of compound, mechanism, and disease level data, and aimed at improving the quality, efficiency, and cost effectiveness of decision making." This approach differentiates from the two previously described by the possibility of including mechanistic thinking and translating physiological and pharmacological knowledge (and related uncertainties) into mathematical models. This is an important feature that allows filling the gap left by incomplete data and/or correcting the errors generated by poor-quality and uninformative studies.

As an example, the use of PK/PD modeling to identify efficacious dose regimens has reduced the need for clinical dose-ranging studies during the development of new antimicrobial agents, allowing more rapid progress to pivotal efficacy studies for substances with a potential to address an unmet medical need (EMA, 2015a, 2016b).

In the case of time-variant systems, when it is possible to implement, pharmacometrics, as described above, carries all of the advantages described above for longitudinal E–R with the additional advantage of being in line with the available knowledge of the disease, the target population, and the drug, all of which add considerable confidence to users of the model for prediction, simulation, and extrapolation.

Pharmacometrics can help predict and define subpopulations where the D–E–R relationship may be altered, supporting regulatory discussions on the need for posology changes, or help identifying uncertainties and associated clinical risks requiring additional studies in these patients. This can be of great importance not only in discussions on Pediatric Investigation Plans but also regarding elderly patients and other special populations. The value of D–E–R characterization for special populations is further discussed in a subsequent section.

As for any type of analysis of clinical data, a model-based approach should be supported with a discussion on sample size and other design features as well as of how they may impact the power to detect and describe a clinically relevant effect (Kang et al., 2005; Ogungbenro et al., 2006; Vong et al., 2012). Efficient methods exist for this purpose. They include clinical trial simulations (Santen et al., 2009; Tannenbaum et al., 2006), optimal design based on the population Fisher information matrix (Ogungbenro et al., 2009), and adaptive and Bayesian adaptive design methods (Antoniou et al., 2016; Lee et al., 2010). This can be of particular importance when practical and/or feasibility issues could hamper data collection in some subgroups of patients. Most model-based analyses presented to the EMA to date have been exploratory in nature, and study designs appear not to be optimized to accommodate confirmatory analyses. There is rarely a discussion of the assumptions associated with the analysis or the power and level of significance. Adherence to the recommendations regarding the analysis of critical dose-finding studies, as addressed above, will increase the regulatory confidence in the methodology.

17.5 Special Populations: PK- or PK/PD-Based Dose Adjustment and B/R Evaluation

Special populations refer to patients with characteristics such as age (pediatrics, geriatrics), pregnancy and breast feeding, comorbidities, or co-medications that may require special consideration during development, B/R assessment, and labeling of medicinal products. Typically, these groups represent only a small proportion of the patient population, and it is often not possible to perform confirmatory studies of efficacy and safety specifically in these patients. These special populations can be generally assigned to two categories: populations where exposure of the drug may be altered, and populations where E–R (safety and/or efficacy) of the drug may be altered.

17.5.1 Populations where exposure of the drug may be altered

In these populations, pharmacometrics can be used either for hypothesis generation or to support posology where dedicated studies are not possible. Examples include drug–drug interactions (DDI), and renal and hepatic impairments.

The effect of impaired renal function on exposure parameters is often evaluated in both Phase I and III studies. If a study with rich data is not feasible, a population pharmacokinetic analysis of sparse data is an alternative. Regardless of design, results from studies evaluating the impact of reduced renal function should be modeled to illustrate the continuous relationship between renal elimination capacity and pharmacokinetics. This model-based evaluation facilitates the assessment of cutoff glomerular filtration (GFR) values that require dose adjustment.

The assessment of impact of liver disease on PK is complicated by the range of symptoms and metrics associated with these conditions. The most commonly used clinical criteria describing liver impairment, the Child–Pugh score, are not necessarily correlated to drug elimination capacity. However, some components of the Child–Pugh score, like serum albumin, prothrombin time, and bilirubin, may be better predictors of drug clearance, and the use of such markers is encouraged.

Guidelines on the investigation of drug interactions emphasize that the worst-case scenario with respect to magnitude of DDI effects should be evaluated. Modeling approaches like physiologically based pharmacokinetics (PBPK) are important tools facilitating the design of optimized studies. In addition, compartmental modeling may be an alternative to non-compartmental analysis (NCA) for the evaluation of DDI studies, particularly for drugs with a long half-life $t1/2$ (EMA, 2012; Svensson et al., 2016).

17.5.2 Populations where E–R (safety and/or efficacy) of the drug may be altered

In fully powered subgroup analyses or dedicated studies, treatment failure or unacceptably high rates of safety concerns provide robust basis for B/R evaluation in these subgroups.

Importantly, however, the subgroup analysis will not identify the cause of the altered outcome. PK/PD modeling could be more informative in this respect and identify appropriate posology, strengthen regulatory confidence of positive B/R assessments, and propose additional investigations in case of a negative B/R assessment in a particular subgroup. In cases where the subgroup analyses are not powered for definitive conclusions or dedicated subgroup efficacy studies are not conducted, PK/PD modeling could still permit B/R evaluation and shift the balance by characterizing uncertainties and clinical risks and could improve posology recommendations. Examples of patients in these categories are not only children and the elderly but also patients with comorbidities that could be determinants of drug efficacy/safety.

At the extremes of the age range, i.e., pediatrics and geriatrics, both PK and PD may be altered in relation to the typical adult patient. Initial pediatric dosing should be guided using an adequately supported adult PK/PD model but taking into account growth and maturation effects on PK and PD. The model needs to be informed not only by data on the chemical entity in question but also from previous developments using systems pharmacology and PBPK. The need for confirmatory pediatric studies other than PK/PD depends on the disease, endpoints, and the quality of the PK/PD model and the confidence in the assumptions associated with the model.

Geriatric patients also tend to be underrepresented in clinical studies and are subject to special consideration during regulatory assessment. This assessment is complicated by the considerable variability in the aging process. While factors associated with aging such as physical and cognitive frailty, comorbidities, and co-medications may be superior to age as predictors of PK and PD in these patients, most subgroup analyses focus on age.

Regardless of the availability of conclusive efficacy/safety data in a subpopulation, a quantitative approach to support optimization of B/R and posology in special populations should encompass a comparison of PK parameters (such as clearance and volume of distribution) and, if relevant, PD parameters (such as EC_{50} or $E_{\max}$). If there is no difference, or if the difference is well characterized, this can be supportive of PK- or PK/PD-based dose adjustment. Again, this type of analysis should be supported by a discussion on the power of the study to identify a relevant difference. In some cases, such as antiretrovirals, PK parameters are known to vary significantly between adults and children. PD parameters, on the other hand, are likely to be similar: a PK-based extrapolation is therefore supported (EMA, 2016a).

17.6   Conclusion

There is significant regulatory interest in dose finding and D–E–R. Assessors use the information gained from well-performed dose-finding studies to evaluate the B/R balance and make recommendations regarding safe and efficacious use across the future patient population. Knowledge of PK-, efficacy-, and safety-associated predictors should also contribute to the planning of postapproval follow-up measures in the Risk Management Plan. Failure to identify the relevant therapeutic window during product development results in considerable uncertainty in the regulatory assessment, potentially causing denial or delay of approval and unnecessary exclusion of subpopulations or concomitant medications in the product label.

The most taxing consequence of suboptimal dosing is an unnecessary risk to patients. The 2014 EMA/EFPIA workshop emphasized the importance of characterization of the D–E–R relationship for successful lifecycle management of medicinal products (EMA/117491/2015). The European regulators welcome discussions on dose selection strategy and D–E–R characterization through scientific advice or the CHMP qualification opinion and are open to novel informative approaches.

Should the dosing rationale still be deemed insufficient during regulatory assessment, the regulatory framework allows for further dose optimization post approval—provided that the overall B/R for the proposed posology is positive. Importantly, this possibility should not encourage deferral of dose optimization studies to postmarketing as dose optimization and characterization of D–E–R should be key deliverables of drug development.

References

Antoniou, M., Jorgensen, A. L., and Kolamunnage-Dona, R., 2016. Biomarker-guided adaptive trial designs in phase II and phase III: A methodological review. *PLOS One*, 11(2):e0149803.

Cross, J., Lee, H., Westelinck, A., Nelson, J., Grudzinskas, C., and Peck, C., 2002. Postmarketing drug dosage changes of 499 FDA-approved new molecular entities, 1980–1999. *Pharmacoepidemiology and Drug Safety*, 11(6):439–446.

European Medicines Agency, 2012. *Guideline on the Investigation of Drug Interactions*. Committee for Human Medicinal Products (CHMP). (CPMP/EWP/560/95/Rev. 1 Corr. 2**). Retrieved from http://www.ema.europa.eu/docs/en_GB/document_library/ Scientific_guideline/2012/07/WC500129606.pdf.

European Medicines Agency, 2015a. Lenvima EPAR. Committee for Human Medicinal Products (CHMP).

European Medicines Agency, 2015b. Report from Dose Finding Workshop, EMA/117491/2015.

European Medicines Agency, 2016a. Guideline on the Clinical Development of Medicinal Products for the Treatment of HIV Infection. Committee for Human Medicinal Products (CHMP). Retervied from http://www.ema.europa.eu/docs/en_GB/document_ library/Scientific_guideline/2016/07/WC500209918.pdf.

European Medicines Agency, 2016b. *Guideline on the Use of Pharmacokinetics and Pharmacodynamics in the Development of Antimicrobial Medicinal Products*. Committee for Human Medicinal Products (CHMP). Retrieved from http://www.ema.europa.eu/docs/ en_GB/document_library/Scientific_guideline/2016/07/WC500210982.pdf.

Food and Drug Administration, 2014. *Guidance for Industry–Exposure-Response Relationships: Study Design, Data Analysis, and Regulatory Applications*. US Food and Drug Administration, Washington, DC. Retrieved from http://www.fda.gov/downloads/ drugs/guidancecomplianceregulatoryinformation/guidances/ucm072109.pdf.

International Conference on Harmonisation of Technical Requirements for Registration of Pharmaceuticals for Human Use (ICH), 1994. *Guidance on Dose-Response Information to Support Drug Registration*, E4. Accessed at http://www.ich.org/fileadmin/Public_Web_ Site/ICH_Products/Guidelines/Efficacy/E4/Step4/E4_Guideline.pdf.

Kang, D., Schwartz, J. B., and Verotta, D., 2005. Sample size computations for PK/PD population models. *Journal of Pharmacokinetics and Pharmacodynamics*, 32(5–6):685–701.

Karlsson, K. E., Vong, C., Bergstrand, M., Jonsson, E. N., and Karlsson, M. O., 2013. Comparisons of analysis methods for proof-of-concept trials. *CPT: Pharmacometrics & Systems Pharmacology*, 2(1):1–8.

Lee, J. J., Gu, X., and Liu, S., 2010. Bayesian adaptive randomization designs for targeted agent development. *Clinical Trials*, 7(5):584–596.

Marshall, S. F., Burghaus, R., Cosson, V., Cheung, S. Y. A., Chenel, M., Della Pasqua, O., Frey, N., Hamren, B., Harnisch, L., Ivanow, F., and Kerbusch, T., 2015. Good practices in model-informed drug discovery and development (MID3): Practice, application and documentation. *CPT: Pharmacometrics & Systems Pharmacology*, 5:93–122.

Ogungbenro, K., Aarons, L., and Graham, G., 2006. Sample size calculations based on generalized estimating equations for population pharmacokinetic experiments. *Journal of Biopharmaceutical Statistics*, 16(2):135–150.

Ogungbenro, K., Dokoumetzidis, A., and Aarons, L., 2009. Application of optimal design methodologies in clinical pharmacology experiments. *Pharmaceutical Statistics*, 8(3):239–252.

Sacks, L. V., Shamsuddin, H. H., Yasinskaya, Y. I., Bouri, K., Lanthier, M. L., and Sherman, R. E., 2014. Scientific and regulatory reasons for delay and denial of FDA approval of initial applications for new drugs, 2000–2012. *JAMA*, 311(4):378–384.

Santen, G., van Zwet, E., Danhof, M., and Della Pasqua, O., 2009. From trial and error to trial simulation. Part 1: The importance of model-based drug development for antidepressant drugs. *Clinical Pharmacology and Therapeutics*, 86(3):248–254.

Svensson, E. M., Acharya, C., Clauson, B., Dooley, K. E., and Karlsson, M. O., 2016. Pharmacokinetic interactions for drugs with a long half-life—Evidence for the need of model-based analysis. *The AAPS Journal*, 18(1):171–179.

Tannenbaum, S. J., Holford, N. H., Lee, H., Peck, C. C., and Mould, D. R., 2006. Simulation of correlated continuous and categorical variables using a single multivariate distribution. *Journal of Pharmacokinetics and Pharmacodynamics*, 33(6):773–794.

Vong, C., Bergstrand, M., Nyberg, J., and Karlsson, M. O. 2012. Rapid sample size calculations for a defined likelihood ratio test-based power in mixed-effects models. *AAPS Journal*, 14(2):176–186.

Index